Active Learning Workbook for

Clinical Practice of the Dental Hygienist

TWELFTH EDITION

Charlotte J. Wyche, RDH, MS
Department of Periodontics and Oral Medicine
University of Michigan School of Dentistry
Ann Arbor, Michigan

Jane F. Halaris, RDH, MA
Department of Periodontics and Oral Medicine
University of Michigan School of Dentistry
Ann Arbor, Michigan

Esther M. Wilkins, BS, RDH, DMD
Department of Periodontology
Tufts University School of Dental Medicine
Boston, Massachusetts

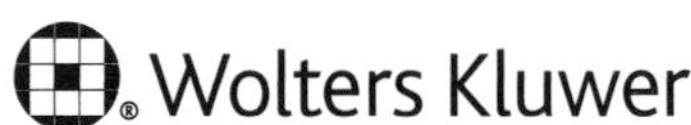

Philadelphia • Baltimore • New York • London
Buenos Aires • Hong Kong • Sydney • Tokyo

Senior Acquisitions Editor: Jonathan Joyce
Senior Product Development Editor: Amy Millholen
Editorial Assistant: Tish Rogers
Senior Marketing Manager: Leah Thomson
Senior Production Product Manager: Alicia Jackson
Design Coordinator: Holly McLaughlin
Manufacturing Coordinator: Margie Orzech
Prepress Vendor: S4Carlisle Publishing Services

Twelfth Edition

Two Commerce Square
2001 Market Street
Philadelphia, PA 19103 USA
LWW.com

Printed in the United States of America

ISBN: 9781451195248

DOH0618

DEDICATION

To instructors who ask open-ended questions and encourage the kind of reflection that helps students discover what they do not yet know. They understand that clinical dental hygiene practice is not a multiple-choice test.

and

To students who struggle to find answers for the open-ended questions their instructors ask them. They will soon discover that reflecting on what they don't know and working to find answers to real questions is what leads to real learning.

Preface

There is no doubt each student learns differently. Therefore, the aim of this workbook is to provide a variety of exercises so you will be able to find something here to help you learn important concepts that are the foundation of the dental hygiene practice. You are always encouraged, of course, to create additional learning experiences and activities that fit with your own learning style.

HOW TO USE THIS WORKBOOK

Some general guidelines for the exercises in the workbook are described here. Exercises in the **Knowledge** sections of the workbook provide lines for you to write your answers. Some chapters include crossword or word search puzzles to help learn terminology. For **Competency**- and **Discovery**-type exercises, a separate computer or handwritten document or a copy of the *Patient-Specific Dental Hygiene Care Plan* template from Appendix B may be required to provide a complete answer.

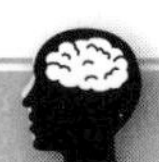

KNOWLEDGE EXERCISES

KNOWLEDGE exercises in each chapter will help you target important information and help you master the introductory material provided in the textbook. You will define terms, concepts, and principles in your own words; list the components of larger ideas; and reorganize information from the textbook in a variety of ways. Knowledge exercises comprise the largest, but by no means the most important, portion of this workbook.

COMPETENCY EXERCISES

COMPETENCY questions are found in each chapter and also in section summary areas of this workbook. Building competence in translating knowledge to practice is an essential component of becoming a professional dental hygienist. These exercises will ask you to use critical thinking skills to apply basic knowledge to clinical situations, analyze patient assessment data, create components of patient care plans, or document patient care activities. Some of the patient scenarios are written in paragraph form so you can learn to isolate important information, and some are formatted using the Assessment Findings section from the Care Plan template.

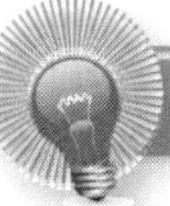

DISCOVERY EXERCISES

DISCOVERY activities are found in some of the chapters and also in each section summary. These exercises will help you learn to think beyond the basic knowledge. The discovery activities will direct you to find and analyze current information about a topic introduced in the textbook by, for example, doing a scientific literature search, a Web-based Internet search, or a dental product analysis.

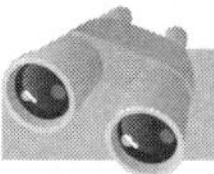

BOX 13-1 MESH TERMS

Medical Subject Heading (MeSH) boxes in each chapter contain some headings related to chapter topics under which journal articles are organized within the PubMed database. Combining the terms you find in the MeSH term box in each chapter with other key words related to your topic of interest will help you initiate efficient and effective literature searches.

Questions Patients Ask

Questions Patients Ask are also intended to encourage you to practice evidence-based decision-making skills. Reflecting on what additional or new knowledge is needed to address patient concerns is a key skill for lifelong learning and ultimately for providing evidence-based, comprehensive, and effective dental hygiene care.

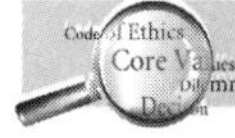

EVERYDAY ETHICS

Everyday Ethics activities will challenge you to reflect on and apply ethical principles. An Everyday Ethics Scenario with "Questions for Consideration" is included in each textbook chapter. Many of these scenarios were created using real-life ethical situations faced by practicing dental hygienists. Each workbook chapter includes an Everyday Ethics box with **individual learning, cooperative learning,** or **discovery** activity prompts that direct you to write about, discuss, or role-play the ethics-related scenario and questions presented in the textbook.

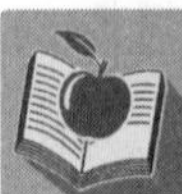

Factors To Teach The Patient

Factors to Teach the Patient cases ask you to outline or develop a patient/provider conversation using motivational interviewing (MI) techniques, patient-appropriate language, and knowledge gained from the textbook. Those brief conversations can then be compared with conversations written by your student colleagues, used for "role-play" exercises, or placed in your portfolio to illustrate your expertise in patient education.

FOR YOUR PORTFOLIO

For Your Portfolio suggestions are located in each section summary and in a few of the chapters. A learning portfolio is a collection of student work and reflection organized in such a way that it demonstrates an increase in student knowledge and professional competence over time. A student portfolio can be compiled simply and creatively using a three-ring binder with tabbed separators to organize the material into appropriate sections. An Internet search will help you locate online portfolio templates that can be used to develop a Web-based portfolio.

Development of a portfolio provides an opportunity for you to reflect on your growth as a dental hygiene professional. A portfolio to highlight your unique talents and provides evidence of special skills, competencies, or learning that goes beyond the requirements of your educational program can be useful during employment interviews or application to graduate education programs.

Answers for the workbook Knowledge questions and rubrics with criteria to help evaluate student responses to Competency exercises are located in the Instructor Resources at http://thepoint.lww.com/Wyche12e. Access to these answers is strictly limited to faculty.

COMPETENCIES FOR THE DENTAL HYGIENIST

The American Dental Education Association (ADEA) competencies outline the areas in which a new graduate dental hygienist is expected to be able to apply knowledge to ensure safe and effective patient care is provided. The title page for each section of this workbook lists specific ADEA competencies supported by learning the information from chapters included in that particular section of the textbook. The complete list of competency statements found in Appendix A will provide a reference point to help you understand why learning specific concepts from each chapter is important for becoming a professional dental hygienist.

As you read the ADEA competency statements, you should note that your school might have adapted them somewhat for use in your dental hygiene program. Your school's competencies may be organized in a slightly different manner but will probably be very similar. You should make a point of receiving a copy of your school's competency statements for reference.

We encourage you to enjoy the process of learning and hope this workbook offers activities that will help you.

Sincerely,
Charlotte J. Wyche, RDH, MS
and
Jane J. Halaris, RDH, MA
Dental Hygiene Educators

Acknowledgments

It takes a team to complete a project as big as this workbook. The publishing team is listed at the front of the book, and of course the "main authors" have their names on the cover. However, it doesn't even begin there. The following people gave their knowledge, expertise, experience, and most of all their time to help us make this edition of the workbook what it is. Thank you all for making this workbook possible. We could not have done it without your dedication and help.

Heather Stack, RDH, BSDH, Renée Ann-Wasylewski Fitzgerald, RDH, BSDH, and **Elizabeth L. Miller, RDH, BS,** graduates of the University of Michigan dental hygiene degree completion e-learning program (2013) who worked together (online) to compile the lists of MeSH terms in each chapter to help provide a "jumpstart" for students just learning to initiate a literature search on PubMed.

Dina L. Korte, RDH, MS (dental hygiene faculty), and **Michelle C. Arnett, RDH, MS** (dental hygiene graduate student), from the University of Michigan, who were instrumental in developing an MI infomap (Appendix D) and the brief motivational interviewing (BMI) patient conversations used in the competency exercises for Chapter 26.

Janet Kinney, RDH, MS (director of dental hygiene), and University of Michigan second-year dental hygiene students who let me visit their class session on MI.

Mary Larsen, BS, freelance editor, for her "eagle eye" and for her work compiling the workbook answer keys.

Marcia Williams, medical and scientific illustrator, who provided the drawings that enhance student learning in some of the chapters.

Contents

3. Dental hygiene interventions play a major role in all levels of prevention of oral disease. Give examples (different from those included in the textbook) of a dental hygienist's role in each level of prevention.

DISCOVERY EXERCISES

1. Initiate a review of literature and an Internet search to further investigate the concept of the dental therapist. Describe the relationship between advanced practice dental hygienists and dental therapists.

2. Review a copy of your state's Dental Hygiene Practice Act. List the services dental hygienists may provide and determine the level of supervision required for each service. Explain how the rules in your state enhance or provide a barrier to access to oral health services.

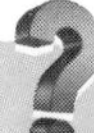

Questions Patients Ask

What sources of information can you identify that will help you answer your patient's questions in this scenario?

Your patient, Jessica Miles, who is a junior in high school, comments, "My mom and I were talking about where I will be going to college after next year. She said to ask you where you went. She thinks what you do would be real cool. What is it that you do, really? Why did you have to take a lot of sciences? Do they have dental chairs and all the equipment right in the school and do people come in for you to learn from? I know you clean our teeth—why do you like working in people's mouths?"

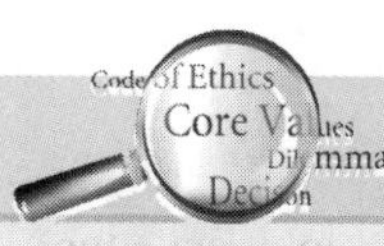

EVERYDAY ETHICS

Before completing the learning exercises below, reread and reflect on the Everyday Ethics Scenario and Questions for Consideration in this chapter of the textbook. It may also be useful to review the Dental Hygiene Ethics discussion in Chapter 1, the Ethical Applications in the introduction pages for each section in the textbook, as well as the Codes of Ethics in textbook Appendices I–IV.

Individual Learning Activity

Imagine that you are the dental hygienist in this scenario. Answer each of the questions for consideration at the end of the scenario in the textbook chapter.

Collaborative Learning Activity

Work as a group to develop a 2- to 5-minute role-play that introduces the everyday ethics scenario described in the chapter (a great idea is to video record your role-play activity). Then develop separate 2-minute role-play scenarios that provide at least two alternative approaches/solutions to resolving the situation. Ask classmates to view the solutions, ask questions, and discuss the ethical approach used in each. Ask for a vote on which solution classmates determine to be the "best."

Factors To Teach The Patient

This scenario is related to the following factors listed in this chapter of the textbook:

- ▷ The role of the dental hygienist as cotherapist with each patient and with members of the dental profession.
- ▷ The moral and ethical nature of becoming a dental hygiene professional person.
- ▷ The patient's potential state of oral health and how it can be improved and maintained.

Sarah, your really good friend, has agreed to be a patient for your first clinical experience as a dental hygiene student. When you call her to remind her of her appointment tomorrow, she asks you a bit about what you will do during the appointment. You excitedly begin to explain the procedures.

Sarah interrupts saying that it all sounds pretty boring to her. She asks you to tell her why you are studying so hard to become a dental hygienist. Write a statement explaining your knowledge and interest in dental hygiene practice to Sarah.

2

Evidence-Based Dental Hygiene Practice

LEARNING OBJECTIVES

Upon successful completion of these exercises, you will be able to:

1. Explain evidence-based dental hygiene practice and identify the skills needed to practice evidence-based dental hygiene care.
2. Discuss research approaches and connect research types to the strength of evidence each provides.
3. Describe a systematic approach to finding science-based information in the health care literature.
4. Describe skills needed for analyzing Internet-based health information.

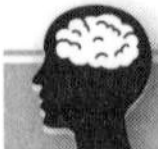

KNOWLEDGE EXERCISES

Write your answers for each question in the space provided.

1. List four factors that interact to direct selection of patient care interventions in an evidence-based dental hygiene practice.

____

____

____

____

2. Place the steps for a systematic approach to evidence-based dental hygiene practice in the correct order by placing the numbers 1 through 6 in the space beside each step.

Order	Description of Step
	___ Develop a researchable question
	___ Evaluate the results
	___ Search for the evidence
	___ Analyze the evidence
	___ Determine the clinical issue
	___ Apply the evidence

3. What is a refereed publication?

4. List four types of research studies.

5. What is the difference between qualitative and quantitative research approaches?

6. What type of research looks at the strength and types of relationships between variables?

7. What is the difference between experimental and quasi-experimental research?

8. What is in vitro research?

9. What is the difference between a case report and a case study?

10. What is a case–control study? What does *retrospective* mean?

11. Randomized controlled double-blind studies help eliminate ___________ by placing study participants randomly in either the experimental or the control group and by "blinding" the researchers to which participant is in which group.

12. Place the levels of evidence in order from the most valuable to support evidence-based practice (1) to less valuable (6) for making decisions related to clinical dental hygiene care.

Order	Type of Evidence
	____ Analysis of all studies that investigate a specific question
	____ Opinions of journal editors or other "expert" practitioners
	____ Prospective studies that follow groups or retrospective studies that compare groups of research subjects
	____ Research that does not include human subjects
	____ RCT studies
	____ Studies that describe or analyze one or more cases of an unusual condition

13. What six actions can help the dental hygiene practitioner to analyze the content of health information found on the Internet for validity and reliability?

14. List two ways to help determine the accuracy of health information found on the Internet?

15. List ways to help determine whether or not a health-related website is providing biased information (checking for objectivity).

16. Informed consent forms and Institutional Review Board approval help protect the rights of ________________ in research studies.

17. What is a PICO question?

____

____

____

____

18. List the components of a PICO question.

____

____

____

____

COMPETENCY EXERCISES

Use paper and pen or create an electronic document to answer these questions.

1. Your patient is a 1-year old child who already has evidence of early childhood caries. You know that in order to help decrease risk for further caries activity and help remineralize white spot lesions, this child needs to be provided with topical fluoride application even at this young age. However, you are unsure whether the topical gel application or the fluoride varnish would be the best choice.
   Part 1: Write a PICO question that will help direct your search for information to support the intervention you select for this very young child.
   Part 2: Identify the MeSH terms you would use to initiate the literature search.
2. Explain why a peer-reviewed journal is more likely than a commercial-based health magazine to contain the type of evidence that is appropriate to support clinical recommendations that a dental hygienist includes in a patient's care plan.

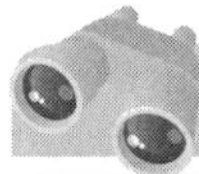

BOX 2-1 MeSH TERMS

Use a combination of MeSH terms and other key words to develop an effective and efficient PubMed literature search strategy.

Evidence-based practice
Evidence-based dentistry
Practice guidelines as topic
Clinical trials as topic
Periodicals as topic
Ethics committees, research
Meta-analysis
Randomized controlled trial
Case-control studies
Cohort studies
Case reports
Qualitative research
Reproducibility of results

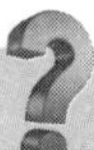

Questions Patients Ask

What sources of information can you identify that will help you answer your patient's questions?

"I just heard about this cool new dental product from my friend! Do you think it is any good?" "Will it clean my teeth as well as what I am doing now?" "I know my situation is different than some other people, so will it work for me?"

Factors To Teach The Patient

This scenario is related to the following factors listed in this chapter of the textbook:

▷ A result from one study doesn't necessarily provide the best answer.

Your patient, Marcus, tells you that he just read a newspaper article citing new research study that contradicts a recommendation you have made for his self-care. How will you respond to his assertion that the research proves that this new technique is probably better than the one that you have recommended?

EVERYDAY ETHICS

Before completing the learning exercises that follow, reread and reflect on the Everyday Ethics Scenario and Questions for Consideration in this chapter of the textbook. It may also be useful to review the Dental Hygiene Ethics discussion in Chapter 1, the Ethical Applications in the introduction pages for each section in the textbook, as well as the Codes of Ethics in textbook Appendices I–IV.

Individual Learning Activity

Identify a situation you have experienced that presents a similar ethical dilemma. What did you learn from how the situation was (or was not) resolved at the time it happened?

Discovery Activity

Ask a friend or relative who is not involved in healthcare to read the scenario and discuss it with you from the perspective of a "patient" who receives services within the healthcare system. Discuss what you learned from the concerns, insights, or difference in perspective that person expressed.

Chapter 2 Word Search Puzzle

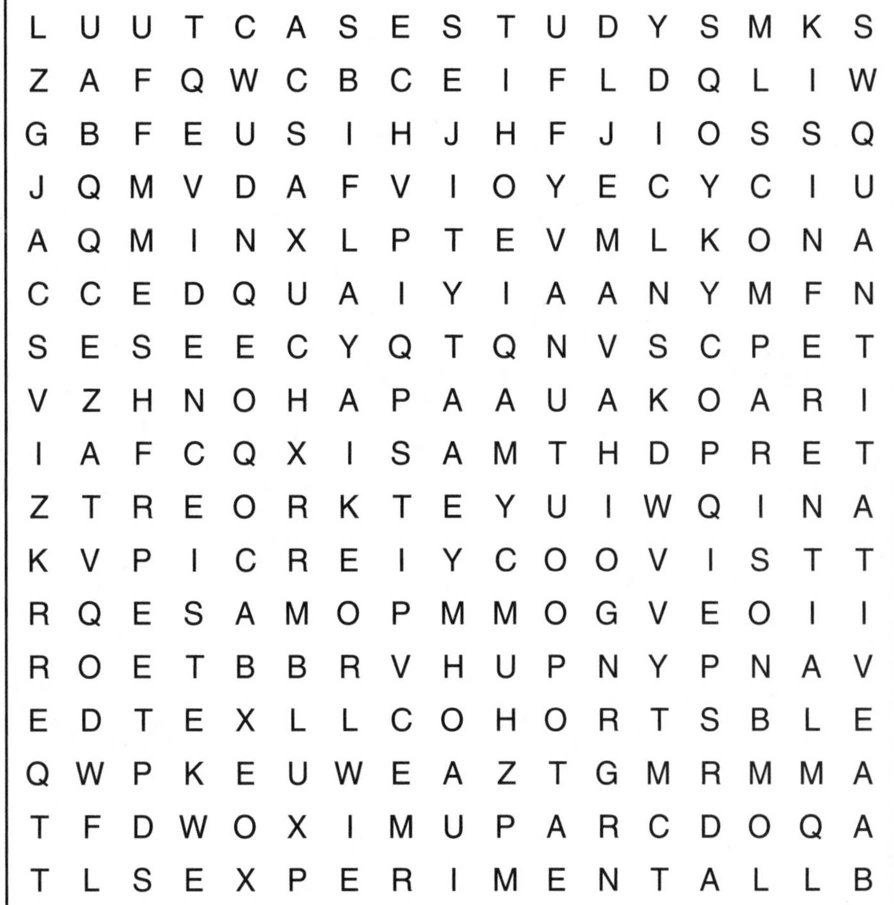

Word Search Puzzle Clues

- A type of study in which the same subjects are followed over time.
- A retrospective study that compares individuals with a condition with others who do not have that condition.
- In-depth description of a number of cases of individuals who have an unusual or complex condition.
- A type of study in which results are reported in numbers.
- The group in a research study that does not receive the intervention.
- A factors that is manipulated and measured during a research study.
- The highest level of evidence to support best-practices.
- Type of statistical analysis that can help determine the frequency with which something exists.
- Type of numerical statistic that allows generalization from a sample to a population.
- Supports efforts to determine or demonstrate the truth.
- Type of study in which intervention variables are manipulated to find the effect of one upon another.
- Acronym sometimes used to indicate a randomized controlled double-blind study.
- A subjective research approach in which study results are reported using a narrative.
- Terms used to index articles in the MEDLINE database; useful for literature search.

3

Effective Health Communication

LEARNING OBJECTIVES

Upon successful completion of these exercises, you will be able to:

1. Discuss the skills and attributes of effective health communication.
2. Identify barriers to effective communication.
3. Explain how the patient's age, culture, and health literacy level affect health communication strategies.

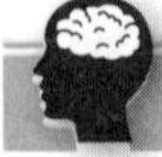

KNOWLEDGE EXERCISES

Write your answers for each question in the space provided.

1. Define health communication in your own words.

____

____

____

____

2. To establish the kind of rapport that enhances communication with a patient of any age, gender, or culture, the dental hygienist will ____________ more than ____________, especially at the beginning of the appointment.

3. List as many as you can of the abilities/attributes of a dental professional who is able to establish rapport with each patient in order to provide effective health communication.

____

____

____

____

____

____

____

____

____

4. What factors contribute to effective health messages?

5. List and briefly define in your own words the three types of communication.

6. What barriers can affect the way health messages are understood during patient's education sessions.

7. The level of a patient's health literacy does not only depend on the individual's reading level, but rather also on the interaction of a complex set of ________________ and ________________ skills, as well as personal health-related knowledge.

8. List some ways the dental hygienist can address health literacy issues in the dental hygiene practice.

9. Match the age group in column 1 with the correct description of a key point related to communicating with that age group in column 2.

Age Group	Communication-Related Description
____ Infants	A. Marked desire to have their viewpoint and needs considered with respect.
____ Toddlers and preschoolers	B. Like to assert independence and maintain control over situations.
____ School age children	C. Physical and cognitive changes may impact ability to communicate.
____ Adolescents	D. Communicate primarily through senses.
____ Older adults	E. Developing ability to relate the impact of external events to themselves.

10. True or False (circle one). Using "*terms of endearment*" to address a frail elderly patient is a communication approach that will put the patient at ease as well as demonstrate the care provider's empathy.

11. True or False (circle one). When communicating with a caregiver who is in the treatment room while you are providing oral hygiene instructions for the patient, maintain eye contact with the caregiver as the primary focus of the conversation so that they don't feel left out.

12. In your own words, describe the effect ethnic or cultural background can have on your patients' health status or the way they respond to your dental hygiene interventions.

13. ________________ (two words) delivery of dental hygiene care, including respect for and responsiveness to the unique culturally related characteristics,

values, and needs of each patient can make a positive difference in oral health outcomes.

14. ______________________ (two words) is a skill that can be developed by exploring and learning to appreciate the wide variety of differences among the individuals who are your patients.

15. ______________________ (two words) is about building relationships that foster understanding.

16. List attributes of a dental hygienist who strives to deliver effective health care for patients of all cultures.

17. List ways to enhance awareness of culture-related needs during patient care.

18. List ways to enhance language-related communication with all patients.

19. List skills that enhance interprofessional communication between healthcare providers.

20. When communicating with a patient while using an interpreter, which one do you speak directly to when asking questions?

21. What factors related to communication and culture are appropriate to document in a patient's permanent record?

BOX 3-1 MeSH TERMS

Use a combination of MeSH terms and other key words to develop an effective and efficient PubMed literature search strategy.

Health communication
Communication barriers
Health literacy
Cultural competency
Nonverbal communication

COMPETENCY EXERCISES

Apply information from the chapter and use critical thinking skills to complete the competency exercises. Write responses on a paper or create electronic documents to submit your answers.

1. Table 3-1 in the textbook list several factors that can interfere with effective communication and describes or defines what each factor means. Provide a brief *example* from your own life experience (not necessarily related to dental hygiene) that illustrates **each of the types of barriers**. For example, an **interpersonal barrier** to effective communication could be illustrated by describing a time when you could only seem to argue, rather than discuss, with a friend who had taken a political stand opposite yours. After you describe the situation, jot down any thoughts you have about how you might have overcome that barrier and been more effective in communicating.

2. Explain the dental hygienist's role in helping patients understand health-related messages and health information available from popular media and Internet-based sources.

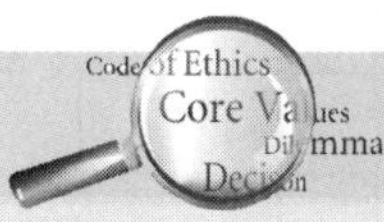

EVERYDAY ETHICS

Before completing the learning exercises below, reread and reflect on the Everyday Ethics Scenario and Questions for Consideration in this chapter of the textbook. It may also be useful to review the Dental Hygiene Ethics discussion in Chapter 1, the Ethical Applications in the introduction pages for each section in the textbook, as well as the Codes of Ethics in textbook Appendices I–IV.

Individual Learning Activity

Imagine the scenario from the patient's perspective. How might the patient's response to the questions following the scenario be different from those of the dental hygienist involved?

Collaborative Learning Activity

Work with a small group to develop a 2- to 5-minute role-play that introduces the everyday ethics scenario described in the chapter (a great idea is to video record your role-play activity). Then develop separate 2-minute role-play scenarios that provide at least two alternative approaches/solutions to resolving the situation. Ask classmates to view the solutions, ask questions, and discuss the ethical approach used in each. Ask for a vote on which solution classmates determine to be the "best."

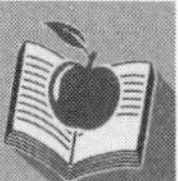

Factors To Teach The Patient

This scenario is related to the following factors listed in this chapter of the textbook:

▷ The dental hygienist's ability to provide quality dental hygiene care is affected by the willingness and ability of the patient to communicate accurate and complete information about health status, needs, and concerns.

Mr. Romine has been a patient in the practice for many, many years. You are a new dental hygienist in the practice who is scheduled to provide his regular dental hygiene care today. You discover that his health history form, which notes some significant health history issues including history of an infectious disease, arthritis, hypertension, and an undefined "heart problem" has not been updated in several years. When you politely ask him to fill out a new one, he angrily states, "Information about my health is my private business."

What are some ways that you might approach Mr. Romaine to help build rapport and establish enough trust to help him share the information you need to provide safe and effective dental hygiene care for him? Share your ideas with student colleagues. Was their approach similar to yours or very different? What did you learn from the discussion?

Chapter 3 Crossword Puzzle

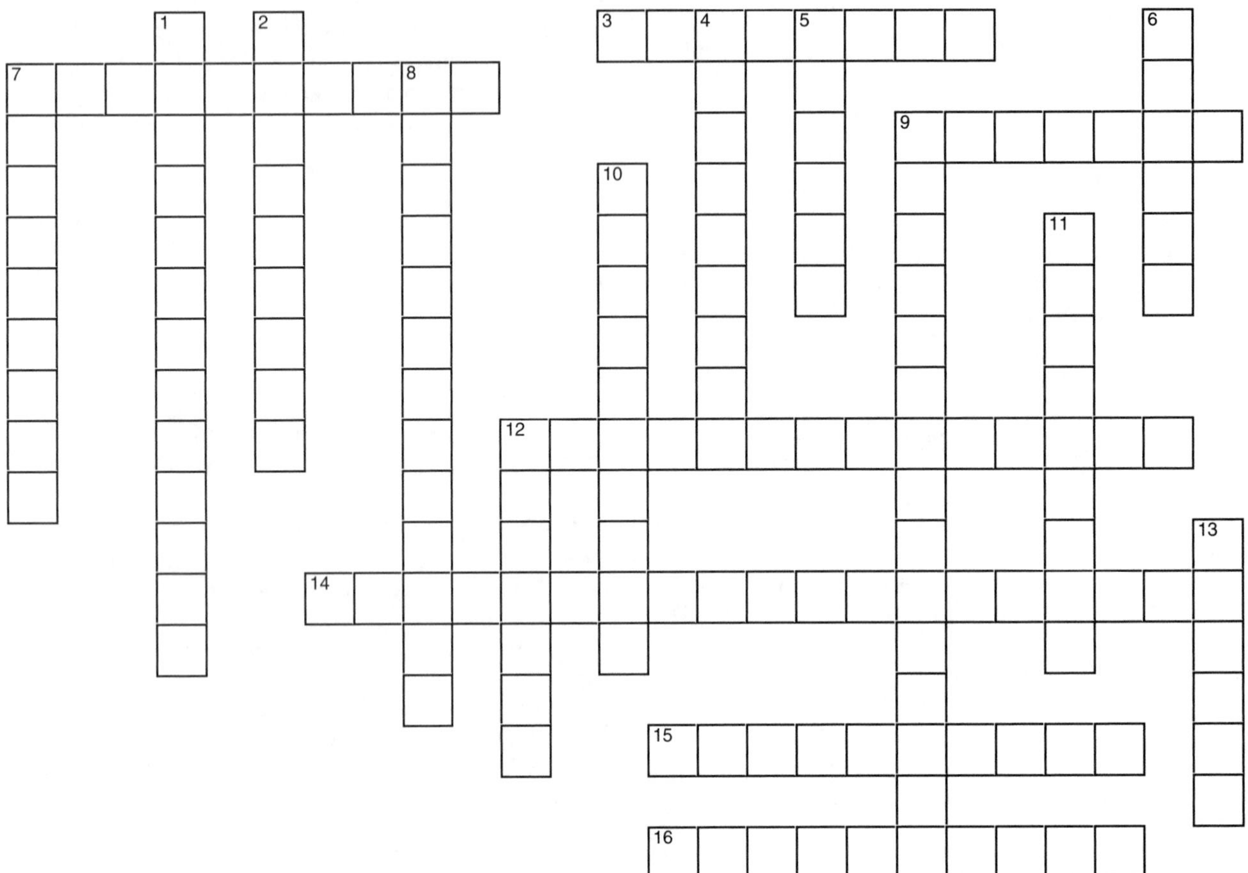

Puzzle Clues

Across

3. Nonword cues that help provide meaning during verbal communication.
7. An attitude or judgment about others that is usually not based on personal experience, but rather, learned from other sources.
9. A common set of learned beliefs, attitudes, values, and behaviors.
12. A set of cognitive and psychosocial skills that determines ability to obtain, understand, and respond to health messages (two words).
14. The process of sharing messages related to health and wellness (two words).
15. The ability to provide health messages for persons with limited English (or other language) proficiency is referred to as ________ competence.
16. An approach to communication with elderly patients that may include baby and using terms of endearment and can be perceived as patronizing or demeaning.

Down

1. Refers to communication with patients from cultures other than one's own (two words).
2. Type of communication that sends wordless messages (two words).
4. If a dental hygienist possesses set of skills that enable effective cross-cultural health-related communication with individuals of another culture, that dental hygienist is considered to be culturally _____.
5. What a dental hygienist should do more often than talking during a health education conversation with a patient.
6. A form of communication based on words.
7. Making an effort to understand behaviors of diverse groups is referred to as being culturally _______.
8. Easy to read written health information (two words).
9. Cultural ___________ that can affect communication or delivery of dental hygiene care are documented in a patient's record.
10. The study of how people use language and the impact of language.
11. Significant differences in health status observed in underserved or minority populations.
12. Communication through touching.
13. Translation of a thought using words, gestures, or signs.

SECTION I Summary Exercises

Orientation to Clinical Dental Hygiene Practice

Chapters 1-3

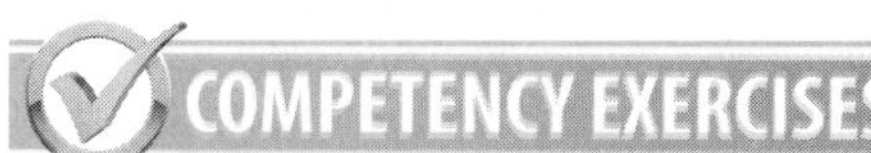

Apply information from Chapters 1-3 and use critical thinking skills to complete the competency exercises. Write responses on paper or create electronic documents to submit your answers.

SECTION I – PATIENT ASSESSMENT SUMMARY

Patient Name: *Christopher Michaels* | Age: *10* | Gender: [M] F | ☑ Initial Therapy ☐ Maintenance ☐ Re-evaluation

Provider Name: *D.H. Student* | Date: *Today*

Chief Complaint:
Toothache and swollen area in lower left jaw. Ulcerated lesion on left upper lip.

Assessment Findings

Health History • No current findings • ASA II and ADL level 0	**At Risk For:** • N/A
Social and Dental History • No dental exam in 5 years • Ulcerated, crusted lesion on left upper lip, spreading to nose. • High sucrose intake (juice, candy) • Poor dental biofilm control	**At Risk For:** • Low health literacy (of parents) • Pain and secondary infection due to active herpetic lesion • Increased incidence of dental caries • Increased risk of periodontal infection
Social and Dental History • Enlarged left submandibular lymph node • Large lesion on mandibular left primary second molar • Numerous small carious lesions • Generalized gingivitis	**At Risk For:** • Secondary infection • Possible endodontic infection and pain from dental caries • Further incidence of dental caries • Gingival infection/periodontal disease
Social and Dental History Gingivitis	**Caries Management Risk Assessment (CAMBRA) Level:** ☐ Low ☐ Moderate ☐ High ☑ Extreme

Read the Section I Patient Assessment Summary to help you answer questions #1 and #2.

1. The clinical issue: The dentist who examines Christopher tells you that the ulcerated lesion you observe on Christopher's upper lip is caused by the herpes virus and is an infectious condition. You are worried that providing treatment for him while the lesion is active can cause the infection to spread or that you could be infected. Write a PICO question that you can use to help guide your search for evidence to help make a decision about providing dental hygiene treatment today.

2. After talking to Christopher and his mother you determine that his habit of drinking juice all day long is a health-related behavior that needs to be changed in order to reduce the risk for additional dental caries. However, Mrs. Michaels insists that he really enjoys drinking the juice and that she gives him at least five containers each day because she believes that juice is a healthy way for him to drink lots of liquids when he is active. Write a short paragraph reflecting on a patient education approach that may begin help her move toward a willingness to change both her and Christopher's behavior. Is simply providing information enough?

3. Core values in dental hygiene practice include autonomy and respect. An example of this value is that you, as the dental hygienist, must respect your patients' right to refuse dental hygiene recommendations or treatment, even when your professional opinion is that doing so may cause deterioration of their oral health status.

   Select another one of the core values in dental hygiene practice and give an example to illustrate it. Discuss your example with student colleagues.

4. Identify an expression, gesture, or movement that you commonly make (see Table 3-3 in Chapter 3 for some ideas). Explain how your action can have unintended meaning or be the cause of a misunderstanding that will have a negative effect on the relationship you are developing with a patient of cultural background that is different than your own.

5. Explain why systematic reviews and meta-analysis articles are considered to constitute the highest level of evidence to support the selection of dental hygiene interventions for patient care.

DISCOVERY EXERCISES

1. Obtain a copy of the rules or laws that govern the practice of dental hygiene in your state or country. Answer the following questions.
   - *What specific services are the dental hygienists in your state or area licensed to provide?*
   - *What type of supervision must dental hygienists have when they provide care for the patients?*
   - *Does your state have any provisions that allow dental hygienists to provide care in a collaborative practice or under reduced supervision to provide direct access care for underserved populations or in any specific kinds of public health settings?*
   - *What are continuing education requirements for dental hygienists who practice in your state or country?*

2. Find a contact person for the dental hygiene professional association nearest to you and ask questions about membership, continuing education, and leadership opportunities.

3. Explore *The Provider's Guide to Quality and Culture* (available at http://erc.msh.org/mainpage.cfm?file=1.0.htm&module=provider&language=English&ggroup=&mgroup=). Click on the "take the Quiz" link at the left-hand side of the page. Take the quiz to identify misconceptions you may have about characteristics common to individuals of other cultures. Return to this website to review more specific information when you are planning care for a patient whose cultural background is different from your own.

4. Explore the Health on the Net Foundation/HONcode website by typing http://www.hon.ch into your browser and then clicking on the Medical Professional link at the top of the page. Click on the "Trustworthy Medical Information" link and then type in the words "dental hygienist" in the search engine to get a list of HONcode-certified websites that provide information about dental hygienists. Try typing other words related to dental hygiene care into the search engine to see what "hits" you receive.

FOR YOUR PORTFOLIO

Use the basic information from the three chapters in Section I of the textbook to write a personal philosophy of dental hygiene practice statement. Describe how you believe yourself to be as a dental hygiene professional. Identify characteristics that describe the way you will provide dental hygiene care. Do this at the beginning of your training just after you complete these chapter and section exercises, and then do it again just before you graduate (don't peek at what you wrote the first time, please). Finally, write a summary of how these two documents reveal your personal growth during your training as a professional.

EVERYDAY ETHICS

Surf health-related websites, government websites, online health literature databases, or any other online resource to find information related to ethics in health care, research, or public health. In particular, topics such as informed consent, HIPAA, public health access, licensure, etc. provide good topics to investigate on the Internet. Identify a URL that others can use to locate the website or resource you discover, and then annotate the citation by writing a brief description, provide an overview of the contents, and explaining how the resource might be helpful for the study of professional ethics.

Combine what you discover with ethics-related materials identified by other student colleagues to develop an annotated bibliography of online resources everyone can use to help further explore the Everyday Ethics scenarios throughout the textbook.

(**Annotate:** *to provide a critical or explanatory description.*)

Section I Puzzle Clues

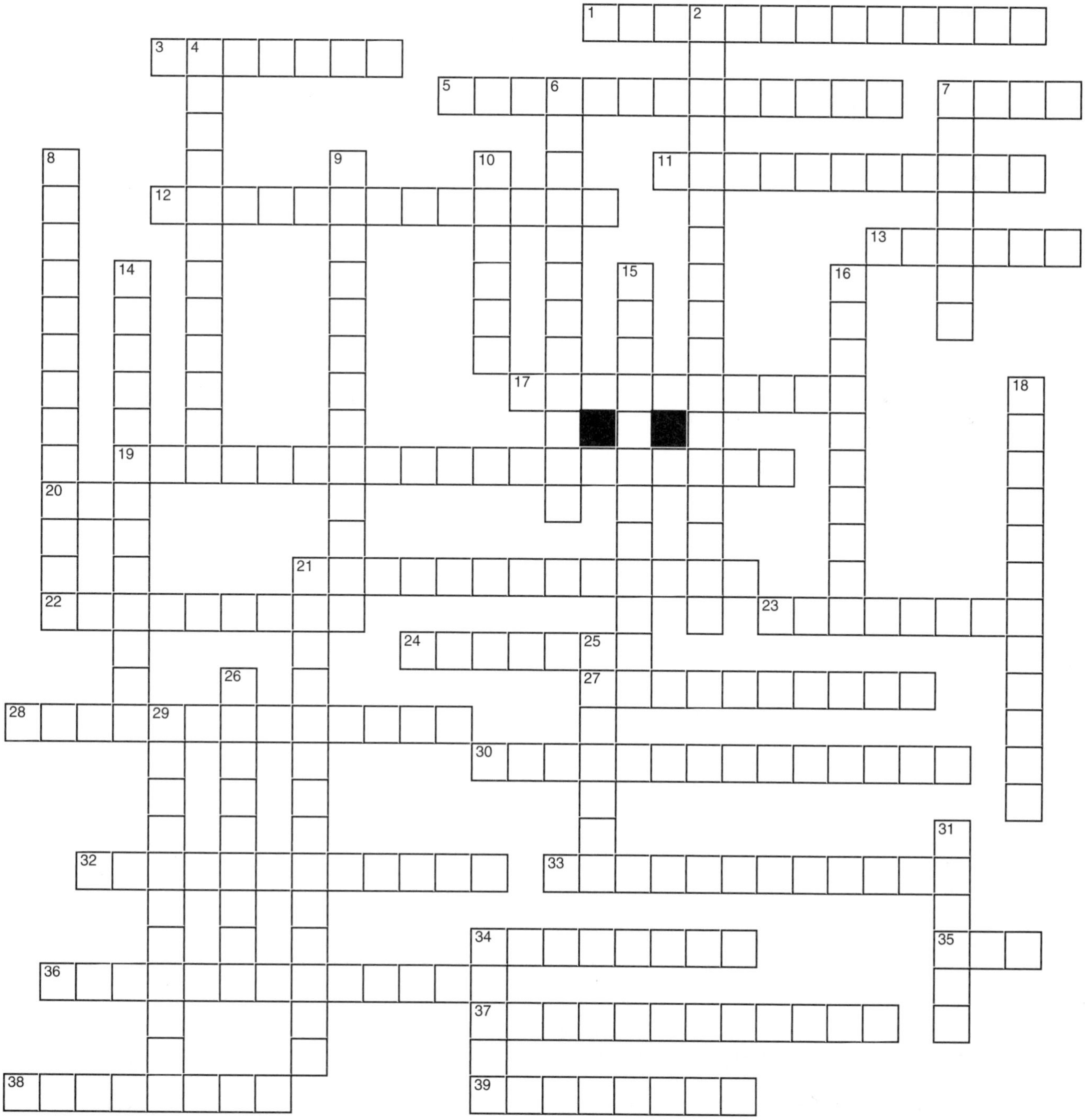

1 2 3 4 5 6 7 8 9 10 11 12 13 14 15 16 17 18 19 20 21 22 23 24 25 26 27 28 29 30 31 32 33 34 35 36 37 38 39

Puzzle Clues

Across

1. The dental hygiene role (often a component of clinical practice as well) that requires the dental hygienist to apply organizational skills and communicate objectives.
3. Communication disorder in which it is difficult to read, write, express or understand language.
5. Research type that helps determine the strength and type of relationship between two or more variables.
7. Acronym for the four components of a good researchable question.
11. The dental hygienist can help patients determine whether this attribute is present in health related websites.
12. An individual who is blind and cannot hear well has a ________ barrier to communicating.
13. Notation indicating the extent to which research results are not due to chance.
17. Self-____________ is an essential element of attaining both personal and professional goals and objectives.
19. Making an effort to understand the language, culture, and behaviors of patients with different backgrounds and beliefs.
20. Continuing Education Unit (acronym).
21. Effective health communication is enhanced if the practitioner is ________ regarding a patient's culturally related health practices and beliefs.
22. Originally identified by Dr. Fones as the primary role of a dental hygienist.
23. A collaborative organization that produces and disseminates a database of systematic reviews and other synthesized research to support clinical decisionmaking.
24. An ethical problem involving two or more morally correct choices or courses of action.
27. Use of inappropriate or simplistic modifications of speech when communicating with an older adult.
28. Affiliated dental hygiene practice relationship in which a consulting dentist provides oversight but not necessarily direct or general supervision. Can also refer to working with an interdisciplinary team of healthcare providers to meet a patient's needs.
30. A set of skills that allow individuals to obtain, process, understand, and respond to health messages (two words).
32. Social __________________ of health are conditions shaped by the distribution of power, money, and resources.
33. ________________ signs for yes and no vary between cultures. (two words).
34. A provider such as a dental therapist or advanced dental hygiene practitioner.
35. A group of individuals within an institution who review research proposals in order to protect the rights and welfare of volunteer research subjects (Acronym).
36. Verbal or written health information that is provided using simplified, clear terminology or pictures.
37. Type of supervision in dental hygiene practice that allows the dental hygienist to plan and initiate dental hygiene treatment without specific authorization of the supervising dentist (two words).
38. This barrier to effective health communication can happen when too much information is provided on too many topics at one time and no written reinforcement is provided.
39. Dental hygiene role related to influencing change in agencies and organizations to resolve problems and improves access to care.

Down

2. Communication between members of an interdisciplinary group of healthcare providers.
4. The skill set related to this health literacy domain include skills and knowledge developed during previous health-related experiences.
6. The ability to build a __________________ with patients is a key attribute of effective health communication.
7. Category of prevention measures initiated so that disease does not occur.
8. The six steps that form the basis for the standards for clinical dental hygiene practice (three words).
9. One of the steps in the dental hygiene process of care that is linked to all of the other steps.
10. Type of supervision in dental hygiene practice that requires an on-site presence of the dentist.
14. Communication with patients from other cultures (two words).
15. Research type in which variables are manipulated to discover cause and effect.
16. A _____________, step-by-step approach to finding applicable and current scientific information is an important component of evidence-based dental hygiene practice.
18. Outlines the responsibilities and duties of each dental hygienist toward patients, colleagues, and society (three words).
21. A core dental hygiene value involving avoidance of harm.
25. Database commonly used by dental hygienists for locating biomedical information related to patient care.
26. A type of communication that can be particularly important to consider if effective health communication is desired with a patient whose culture differs from that of the care provider.
29. When the patient perceives a lack of respect on the part of the care provider, an ___________ barrier to communication may exist.
31. The general standards of right and wrong that guide the behavior of members of a profession.
34. Communication type that uses technology to convey information to individual patients as well as a larger target audience.

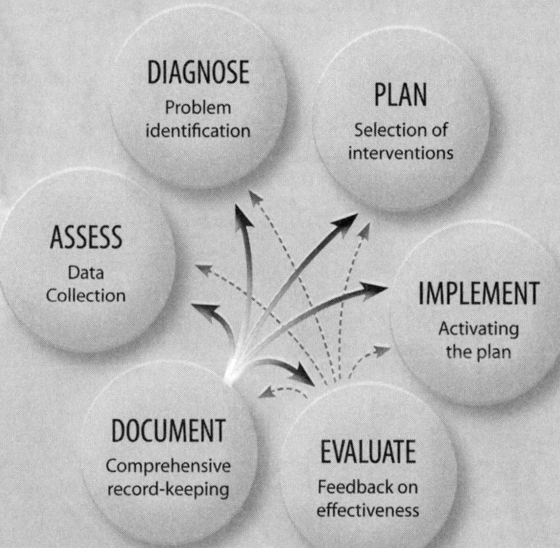

SECTION II

Preparation for Dental Hygiene Practice

Chapters 4-8

SECTION II LEARNING OBJECTIVES

Completing the exercises in this section of the workbook will prepare you to:

1. Apply concepts of infection/exposure control to protect the safety of self and patient during the dental hygiene appointment.
2. Position self, patient, and equipment to promote comfort, safety, and efficiency during the dental hygiene appointment.
3. Prevent and respond to emergency situations during patient care.

COMPETENCIES FOR THE DENTAL HYGIENIST (APPENDIX A)

Competencies supported by the learning in Section II

Core Competencies: C2, C3, C4, C5, C6, C9, C11, C12, C14

Health Promotion and Disease Prevention: HP2, HP4, HP6

Patient/Client Care: PC2, PC3, PC4, PC5

4

Infection Control: Transmissible Diseases

LEARNING OBJECTIVES

Upon successful completion of these exercises, you will be able to:

1. Identify and define key terms and concepts related to control of infectious diseases.
2. Explain the infectious process and discuss methods of preventing transmission of infection.
3. Identify and distinguish pathogens transmissible by the oral cavity.
4. Identify oral lesions related to various infectious agents.

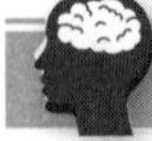

KNOWLEDGE EXERCISES

Also refer to Sections I, II, and IXK in the CDC Guidelines for Infection Control in Dental Healthcare Settings (Appendix V in the textbook) as you complete the exercises for this chapter.

Tables 4-1 to 4-3 in Chapter 4 of the textbook provide an excellent summary of details related to a variety of infectious agents that are of special concern for healthcare providers. You should study these tables carefully. Ask your instructor to tell you how thoroughly (or to what level of detail) you will need to study the information in these tables at this point in your dental hygiene program.

Write your answers for each question in the space provided.

1. Standard precautions apply regarding direct contact with:

   ____

   ____

2. List additional precautions healthcare providers are required to address.

   ____

   ____

   ____

   ____

3. In your own words, define cross-contamination.

   ____

   ____

4. List six factors that are necessary for transmission of disease.

   ____

   ____

   ____

   ____

5. Preventing disease from infectious agents requires breaking the chain of transmission. The use of standard precautions during patient care breaks the chain at every point. Identify additional ways that the dental team can break the chain and prevent transmission of infection.

6. Identify items in the dental setting that can serve as reservoirs for infectious agents.

7. Identify three ways infectious particles can be airborne in the dental setting.

8. Identify ways of controlling airborne transmission of infection in the dental setting.

9. Chapter 2 and Section IXK of the CDC recommendations (see textbook Appendix V) both mention tuberculosis as an infectious disease that is of concern for dental healthcare providers. Identify the microorganism that causes tuberculosis.

10. In what way is tuberculosis infection most commonly transmitted?

11. Describe XDR-TB.

INFOMAP 4-1 HEPATITIS INFECTIONS

HEPATITIS TYPE	VIRUS	MODE OF TRANSMISSION	METHOD FOR PREVENTION
"Infectious" hepatitis			Not discussed in this textbook, but use of careful handwashing and standard precautions is a very good start
"Serum hepatitis"			
Type C hepatitis			
Delta hepatitis			
Type E hepatitis			See the note below for hepatitis A

Note: Use information from Table 4-1 and the textbook information about viral hepatitis to compare modes of transmission and methods for preventing transmission of each type in the dental office setting.

12. What course of action does CDC recommend if a patient with symptoms or history suggestive of tuberculosis presents for elective dental services, such as dental hygiene care?

13. What is the significance of HbsAg? (see Table 4-2)

14. What is the significance of anti-HBs?

15. Which type of virus can be found in periodontitis pockets with relatively high prevalence?

16. Which of the herpes viruses can establish a latent infection in the trigeminal nerve ganglion that can reactivate and erupt in a surface lesion later?

17. Which virus type is associated with lesions on hands and eyes?

18. What clinical management protocol applies for a patient with an active HSV-1 lesion?

19. AIDS is associated with infection by the ______________________ virus.

20. List the ways the HIV virus can be transmitted from on individual another.

INFOMAP 4-2 HERPESVIRUS INFECTIONS

VIRUS	ACRONYM	MODE OF TRANSMISSION	ASSOCIATED OROFACIAL CONDITIONS
Herpes simplex virus Type 1			
Herpes simplex virus Type 2			
Varicella–zoster virus			
Epstein–Barr virus			
Cytomegalovirus			
Herpes lymphotropic virus			
Human herpesvirus 7			
Kaposi's sarcoma–related virus			

Note: Many herpes virus infections are associated with intraoral findings. Use the information in Tables 4-1 and 4-3 as well as the text to complete the INFOMAP 2. Include the acronym, mode of transmission and associated orofacial conditions for each herpesvirus listed.

21. A count of which serologic marker is most often used to evaluate and monitor the progression of HIV infection.

____

____

22. In HIV disease, the number of CD4+ T lymphocytes _______________ as the infection and symptoms become more severe.

23. At what level does the CD4+ T cell count indicate late stage disease or AIDS infection?

____

24. As the count of indicator cells decreases, the symptoms of disease and the incidence of oral infections or oral lesions related to the HIV infection _______________.

25. What are the most common oral lesions associated with HIV infection?

____

____

____

____

____

____

____

____

____

____

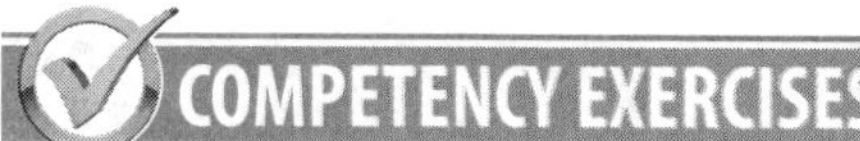

COMPETENCY EXERCISES

Apply information from the chapter and use critical thinking skills to complete the competency exercises. Write responses on a paper or create electronic documents to submit your answers.

1. The very first section of CDC Guidelines for Infection Control in Dental Health Care Settings (Appendix V in the textbook), which is titled Recommendations, provides a description of the evidence-based categories used to support each recommendation made in the report. Discuss, in your own words, what each of the recommendation categories means.

2. In your own words, write a paragraph or two summarizing the recommendations (in Section II of CDC Guidelines) for preventing transmission of bloodborne pathogens. In general, indicate the category of evidence that supports these recommendations.

3. In your own words, identify clinical management procedures to follow if your patient's medical history raises concerns about tuberculosis infection (section IVK of the CDC Guidelines can provide guidance).

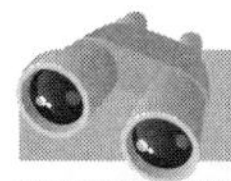

BOX 4-1 MeSH TERMS

Use a combination of MeSH terms and other key words to develop an effective and efficient PubMed literature search strategy.

Communicable diseases	Herpes labialis
Hepatitis	Herpesvirus 1, human
Hepatitis, viral, human	Herpesvirus 2, human
HIV	Herpesvirus 3, human
Tuberculosis	Herpesvirus 4, human
Methicillin-resistant staphylococcus aureus	Herpesvirus 6, human
	Herpesvirus 7, human
Herpes simplex	Herpesvirus 8, human

EVERYDAY ETHICS

Before completing the learning exercises below, reread and reflect on the Everyday Ethics Scenario and Questions for Consideration in this chapter of the textbook. It may also be useful to review the Dental Hygiene Ethics discussion in Chapter 1, the Ethical Applications in the introduction pages for each section in the textbook, as well as the Codes of Ethics in textbook Appendices I–IV.

Individual Learning Activity

Imagine the scenario from the patient's perspective. How might the patient's response to the questions following the scenario be different from those of the dental hygienist involved?

Discovery Activity

Ask a dental hygienist who has been practicing for a year or more to read the scenario. Provide them with a copy of the Code of Ethics as well. Share the responses you have made to answer each question and ask that person to discuss the situation with you. What insights did you have or what did you learn during this discussion?

Factors To Teach The Patient

- ▷ Reasons for postponing an appointment when a herpes lesion (fever blister or cold sore) is present on the lip or in the oral cavity.
- ▷ Importance of not touching or scratching the lesion because of self-infection to the fingers or eyes, for example.
- ▷ How the viruses can survive on objects and transfer infection to other people.

Your patient, Ms. Janette Whitlow, arrives just on time for her dental hygiene appointment, and you greet her cheerfully. As you update her health history, she mentions that she is grumpy because she is getting another cold sore and her lip itches and burns. You look closely and observe a reddened, slightly swollen area on her lower lip that is just beginning to get small bumps. As she talks, Janette slowly rubs her hand up across her face and eyes and up into her hair.

Write the outline that contains the main points you will cover in a conversation explaining to Janette why you recommend postponing her appointment until another day. Also explain why she should not touch or scratch the sore area on her lip.

Ask a student colleague or dental hygiene instructor to give feedback on the conversation you create, and then modify the conversation based on what you learned from the feedback.

Chapter 4 Crossword Puzzle

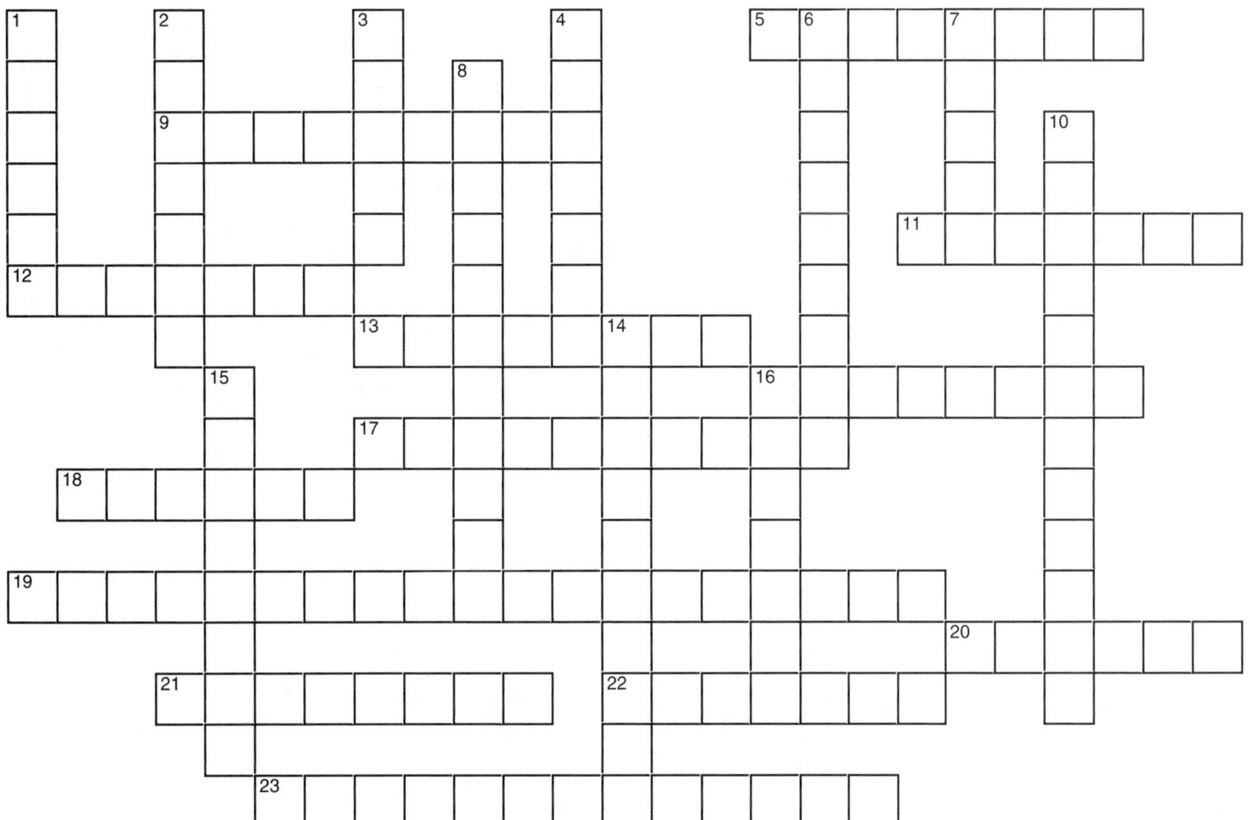

Puzzle Clues

Across

5. Widespread occurrence of more than the usual number of cases of a particular disease.
9. A latent viral infection that reactivates at a later date.
11. Someone who harbors a specific infectious agent but shows no clinical signs of disease.
12. Constant presence of a disease within a geographic area.
13. A natural or an acquired resistance against disease.
16. A widespread, extensive, or worldwide epidemic.
17. A path of entry through a mucous membrane.
18. The type of infection in which the causative agent remains inactive for a period of time within certain body cells.
19. An infection control approach that protects both healthcare providers and patients from pathogens (two words).
20. A carrier that transfers an infectious microorganism from one host to another.
21. Produced and secreted by body cells in response to, and able to bind to, a specific antigen.
22. Another term used for jaundice.
23. A pathogen that causes infection only when the host's resistance is lowered.

Down

1. An inanimate object on which disease-producing agents can be conveyed.
2. An individual who harbors a specific infectious agent with no discernible clinical signs or symptoms.
3. A genetic entity that contains either DNA or RNA or both; replicates inside living cells.
4. A substance that induces an immune response.
6. Early or premonitory symptom (adjective).
7. A laboratory test to detect antibody in the blood serum.
8. The factor that identifies a specific disease in a laboratory blood test (two words).
10. Continuous observation of the patterns of a disease in order to try to control it.
14. The period of time between initial contact with an infectious agent and the appearance of clinical symptoms of the disease.
15. The presence of a virus in certain body secretions, excretions, or surface lesions.
16. The type of immunity that is transferred from the mother or acquired by inoculation of protective antibodies.

5

Exposure Control: Barriers for Patient and Clinician

LEARNING OBJECTIVES

Upon successful completion of these exercises, you will be able to:

1. Identify and define key terms and concepts related to exposure control, clinical barriers, and latex allergies.
2. Apply and remove clinical barrier materials without cross-contamination.
3. Identify and explain the rationale for hand washing and other exposure-control techniques used during patient care.
4. Identify criteria for selecting appropriate protective barrier materials.

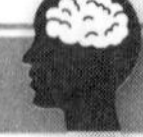

KNOWLEDGE EXERCISES

Write your answers for each question in the space provided.

Also refer to Sections III, IV, and V in the CDC Guidelines for Infection Control in Dental Healthcare Settings (Appendix V in the textbook) as you complete the exercises for this chapter.

1. An organized system for exposure control that treats body fluids of all patients as though they were infectious is a description of ______________________.

2. Identify the term or concept related to each of the following statements.
   - Physically blocks exposure to bodily fluids to prevent disease transmission.

     ____
   - A specific, potentially health-threatening bodily contact with infectious material while you are providing dental hygiene care.

     ____
   - Contact with infectious material that is reasonable to expect as a component of providing dental hygiene care.

     ____

3. List three purposes for having a written exposure control plan.

   ____

   ____

   ____

4. Define the following terms in your own words.
   - *Immunization*
   - *Inoculation*
   - *Toxoid*
   - *Vaccine*
   - *Vaccination*
   - *HCP*
   - *DHCP*

5. Unscramble the following words; definitions are included to help you.
   - hiiinrts (inflammation of the mucous membrane of the nose)
   - toxmanu (a test for the presence of active or inactive tuberculosis)
   - bcMytaercoiumr cykitbreysos (droplet nuclei, ranging from 0.5 to 1 μm, that are a risk in healthcare settings)

6. Updating immunizations against a number of diseases is an important protective factor for DHCP. What is a booster immunization?

7. List the basic immunizations recommended for DHCP.

8. List the factors that describe an appropriate clinic gown or uniform.

9. During patient care, long hair should be fastened back, and facial hair should be covered by ______________________.

10. List the essential characteristics of an ideal face mask.

11. Particles in aerosols smaller than ____________ can remain suspended up to 24 hours.

12. What size particle can penetrate to the alveoli of lungs when inhaled?

13. What size are the tuberculosis-causing bacterium particles?

14. When should a clinician wear a face shield over a regular mask?

15. How is a contaminated mask removed from your face?

16. Who wears protective eyewear during dental hygiene care?

17. List types of eyewear appropriate for wear during patient care.

18. List the features of acceptable eyewear.

19. List three steps you can use to disinfect and provide care for eyewear worn during patient care.

20. List glove safety factors that are important for both the patient and the dental hygienist during dental hygiene care.

21. When you are selecting the type of gloves to use during patient care, which glove factor is important for clinician comfort?

22. The cuffs of your gloves should _______________ the cuffs of your long-sleeved clinic wear to provide a complete barrier to contamination.

23. After positioning your gloves before patient care, you should touch only:

24. List factors that can affect the ability of gloves to provide a complete aseptic barrier.

25. When are heavy-duty utility gloves used?

26. During clinical practice, you will wash your hands many, many times each day. List the indications for washing your hands.

27. In your own words, describe the characteristics of an ideal sink for hand washing before patient care.

28. List the sequence of steps used for the antiseptic handwashing procedure you will perform before patient care.

29. Match each term with the correct description. Write the letter of the appropriate description in the space next to the term it refers to.

Term	Description
____ Standard mask filtration	A. Relatively stable on skin; reduced by washing
____ Surgical soap	B. Blocks particles with greater than 95% efficiency
____ Antiseptic hand wash	C. Used before patient care
____ Handwashing	D. Most important in preventing cross-contamination
____ Wide-coverage eyewear	E. Never at the sink used for patient care handwashing
____ Resident bacteria	F. Used by both clinician and patient
____ Transient bacteria	G. Contains antimicrobial agent
____ Skin integrity	H. Contaminates skin if contacted; reduced by washing
____ Gloves	I. Available in nonsterile and presterilized forms
____ Glove integrity	J. Affected by many things, including length of time worn
____ Eyewash station	K. Can be protected by covering abrasions with a liquid bandage

30. In your own words, define the following terms related to a latex allergic response.

- *Allergen*
- *Hypoallergenic*
- *Atopy*
- *Type I hypersensitivity reaction*
- *Type IV hypersensitivity reaction*

31. List five pieces of equipment used when providing dental hygiene care (other than gloves) that may contain latex.

32. List factors that increase risk for latex sensitivity.

33. What actions, taken prior to patient care for an at-risk patient, can reduce the risk of a latex allergy related emergency?

34. Refer to Appendix V in the textbook (CDC Guidelines for Infection Control in Dental Healthcare Settings) as you answer the following questions.
    - In the CDC 2003 guidelines, Section III, an alternative hand hygiene method for hands that are not visibly soiled, is given the highest category (IA) recommendation. What is the method recommended for hands that are not visibly soiled?
    - What is the recommendation included in the CDC 2003 guidelines regarding hand jewelry and what does the category II and the numbers (in parentheses at the end of the statement) included in the recommendation mean?
    - If your gloves become torn, cut, or punctured during patient care, what should you do?
    - The CDC guidelines recommend changing a mask between patients or during patient care if the mask becomes ________________.
    - If your protective covering (clinic gown) becomes visibly soiled during patient care, what should you do?

INFOMAP 5-1

METHOD	PREPARATION	LATHERING METHOD	SITUATION IN WHICH THE TECHNIQUE IS RECOMMENDED
Routine handwash			
Antiseptic handwash			
Surgical antisepsis			
Antiseptic hand rub			

Note: Fill out to compare the methods of handwashing. Then use the information in the Infomap to verbally describe the differences between the methods to a fellow student or a patient.

COMPETENCY EXERCISES

Apply information from the chapter and use critical thinking skills to complete the competency exercises. Write responses on paper or create electronic documents to submit your answers.

1. Use the information in Chapter 5 to develop a step-by-step checklist, in proper sequence, for getting ready to provide patient care. Consider the sequence for handwashing as well as applying all of the personal protective barriers that you use in your clinic. Pay careful attention to creating a detailed system that minimizes the possibility of cross-contamination.

2. Compare your checklist to the lists that other student colleagues have created or to one provided by your instructor. Refine your list and use it as part of your own personal written exposure control plan.

3. Describe at least three ways you can prevent cross-contamination during handwashing in the clinic at your school.

4. Practice removing gloves using the system illustrated in Figure 5-4 in the textbook. Explain how this procedure will prevent cross-contamination.

5. Explain why it is necessary to document a latex allergy on the patient's permanent record. Identify how that information is recorded in the patient records at your school.

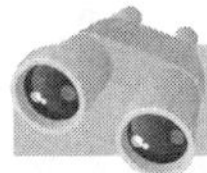

BOX 5-1 MeSH TERMS

Use a combination of MeSH terms and other key words to develop an effective and efficient PubMed literature search strategy.

Communicable disease control
- Hand hygiene
- Hand disinfection
- Infection control
- Universal precautions

Masks

Aerosols

Gloves, protective

Gloves, surgical

Hypersensitivity
- Hypersensitivity, delayed
- Hypersensitivity, immediate
- Latex hypersensitivity

Questions Patients Ask

What sources of information can you identify to help you answer your patient's questions in this scenario?

How do I know this room was cleaned after the last patient was in here? Did you wash your hands? Is everything you use brand new for each patient? How do I know that I won't be exposed to an infectious disease during my dental hygiene treatment?

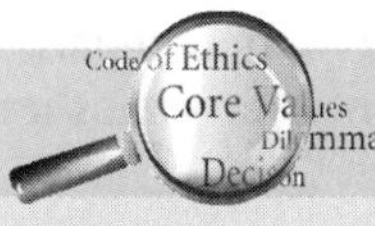

EVERYDAY ETHICS

Before completing the learning exercises below, reread and reflect on the Everyday Ethics Scenario and Questions for Consideration in this chapter of the textbook. It may also be useful to review the Dental Hygiene Ethics discussion in Chapter 1, the Ethical Applications in the introduction pages for each section in the textbook, as well as the Codes of Ethics in textbook Appendices I–IV.

Individual Learning Activity

Imagine that you are the dental hygienist in this scenario. Answer each of the questions for consideration at the end of the scenario.

Collaborative Learning Activity

Work with a small group to develop a 2- to 5-minute role-play that introduces the everyday ethics scenario described in the chapter (a great idea is to video record your role-play activity). Then develop separate 2-minute role-play scenarios that provide at least two alternative approaches/solutions to resolving the situation. Ask classmates to view the solutions, ask questions, and discuss the ethical approach used in each. Ask for a vote on which solution classmates determine to be the "best."

Factors To Teach The Patient

- ▷ Purposes for use of barriers (face mask, protective eyewear, and gloves) by the clinician for the benefit of the patient.
- ▷ Importance of eye protection.

Mrs. Johnson is bringing her 3-year-old son, Jimmy, in for his first dental hygiene appointment. She states that he is frightened by the mask and asks you not to wear it during the appointment. She is also concerned because she has never been asked to wear glasses during previous dental hygiene appointments at another dental office. She states that Jimmy will probably protest at having to wear the child-size glasses you have ready.

Write a paragraph you will use to explain to Mrs. Johnson the importance of, and the rationale for, using these barriers. Include some comments that will help explain their use to Jimmy.

6

Infection Control: Clinical Procedures

LEARNING OBJECTIVES

Upon successful completion of these exercises, you will be able to:

1. Identify and define key terms and concepts related to clinical procedures for infection control.
2. Identify basic considerations, guidelines, procedures, and methods for prevention of disease transmission.
3. Describe characteristics of an optimal treatment room and instrument-processing center.
4. Select appropriate disinfection, sterilization, and storage methods for clinical instruments and materials.
5. Identify procedures for management of an exposure incident.

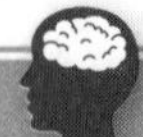

KNOWLEDGE EXERCISES

Write your answers for each question in the space provided.

1. Define *asepsis* in your own words.

2. What does *infection control* mean?

3. What is the purpose of maintaining proper infection control when you are providing dental hygiene care.

4. List three infection-control components that are all necessary for preventing transmission of infection and eliminating cross-infection.

5. What objects or features of a dental hygiene treatment room are important to consider when discussing infection control measures?

6. In your own words, describe the two processing steps to implement before sterilizing instruments used for patient care.

7. List the three basic methods for precleaning instruments prior to sterilization.

8. What procedures will protect you and others during manual scrubbing of instruments?

9. Identify three approved sterilization methods and list the time requirement that ensures adequate sterilization for each method.

10. Which method of sterilization processes instruments at the highest temperature?

11. List three types of tests used to determine whether or not sterilization has been achieved.

12. Describe a type of chemical indicator used each time on packaging to identify instruments that have been processed.

13. What microorganism is used as a biologic monitor for a steam autoclave system.

14. How frequently is biological monitoring of sterilization procedures recommended in the dental office setting?

15. Which type of autoclave sterilizes instruments the fastest?

16. Identify contraindications or special considerations to think about before using steam autoclaving as a method for sterilization.

17. What is the effect of pressure generated by an autoclave sterilizer?

18. List actions that can enhance the penetrability of the steam during an autoclave cycle.

____

____

____

____

____

____

19. During a dry heat sterilization cycle, a temperature of ____________ is maintained for 2 hours.

20. List two disadvantages of the dry-heat method of sterilization.

____

____

____

____

21. Chemical vapor sterilization cannot be used for materials and objects that ______________; it also cannot be used for heavy, tightly wrapped packages that ________________.

22. Chemical vapor sterilization systems should not be used in a small room because ________________ is required for safe use.

23. A chemical vapor sterilization system is tested weekly with biologic indicator strips containing ____________________________.

24. When is spore testing done?

____

____

____

____

25. Briefly describe a system for remembering to regularly monitor sterilization effectiveness.

____

____

____

____

26. To keep your instruments contamination free after sterilizing, you can store them in the ________________________.

27. List three uses for chemical disinfectants.

____

____

____

28. Describe the three levels of chemical disinfectants.

____

____

____

____

____

____

29. List the factors you will consider when selecting a chemical disinfectant for use in your dental hygiene treatment room.

____

____

____

____

____

____

____

____

____

30. What information on a product label tells you about the effectiveness of the chemical agent you use for disinfection?

____

____

____

____

31. List the product label items to look for when you prepare and use a chemical disinfectant.

____

____

____

____

____

____

32. Define each of the following types of waste.
    - Infectious waste
    ____
    - Contaminated waste
    ____
    - Hazardous waste
    ____
    - Toxic waste
    ____
    - Regulated waste
    ____

33. Items such as needles are disposed of in a ________.

34. Correctly number the sequence of steps for disinfecting environmental surfaces in the treatment room by placing the numbers 1–4 in the space provided.

Step #	Description of Step
______	Spray surfaces and allow to air dry
______	Put on PPE, including heavy-duty household gloves
______	Scrub surfaces with gauze sponges or paper towels
______	Spray all surfaces liberally and completely

35. According to CDC recommendations, water lines should be flushed for ______________ at the beginning of the day and for ______________ between patients to reduce microbial counts.

36. Identify two oral procedures that can reduce microbial counts before dental hygiene treatment.

____

37. What additional patient-related factors can be included as standard procedures that will help manage infection control during treatment?

____

38. Describe how a permucosal exposure to blood or other body fluids might occur.

____

39. What basic procedures are followed when a clinician experiences a percutaneous exposure to blood or contaminated body fluids?

____

40. Why is it important to clean the exposed parts of your face regularly during your clinical day?

____

41. What three components regarding infection control are included in an office policy manual?

____

Refer to Appendix V in the textbook (CDC Guidelines for Infection Control in Dental

Healthcare Settings) as you answer the following three questions.

CDC 1 Section VIA of the CDC guidelines recommend that you use only FDA-cleared medical devices and that you follow manufacturer's instructions for sterilization. The category for this recommendation is IB. What does a category IB recommendation mean?

CDC 2 What procedure does Section VIF of the CDC guidelines recommend in the case of a positive spoor-monitoring test?

CDC 3 The CDC guidelines, Section VII, recommends the use of ______________-level chemical disinfectants on clinical contact surfaces that are visibly contaminated with blood.

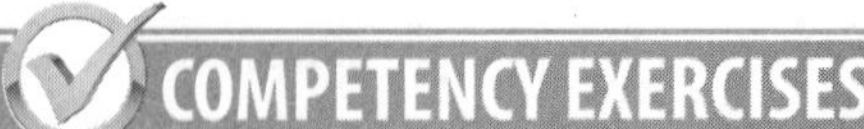

COMPETENCY EXERCISES

Apply information from the chapter and use critical thinking skills to complete the competency exercises. Write responses on paper or create electronic documents to submit your answers.

1. *Putting it all together:* Review both Chapters 5 and 6 to answer this question. Write brief statements or lists to summarize all of the procedures you can follow every day to maintain the chain of asepsis and prevent disease transmission in each of the following categories.
   - You and your colleagues
   - Your patient
   - The clinic
   - During treatment
   - Post-treatment.
2. Explain the difference between decontamination, disinfection, and sterilization.
3. Identify specific ways planning ahead prior to seating a patient in the dental chair can ensure you will maintain asepsis and eliminate cross-contamination during patient treatment.
4. The textbook describes features of dental treatment room equipment that facilitate optimum infection control. Describe the features in your school clinic that meet these criteria.

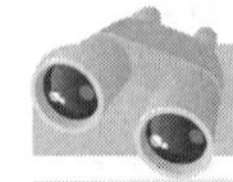

BOX 6-1 MeSH TERMS

Use a combination of MeSH terms and other key words to develop an effective and efficient PubMed literature search strategy.

Infection control, dental	Sterilization
Universal precautions	Dental waste

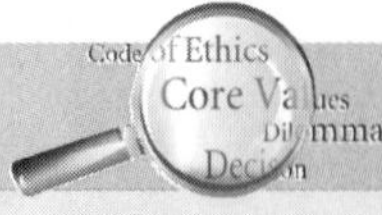

EVERYDAY ETHICS

Before completing the learning exercises below, reread and reflect on the Everyday Ethics Scenario and Questions for Consideration in this chapter of the textbook. It may also be useful to review the Dental Hygiene Ethics discussion in Chapter 1, the Ethical Applications in the introduction pages for each section in the textbook, as well as the Codes of Ethics in textbook Appendices I–IV.

Individual Learning Activity

Imagine that you are the dental hygienist in this scenario. Answer each of the questions for consideration at the end of the scenario.

Collaborative Learning Activity

Ask a dental hygienist who has been practicing for a year or more to read the scenario. Share the responses you have made to answer each question and ask that person to discuss the situation with you. What insights did you have or what did you learn during this discussion?

4. A treatment room that is completely prepared when each patient arrives demonstrates professionalism and inspires patient confidence. The dental hygiene instruments are arranged for each patient, with the sterile packaging sealed until the patient is seated and the appointment has started. Explain how your body language can affect a patient's impression of your professionalism as you welcome him or her into your treatment room.

5. Mrs. Virginia Weatherbee, a 50 year old with a charming smile, has been a patient in your clinic for many years. In a previous appointment with you, Mrs. Weatherbee has said that you may call her Ginny. Right after you get your patient settled in the dental chair, Samantha, who is in her first year of college and working for the summer as the dental hygiene assistant, peeks in to ask you a question. Discuss several reasons why it might be important to introduce your patient to Samantha as "Mrs. Weatherbee" prior to, or even instead of, explaining that she has asked you to call her Ginny.

DISCOVERY EXERCISES

Ask a student colleague to observe you periodically as you provide care for a patient or practice instrumentation during your preclinic labs. What risk factors for physical occupational disorders does your colleague identify in the way you are positioning yourself during instrumentation? What steps will you need to take to help maintain personal wellness throughout your career?

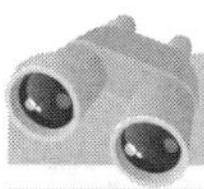

BOX 7-1 MeSH TERMS

Use a combination of MeSH terms and other key words to develop an effective and efficient PubMed literature search strategy.

Bursitis	Orthostatic hypotension
Carpal tunnel syndrome	Supine position
Cumulative trauma disorders	Tendinopathy
Head-down tilt	Thoracic outlet syndrome

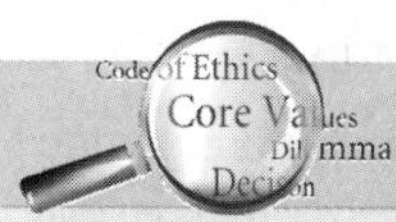

EVERYDAY ETHICS

Before completing the learning exercises below, reread and reflect on the Everyday Ethics Scenario and Questions for Consideration in this chapter of the textbook. It may also be useful to review the Dental Hygiene Ethics discussion in Chapter 1, the Ethical Applications in the introduction pages for each section in the textbook, as well as the Codes of Ethics in textbook Appendices I–IV.

Individual Learning Activity

Imagine that you are the dental hygienist in this scenario. Answer each of the questions for consideration at the end of the scenario.

Discovery Activity

Ask a dental hygienist who has been practicing for a year or more to read the scenario. Provide them with a copy of the Code of Ethics as well. Share the responses you have made to answer each question and ask that person to discuss the situation with you. What insights did you have or what did you learn during this discussion?

Factors To Teach The Patient

This scenario is related to the following factors listed in this chapter of the textbook:

▷ How patient cooperation makes it possible for the dental hygienist to practice with less stress and strain to prevent musculoskeletal discomfort and pain, and deliver better patient care

The patient in your chair today is a curious and very fidgety 10-year-old boy named Nathan. Even before you get him seated in the dental chair, he starts asking you questions about how things work and the function of each button and switch. He just can't seem to sit still.

Use the motivational interviewing approach (Chapter 26) to write a statement explaining the dental chair and how it helps keep both Nathan and you safe and comfortable. Use the conversation you create to role play this situation with a fellow student. If you are the patient in the role play, be sure to ask questions. If you are the dental hygienist in the role play, try to anticipate questions and answer them in your explanation—and remember as you talk that Nathan is only 10 years old.

8

Emergency Care

LEARNING OBJECTIVES

Upon successful completion of these exercises, you will be able to:

1. Identify and define key terms, abbreviations, and concepts related to emergency care.
2. List factors and procedures essential for preventing and preparing for a medical emergency in a dental setting.
3. Recognize signs and symptoms of a medical emergency, and identify an appropriate response.

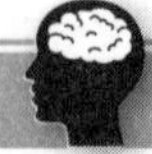

KNOWLEDGE EXERCISES

Write your answers for each question in the space provided.

1. Identify the patient assessment components that will help you know enough about your patient to help prevent an emergency during dental hygiene treatment.

2. Identify five **patient-related** factors that contribute to increased risk for medical emergency in a dental setting. (*Hint*: These are identified in several places throughout Chapter 8 in the textbook; some are psychosocial and some are specific to patient health status.)

3. Identify at least two dental treatment–related factors that contribute to greater risk for emergencies.

Recognizing the signs of patient stress is one impor- ıt way to prevent medical emergencies. Identify vou can reduce your patient's stress during den- ta. ne treatment.

5. Where in the patien. .tal record is medical information indicating that e patient is predisposed to medical emergencies liste l?

6. What additional information should you document in the patient record about your patient's risk for medical emergency?

7. What information must be clearly posted by the telephone in a dental clinic?

8. What does EMS stand for?

9. When a medical emergency happens in the dental setting, it is essential to document all pertinent information as well as everything that happens during the event and as well as in the patient's record after the event. Why?

10. In a medical emergency, your patient is "compensating" if the vital signs are:

11. In your own words, describe what happens if your patient goes into shock.

12. When a patient is in shock, he or she is often placed in the Trendelenburg position. What does this mean?

13. If an emergency situation occurs, you will first quickly ___________ the situation and then ___________ promptly but not hastily to provide basic life support as indicated.

14. Define *dyspnea*.

15. Describe the actions of a patient with a "mild" airway obstruction.

16. What are the signs of a "severe" airway obstruction?

17. If your patient is in distress and coughing but he or she appears to have good air exchange, what should you do?

18. Describe the difference between hypoxia and hypoxemia?

____

____

____

____

19. Direct delivery of oxygen is useful in most emergencies, but it is contraindicated in which two situations?

____

____

____

____

20. If your patient is not breathing, _______________ oxygen delivery is indicated, and a bag mask or _______________ is used to deliver _______________ percent oxygen.

21. If a regular face mask oxygen delivery system is used, _______________ L/min and _______________percent oxygen is delivered to the patient.

22. If the patient is breathing and needs only low levels of oxygen, the use of a _______________ device is indicated. Supplemental oxygen is started at _______________ L/min.

23. If a bag mask device is used, the bag is compressed at _______________ second intervals for an adult and _______________ second intervals for a child.

24. What will you do if your patient's chest does not rise and fall after applying an oxygen delivery system?

____

____

25. Place the steps for turning on an oxygen tank and using an oxygen delivery system in the correct order by placing numbers 1–4 in the space beside each step.

Order	Description of Step
_____	Attach delivery system to the patient
_____	Attach the delivery system to the tank
_____	Read and adjust the flow (turning knob in direction the arrow indicates)
_____	Turn the key counterclockwise

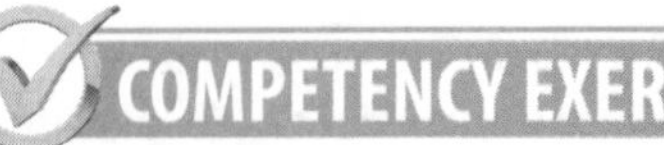

COMPETENCY EXERCISES

Apply information from the chapter and use critical thinking skills to complete the competency exercises. Write responses on paper or create electronic documents to submit your answers.

1. The only real way to become competent in responding to emergencies in the dental setting is to practice, practice, practice, and then practice some more. This exercise should be ongoing and include everyone in your dental clinic.

First, all students, faculty, and support personnel should *study Tables 8-3 and 8-4 in the textbook and be able to list the procedure to follow in each emergency*. Next, refer to Figure 8-2 in the textbook and write the list of duties assigned to each emergency team member on three small cards. (Or use your school's already established emergency protocols and procedures instead.) Finally, write the signs and symptoms of each emergency health situation listed in Tables 8-3 and 8-4 on a 3 × 5 inch card. If you'd like, write the list of procedures to follow for each emergency on the back of each signs and symptoms card so that you will have a handy reference for evaluating everyone's response to that situation.

When everything is ready, randomly give three people one of the three emergency team member cards and one person one of the emergency situation cards. The person who receives the emergency situation card is the patient and acts out the signs and symptoms listed. The emergency team must respond appropriately to the situation.

It is a great idea to practice this in your clinic setting, if possible. Try to initiate a round of this game when it is not expected, to add to the reality of the situation. When you and your colleagues become proficient at responding, try doing this role-play when patients are in the clinic receiving treatment. If you do this, talk quietly to each patient and make sure he or she knows what is going on; you will find that the patients are delighted to see you are practicing your emergency response. Some of them might even be willing to participate by pretending to be the patient who is experiencing the emergency!

DISCOVERY EXERCISE

1. Locate the emergency cart or kit in your school clinic. Use the emergency equipment list in Table 8-1 in the textbook to identify what items are included in the kit.
2. Does your school have a written plan for medical emergencies in the dental clinic? Is the procedure outlined similar to or different from the example in Figure 8-3 in the textbook? In what ways is your school's emergency report form similar to or different from Figure 8-1 in the textbook?
3. Determine how emergency medical services are activated in your school and/or in your community.

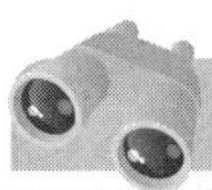

BOX 8-1 MeSH TERMS

Use a combination of MeSH terms and other key words to develop an effective and efficient PubMed literature search strategy.

Advanced Cardiac Life Support
Cardiopulmonary Resuscitation
Defibrillators
Airway Management
Heimlich Maneuver
Emergency Medical Service Communication Systems

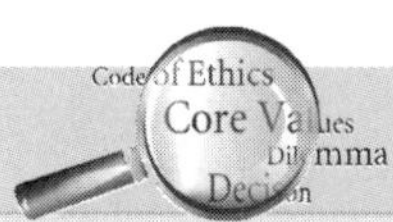

EVERYDAY ETHICS

Before completing the learning exercises below, reread and reflect on the Everyday Ethics Scenario and Questions for Consideration in this chapter of the textbook. It may also be useful to review the Dental Hygiene Ethics discussion in Chapter 1, the Ethical Applications in the introduction pages for each section in the textbook, as well as the Codes of Ethics in textbook Appendices I–IV.

Individual Learning Activities

Imagine that you are the dental hygienist in this scenario. Answer each of the questions for consideration at the end of the scenario.

Identify a situation you have experienced that presents a similar ethical dilemma. Write about you would do differently now than you did at the time the incident happened—support your discussion with concepts from the dental hygiene codes of ethics.

Factors To Teach The Patient

This scenario is related to the following factors listed in this chapter of the textbook:

▷ Stress minimization to prevent emergencies.

It is clear that Mr. Montgomery is an extremely anxious dental patient. He is scheduled with you today for presentation of the dental hygiene care plan you have developed. His health history indicates that he has Type-2 diabetes, hypertension, and angina. He has a past history of alcohol abuse, and he still uses tobacco.

Mr. Montgomery is extremely overweight and has trouble catching his breath after walking from the reception area to your treatment room. His periodontal status is poor, and he will require multiple appointments for scaling and root planing. In your dental hygiene care plan, there are several dental hygiene diagnosis statements that address his risk for medical emergencies during treatment.

To minimize the risk of a medical emergency, you plan to educate Mr. Montgomery carefully about how his treatment will proceed. Use a motivational interviewing approach as a guide to develop a conversation to use when you are talking to Mr. Montgomery about ways to reduce his stress during his dental hygiene treatment.

SECTION II Summary Exercises

Preparation for Dental Hygiene Practice

Chapters 4-8

COMPETENCY EXERCISES

Apply information from the chapter and use critical thinking skills to complete the competency exercises. Write responses on paper or create electronic documents to submit your answers.

1. Prior to seating the patient, you are handed the information in the Assessment Summary, received during a preappointment telephone call. This is a first-ever dental appointment for young Jean Luc Aristide who has recently arrived in this country from Haiti to live with a foster family while he receives treatment for his disease. He speaks very little English, but his bright smile and curious gaze capture your attention and make you smile back at him. Marge Black, a social worker who is arranging access to healthcare services, accompanies him to the dental appointment. What questions will you need to ask his guardian in order to determine Jean Luc's health status before providing dental hygiene care?
2. What steps will you take to protect both Jean Luc and yourself while you collecting the rest of your assessment data and providing oral hygiene instructions during this first appointment?
3. Identify any potential for emergency situations that could happen during Jean Luc's dental visit. What would be your response to any situation you have identified?
4. Examine the personal protective barrier equipment (protective eyewear, masks, gloves, etc.) you have

SECTION II – PATIENT ASSESSMENT SUMMARY			
Patient Name: *Jean Luc Aristide*	Age: *11*	Gender: [M] F	☑ Initial Therapy ☐ Maintenance
Provider Name: *yD.H. Student*	Date: *Today*		☐ Re-evaluation
Chief Complaint: *According to a preappointment telephone conversation with a social worker, there are no immediate dental problems. The social worker is trying to help the foster family provide the child with dental care.*			
Assessment Findings			
Health History • HIV positive status.	**At Risk For:** • Risk status is unclear without further medical information.		
Social and Dental History • Pt is newly emigrated to the United States and has never been to the dentist.	**At Risk For:**		

selected for your own use in clinic and describe how they meet the characteristics of acceptable exposure-control barriers.

5. Locate the eyewash station in your clinic that is nearest to your treatment area. Practice using the eyewash.

6. Plan and initiate an Emergency Situation Practice Session such as that outlined in Competency Exercise #1 in Chapter 8 of this workbook.

DISCOVERY EXERCISES

1. Search online or in the library to discover the purpose and function of each of the following federal, state, and local government organizations and discuss how they relate to the practice of dental hygiene.
   - *CDC*
   - *EPA*
   - *FDA*
   - *OSAP*
   - *OSHA*
   - *Department of Community Health*

2. The CDC Guidelines for Infection Control in Dental Healthcare Settings that you will find in Appendix V in the textbook contains only the outlined recommendations, not the full text of the report. You can access the complete report in your library by looking for the Centers for Disease Control and Prevention's *Guidelines for Infection Control in Dental Health Settings—2003 (MMWR 2003;52, no. RR-17)* or online at http://www.cdc.gov/mmwr/preview/mmwrhtml/rr5217a1.htm. Scroll down to explore the full report to find and read the section titled "Contact Dermatitis and Latex Hypersensitivity." Write a brief summary of what you learned. When you have time, explore the information in other sections of the report.

3. Investigate the sterilization methods and procedures used at your school clinic.

4. Investigate to determine your school clinic's protocol for procedures to follow if you experience a percutaneous or permucosal exposure to blood or other bodily fluids in the clinic.

5. Imagine that you have been asked to select a new handwashing soap that will be used in your clinic. Search for scientific evidence of effectiveness of antibacterial agents commonly used in handwashing soaps that are available for use by dental hygienists. Select the best alternative, and explain why you made your selection. (*Hint:* Check the soap currently in use in your clinic as well as some dental supplier catalogs to find the most commonly used antibacterial agents, and then develop a PICO question to help you review the scientific literature for research evidence of effectiveness.)

6. Investigate dental supply catalogs to determine the types of gloves available for use in dental clinics and the cost of each type. What scientific evidence is available to help you determine which type of glove provides the most effective barrier to microorganisms you are likely to encounter during patient care?

FOR YOUR PORTFOLIO

1. Develop a personal, written exposure-control plan. Don't forget to include an appropriate reference list to indicate that you have based your personal plan on scientific evidence. Consider making the plan in a format that could be easily updated and adapted to any setting later on when you are a practicing dental hygienist.

2. List your personal selections/recommendations for handwashing soap, gloves, and any other infection-control supplies used in dental hygiene care. Support each recommendation with a brief written summary of product characteristics and how the product meets criteria for acceptability.

3. Develop a personal, written long-term plan to avoid cumulative trauma injuries related to dental hygiene practice. Update this plan yearly as you learn more about working conditions that compromise your comfort and effectiveness when you are providing dental hygiene care.

4. Compile a personal immunization log. Identify any missing immunizations and make arrangements to receive them.

Crossword Puzzle

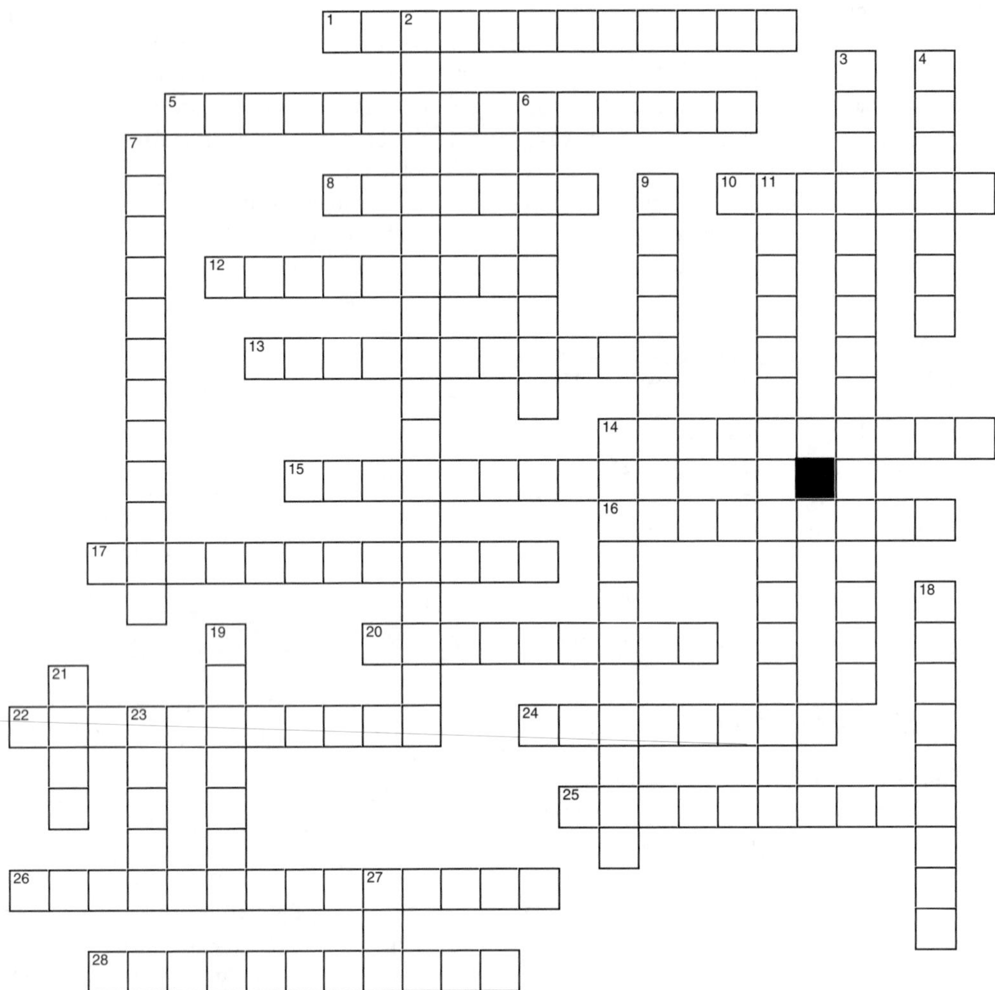

Puzzle Clues

Across

1. Refers to exposure to disease that may result from the performance of one's usual duties.
5. Carpal tunnel syndrome is a ________________ disorder that commonly affects dental hygienists.
8. Labored or difficult breathing.
10. Particles suspended in air.
12. A type of dental hygiene practice that includes attention to equipment, work layout, and work processes that decrease strain and fatigue and protect the functional health and well-being of both the clinician and the patient (two words).
13. A state that can occur if a patient is suddenly brought upright after being in a supine position for a long period of time.
14. Refers to the people, equipment, and other materials identified as a link in the chain of disease transmission.
15. Agent that can be used to reduce surface pathogens on mucosa or skin.
16. Kill all forms of life, as with an autoclave.
17. Refers to the period of time when an infectious agent can be transferred from an infected person to another person.
20. A substance contaminated with biomaterial that has the potential to transmit infection.
22. Process of introducing a substance into the body to produce immunity to a specific disease.
24. A virus, microorganism, or other substance that causes disease or infection.
25. Abnormal heartbeat rhythm.
26. Position in which the patient is supine on an inclined surface with heart higher than the head.
28. Orthostatic __________ is a drop in blood pressure related to a rapid change in position from lying back to standing.

Down

2. Transmission of potentially infectious agents between from one place or person and another person or place (two words).
3. Patient is placed on one side with top leg bent at hip and knee and arm closest to the floor is outstretched above the head.
4. Diminished oxygen in body tissues.
6. A preventive, functional-movement strategy that, performed daily, can help reduce the dental hygienist's risk for musculoskeletal injury and prevent pain.
7. Involuntary muscular contraction; in the heart muscle can be a cause of cardiac arrest.
9. To apply substances that destroy most (but not all) infective organisms onto an inanimate object or surface.
11. Eye, mouth, mucous membrane, nonintact skin, or parenteral contact with blood or other potentially infectious material (two words).
14. Repetitive movements, use of a forceful grasp, and vibration are commonly recognized ergonomic ______________ (two words).
18. A chemical ____________ is used to change the color of a marker on autoclave tape to indicate that the package has been brought to a specific temperature.
19. Temporary loss of consciousness caused by sudden fall in blood pressure.
21. Useful for protecting face and respiratory system from aerosols when providing dental hygiene treatment.
23. Wiping, scrubbing, or other process that reduces bioburden, but does not completely eliminate contamination on clinical instruments or surfaces.
27. Emergency cardiac care that supports ventilation and maintains blood flow (acronym).

SECTION III

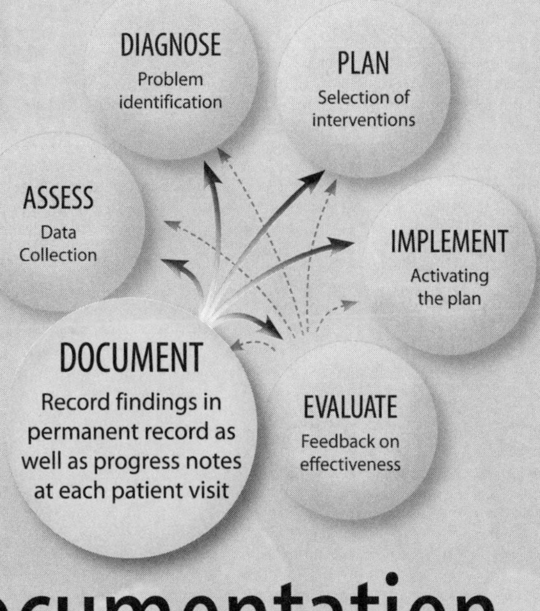

Documentation

Chapter 9

SECTION III LEARNING OBJECTIVES

Completing the exercises in this section of the workbook will prepare you to:

1. Document all aspects of dental hygiene care.

COMPETENCIES FOR THE DENTAL HYGIENIST (APPENDIX A)

Competencies supported by the learning in Section III

Core Competencies: C2, C5, C11

Patient/Client Care: PC1, PC13

9

Documentation for Dental Hygiene Care

LEARNING OBJECTIVES

Upon successful completion of these exercises, you will be able to:

1. Identify and define key terms and concepts related to written and computerized dental records and charting.
2. Describe concepts related to ensuring confidentiality and privacy of patient information.
3. Compare three tooth-numbering systems.
4. Discuss the various components of the patient's permanent, comprehensive dental record.
5. Recognize and explain a systematic method for documenting patient visits.

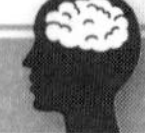

KNOWLEDGE EXERCISES

Write your answers for each question in the space provided.

1. Why do dental professionals document patient care activities and maintain a permanent, comprehensive patient record?

2. What actions regarding a patient record are essential to ensure accurate documentation of patient care in case the record is needed during a legal action?

3. List five types of documentation discussed in this chapter that comprise a permanent, comprehensive patient record.

4. List four types of information that are *never* included in a patient record.

5. Identify the important components of the patient record.

6. Handwritten records are recorded legibly and written in ______________.

7. What does the acronym HIPAA stand for?

8. What are the components of the current HIPAA law?

9. List patient rights that are protected by HIPAA.

10. List HIPAA-designated responsibilities of healthcare providers, employers, and facilities.

11. Identify the purposes for maintaining complete and accurate periodontal and dental records for each patient.

12. Identify the types of chart forms that can be used to record your patient's dental charting.

13. Define systematic procedure as it relates to dental charting.

14. In your own words, briefly describe the following clinical observations included in your patient's periodontal charting.
    - Gingival changes
    - Items charted
    - Deposits
    - Factors related to occlusion
    - Radiographic findings

15. What items are documented in a dental charting record?

16. What factors are included in a patient progress note?

17. Briefly *describe* each of the components in the SOAP note method for documenting patient visits.

18. Because different tooth numbering systems are used in dental offices and clinics, it is necessary for you to be familiar with all of them. Refer to Figures 9-1–9-3 in the textbook to provide guidance as you complete the Infomap below. Completing this exercise will help you compare the three types of tooth numbering systems.

INFOMAP 9-1

TOOTH NUMBERING SYSTEM	ORGANIZATION (ARCHES OR QUADRANTS)	PERMANENT DENTITION	PRIMARY DENTITION	ADDITIONAL FEATURES	EXAMPLE: MAXILLARY RIGHT CENTRAL INCISOR
Palmer system tooth numbering					
International tooth numbering (FDI)					
Universal tooth numbering (American Dental Association)					

COMPETENCY EXERCISES

Apply information from the chapter and use critical thinking skills to complete the Competency exercises. Write responses on paper or create electronic documents to submit your answers.

1. Caroline Lacy arrives for your 10:00 appointment. She is 3 years old. Identify the correct tooth number for the two teeth listed below using each of the tooth numbering systems.

	Mandibular Left Primary First Molar	Maxillary Left Primary First Molar
Palmer		
FDI		
Universal		

2. The dental practice where you work has decided to change from a charting system that uses anatomic drawings of the complete teeth to one that contains only geometric diagrams. The plan is to chart both restorative and periodontal findings on the new form. You are asked for your opinion at the staff meeting. What is your response? Make sure to state your opinion of the benefits and limitations of each type of form.

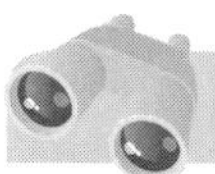

BOX 9-1 MeSH TERMS

Use a combination of MeSH terms and other key words to develop an effective and efficient PubMed literature search strategy.

Dental records	Confidentiality
Health records, personal	Informed consent
Electronic health records	Patient access to records

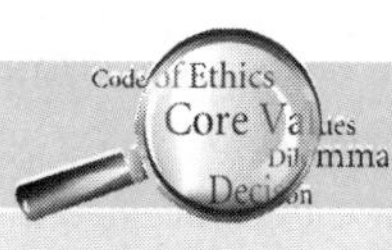

EVERYDAY ETHICS

Before completing the learning exercises below, reread and reflect on the Everyday Ethics Scenario and Questions for Consideration in this chapter of the textbook. It may also be useful to review the Dental Hygiene Ethics discussion in Chapter 1, the Ethical Applications in the introduction pages for each Section in the textbook, as well as the Codes of Ethics in textbook Appendices I–IV.

Discovery Activities

Ask a dental hygienist who has been practicing for a year or more to read the scenario. Provide a copy of the Code of Ethics as well. Share the responses you have made to answer each question and ask that person to discuss the situation with you. What insights did you have or what did you learn during this discussion?

Ask a friend or relative who is not involved in health care to read the scenario and discuss it with you from the perspective of a "patient" who receives services within the healthcare system. Discuss what you learned from the concerns, insights, or difference in perspective that person expressed.

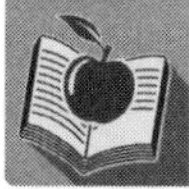

Factors To Teach The Patient

▷ Interpretation of all recordings; meaning of all numbers used, such as for probing depths.

You have just completed the periodontal and dental charting during a patient's initial appointment. The patient asks you to explain all those numbers and letters you were calling out to the dental assistant who was writing everything down for you.

List the main points you would want to cover in a conversation that explains the all of the kinds of numbers and letters that are used to document periodontal and dental conditions.

SECTION III Summary Exercises

Documentation

Chapter 9

COMPETENCY EXERCISE

1. Examine the past progress notes from a patient chart in your school clinic. Analyze each to determine whether the SOAP components have been included in each entry. Table 9-1 and Box 9-3 in the chapter should provide some guidance for this exercise. What, if any, information missing from any of the progress notes you sample?

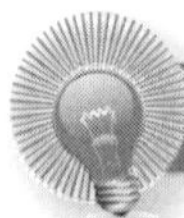

DISCOVERY EXERCISE

1. Examine the HIPAA documents provided for each patient in your school clinic. Interview several patients who have just received the documents to determine their level of understanding about their rights related to their medical records. What questions did patient have related to their right to confidentiality and privacy of their patient records? What questions did they have about their right to access their own information? What questions did they have related to security of their health information? Explain how this exercise might change your approach to presenting these documents to patients in the future.

Section III Summary Word Search Puzzle

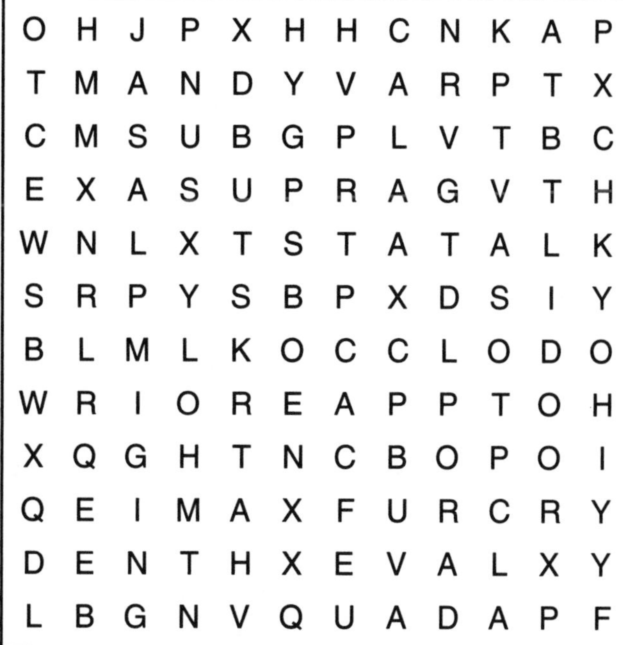

O H J P X H H C N K A P
T M A N D Y V A R P T X
C M S U B G P L V T B C
E X A S U P R A G V T H
W N L X T S T A T A L K
S R P Y S B P X D S I Y
B L M L K O C C L O D O
W R I O R E A P P T O H
X Q G H T N C B O P O I
Q E I M A X F U R C R Y
D E N T H X E V A L X Y
L B G N V Q U A D A P F

Do you know the ADA abbreviations for the following terms used to document patient information? Appendix VIII in the textbook may help you find the answers in the puzzle.

- Clinical attachment level
- Bleeding on probing
- Bite wing radiograph
- Check or observe
- Dental history
- Evaluate
- Examination
- Asidulated phosphate fluoride
- Furcation
- Gingival
- Health history
- Hypertension
- Dental hygiene
- Lidocaine
- Xylocaine
- Vasoconstrictor
- Mandibular
- Maxillary
- No known allergies
- Next visit
- Occlusal or occlusion
- Oral hygiene instruction
- Over the counter
- Prognosis
- Patient
- Quadrant
- Lower right quadrant
- Reappoint
- Scaling and root planing
- Prescription
- Immediately
- Subgingival
- Supragingival
- Toothbrush
- Treatment
- Varnish
- Within normal limits
- Systolic blood pressure

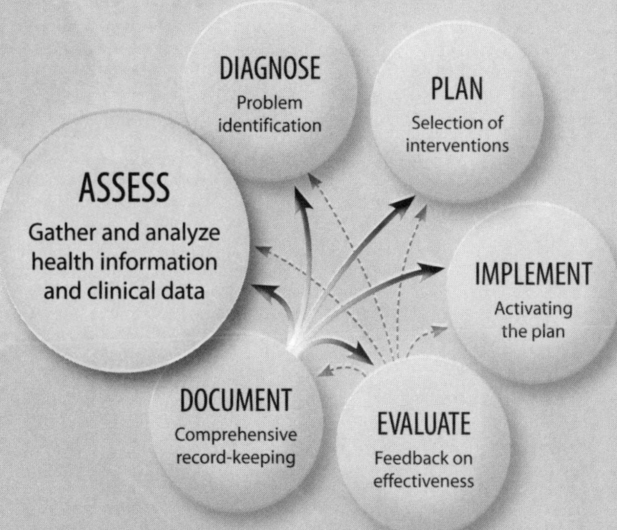

SECTION

IV

Assessment

Chapters 10-23

SECTION IV LEARNING OBJECTIVES

Completing the exercises in this section of the workbook will prepare you to:

1. Identify components of a complete patient assessment.
2. Apply a variety of assessment methods to gather data and document the patient's health status.
3. Determine individual and community oral health status using a variety of dental indices.
4. Document assessment findings.

COMPETENCIES FOR THE DENTAL HYGIENIST (APPENDIX A)

Competencies supported by the learning in Section IV

Core Competencies: C5, C10, C12, C13

Health Promotion and Disease Prevention: HP2, HP3, HP4, HP5, HP6

Community Involvement: CM1, CM2, CM6

Patient/Client Care: PC1, PC2, PC3, PC4

10

Personal, Dental, and Medical Histories

LEARNING OBJECTIVES

Upon successful completion of these exercises, you will be able to:

1. Identify and define key terms and concepts related to preparing patient histories.
2. Discuss the purposes of the personal, medical, and dental histories.
3. List and discuss the types, systems, forms used, question types, and styles used to collect patient-history data.
4. Recognize considerations for patient care that are identified by various items recorded on the patient history.

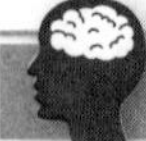

KNOWLEDGE EXERCISES

Write your answers for each question in the space provided.

1. In your own words, explain why taking a complete and accurate patient history is necessary prior to providing dental hygiene care.

2. In your own words, list the purposes of taking personal, medical, and dental histories during patient assessment.

3. List and briefly describe each of the systems for obtaining the patient's history.

4. List the characteristics of an adequate patient-history form.

____

____

____

____

____

5. What factors can affect the accuracy of a patient history?

____

____

____

____

____

6. List factors that can contribute to success in gaining patient cooperation during the history interview.

____

____

____

____

____

____

7. Describe each type of patient-history questionnaires in your own words.

System oriented

____

____

Disease oriented

____

____

Symptom oriented

____

____

Culture oriented

____

____

8. Identify the advantages associated with each method of collecting patient data.

Methods of Data Collection	Advantage
Each answer may be used more than one time. A. Questionnaire B. Interview	______ Legal written record with patient's signature ______ Consistent ______ Development of rapport ______ Time saving ______ Flexibility for individual needs

9. Why is it important to record contact information for the patient's physician in the personal history?

____

____

____

10. List three types of medical consultation related to the development of the patient history.

____

____

____

11. Which health conditions require that a patient receive antibiotic premedication prior to some dental and dental hygiene procedures?

____

____

____

12. Dental hygiene procedures that require antibiotic premedication for a patient at risk for endocarditis include those involving _______________ of gingival tissue or _______________ of oral mucosa.

13. State the standard antibiotic premedication regimen prescribed for at risk adult patients prior to dental procedures.

____

____

____

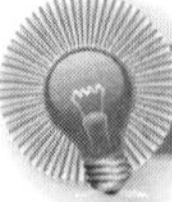

COMPETENCY EXERCISES

Apply information from the chapter and use critical thinking skills to complete the competency exercises. Write responses on paper or create electronic documents to submit your answers.

Review the patient-history questionnaire forms used in your practice setting (either your dental hygiene program clinic or the dental practice where you receive care). Use the information in the "Considerations for Appointment Procedures" column of Tables 10-1, 10-2, and 10-3 to identify the reason for including each of the items included on the form.

Compare the patient-history form used in your practice or school clinic with the ADA form included in the textbook chapter. What are the similarities and differences between the forms?

Using the format required in your dental hygiene program clinic, document an imaginary patient appointment during which personal, dental, and medical histories are obtained.

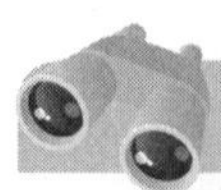

DISCOVERY EXERCISE

Search online to find patient health history questionnaires in languages other than English.

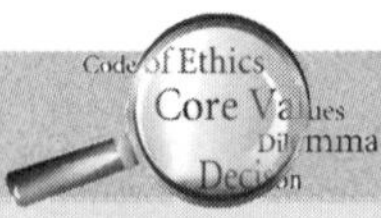

BOX 10-1 MeSH TERMS

Use a combination of MeSH terms and other key words to develop an effective and efficient PubMed literature search strategy.

Dental records	Electronic medical records
History taking	Medical history taking
Health records, personal	Antibiotic prophylaxis

EVERYDAY ETHICS

Before completing the learning exercises below, reread and reflect on the Everyday Ethics Scenario and Questions for Consideration in this chapter of the textbook. It may also be useful to review the Dental Hygiene Ethics discussion in Chapter 1, the Ethical Applications in the introduction pages for each section in the textbook, as well as the Codes of Ethics in textbook Appendices I–IV.

Individual Learning Activity

Imagine that you are the dental hygienist in this scenario. Answer each of the questions for consideration at the end of the scenario.

Discovery Activity

Ask a dental hygienist who has been practicing for a year or more to read the scenario. Provide a copy of the Code of Ethics as well. Share the responses you have made to answer each question and ask that person to discuss the situation with you. What insights did you have or what did you learn during this discussion?

Factors To Teach The Patient

This scenario is related to the following factors listed in this chapter of the textbook:

- The need for obtaining the personal, medical, and dental history before performing dental and dental hygiene procedures and the need for keeping the histories up to date.
- The assurance that recorded histories are kept in strict professional confidence.
- The relationship between oral health and general physical health.
- The interrelationship of medical and dental care.

You are just starting to treat Jon Wojeckick, who is 37 years old. You begin to ask questions about his medical history. You notice that he has stopped making eye contact and is hesitating over some of the answers. You have a feeling that he is not giving you accurate information, and you want to be sure you are obtaining all the data you need to provide optimum safe care. You know from studying Tables 10-1, 10-2, and 10-3 in the textbook that items from the patient history have a connection to how you provide dental hygiene care for your patient.

Use the Motivational Interviewing approach outlined in Appendix D of this workbook as a guide to write a statement explaining the relationship between oral health and physical health. Explain the need for accurate information to facilitate treatment planning. Include at least three examples of appointment considerations that are linked to items in the patient history. Be sure to assure Mr. Wojeckick that recorded histories are kept in strict professional confidence.

11

Vital Signs

LEARNING OBJECTIVES

Upon successful completion of these exercises, you will be able to:

1. Identify and define key terms and concepts related to recording vital signs.
2. Identify four vital signs and describe the range of expected values.
3. Describe procedures for determining and recording a patient's temperature, pulse, respiration, and blood pressure.
4. Discuss the importance of regular determination of vital signs for a patient receiving dental hygiene care.

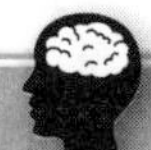

KNOWLEDGE EXERCISES

Write your answers for each question in the space provided.

1. Describe how you will position your patient to explain and record vital signs.

2. If your patient's vital signs are not within normal range, what should you do?

3. What are the normal adult ranges for each of the vital signs?

4. What factors should you consider when you are deciding whether to take your patient's temperature?

5. Normal average temperature varies among individuals, but in general, the average temperature of an adult over 70 years old is slightly ____________ than the adult average, and the temperature of a child under 5 years old may be slightly____________.

6. List the factors that can increase body temperature.

7. The most common location for taking a temperature is the mouth. What contraindications would lead you to select another method?

8. What emergency situations may cause your patient to exhibit an increased pulse rate? (*Hint*: See Tables 8-4 and 8-5 in the Emergency Care chapter of the textbook)

9. In your own words, describe how to obtain and record your patient's pulse.

10. Define a respiration.

11. Describe the factors to observe while you are counting your patient's respiration rate.

12. The count of respirations is taken immediately after counting the pulse. The fingers used to count the pulse remain positioned. Why is this procedure followed?

13. What emergency situations can cause a change in your patient's respiration?

14. What physical factors determine the maintenance of blood pressure?

15. Emergencies such as fainting, blood loss, and shock will cause blood pressure to ____________.

16. What action should you take if your patient's blood pressure is at a prehypertension level or above?

17. How frequently should your patient's blood pressure be taken and recorded?

COMPETENCY EXERCISES

Apply information from the chapter and use critical thinking skills to complete the competency exercises. Write responses on paper or create electronic documents to submit your answers.

1. You have just seated Maura Kennedy in the dental chair for her dental hygiene maintenance appointment. You read in her patient record that she is 33 years old, has no remarkable health problems, and is taking no medications. She reports that the only change in her health history today is that she has had a sinus infection for the last 2 weeks. She reports that she started taking antibiotics the day before yesterday and is feeling a bit better, but her nasal passages are still all stuffed up. Write a brief statement that you will use to inform Maura that you are going to determine and record her vital signs.

2. When you take Maura's temperature, you find that it is normal. Her pulse rate is 70 beats/minute; while you still have your fingers on her wrist, you count her respirations. Her respiration is slightly fast, 20/minute, and you note that she takes several shallow breaths, followed by one or two gulps of air and that she wheezes a bit when she exhales. However, you note that her color is good, so she must not be having any real problem with air exchange, and her breathing problems may just be the result of her stuffy nose. You wrap the blood pressure cuff around her right arm, pump it up, and place the stethoscope. You hear the sounds begin at the 122 mark on the manometer, and the last sound you hear is at 83. After a discussion with Maura and with Dr. Ichero, you all decide to reschedule Maura for her maintenance visit in a couple of weeks when her sinus infection is gone.

   Using your institution's guidelines for writing in patient records, document that you assessed Maura's vital signs at this appointment and rescheduled her appointment for a future date.

3. Create a brief step-by-step guide for determining and recording all of the vital signs on a 3 × 5-inch card (this is sometimes called a "job aid"). If you can laminate your job aid, you will be able to disinfect it to use during patient care. Practice using your step-by-step guide to determine and record vital signs for family members, friends, or student colleagues. If you practice with a dental hygiene instructor as your patient, you can receive valuable feedback on your techniques!

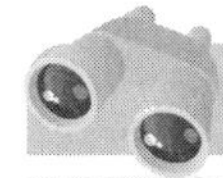

BOX 11-1 MeSH TERMS

Use a combination of MeSH terms and other key words to develop an effective and efficient PubMed literature search strategy.

Vital signs	Respiration
Blood pressure	Blood pressure determination
Body temperature	Sphygmomanometer
Heart rate	Stethoscopes
Respiratory rate	Auscultation
Pulse	

EVERYDAY ETHICS

Before completing the learning exercises below, reread and reflect on the Everyday Ethics Scenario and Questions for Consideration in this chapter of the textbook. It may also be useful to review the Dental Hygiene Ethics discussion in Chapter 1, the Ethical Applications in the introduction pages for each section in the textbook, as well as the Codes of Ethics in textbook Appendices I–IV.

Individual Learning Activity

Identify a situation you have experienced that presents a similar ethical dilemma. What did you learn from how the situation was (or was not) resolved at the time it happened?

Collaborative Learning Activity

Answer each of the questions for consideration at the end of the scenario in the textbook. Compare what you wrote with answers developed by another classmate and discuss differences/similarities

Factors To Teach The Patient

This scenario is related to the following factors listed in this chapter of the textbook:

- ▷ How vital signs can influence dental and dental hygiene appointments.
- ▷ The importance of having a blood pressure determination at regular intervals.

Mr. Borman Gorbachov, the CEO of a large manufacturing firm, is always in a hurry. He simply cannot seem to sit still for his whole appointment and is always chiding you that you should work faster so that he can be done and get back to work. Today he sighs heavily and then protests loudly when you tell him that you are going to take and record his vital signs. He states that he just had his blood pressure taken a month or so ago at his doctor's office and there is nothing wrong with him. You look in his patient record to discover that the previous blood pressure, taken almost 2 years ago, was normal.

Use a motivational interviewing approach as a guide to prepare a conversation you can use to educate Mr. Gorbachov about the reasons you determine a patient's vital signs at each appointment. Use the conversation you create to educate a patient or friend, and then modify it based on what you learned from the interaction.

Word Search Puzzle

V	H	U	O	Q	S	E	O	P	E	N	Y	N	Z	K	R	H
A	C	A	R	O	T	I	D	W	S	O	O	S	Q	S	T	C
B	J	U	Y	B	A	V	J	S	Z	R	Q	P	I	Y	Y	I
D	Y	S	E	A	F	P	G	O	U	M	F	H	E	S	M	H
T	G	C	H	P	P	D	N	T	M	O	V	Y	B	T	P	Y
Y	Y	U	Y	H	U	N	K	B	W	T	T	G	R	O	A	P
E	Q	L	P	B	Z	L	E	U	A	E	A	M	A	L	N	O
A	A	T	E	B	I	D	S	A	R	N	C	O	C	E	I	T
H	A	A	R	R	B	I	X	E	H	S	H	M	H	K	C	H
A	P	T	T	A	K	A	V	C	Y	I	Y	A	I	K	C	E
N	Y	I	E	D	R	S	I	K	T	V	C	N	A	S	J	R
O	R	O	N	Y	F	T	T	O	H	E	A	O	L	W	B	M
X	E	N	S	C	E	O	A	R	M	Q	R	M	J	R	Y	I
I	X	V	I	A	D	L	L	O	M	K	D	E	A	S	Q	A
A	I	O	O	R	D	E	S	T	E	P	I	T	C	S	D	G
Z	A	K	N	D	X	Y	I	K	R	C	A	E	R	T	U	K
T	R	A	D	I	A	L	G	O	C	N	G	R	K	I	C	C
S	G	L	Z	A	M	K	N	F	U	I	Y	C	U	F	F	Y
E	F	I	D	T	J	N	S	F	R	X	T	R	E	B	P	O
S	I	Z	G	E	M	Q	B	F	Y	L	B	J	S	T	Z	E

Puzzle Clues

- All four; body temperature, pulse, respiratory rate, and blood pressure (two words).
- Artery in the neck that is the site for taking a pulse during cardiopulmonary resuscitation.
- Device for determining blood pressure.
- A contraction of the heart ventricles during which blood is forced into the aorta and the pulmonary artery.
- A count of heartbeats; can also refer to the pressure that is the difference between systolic and diastolic blood pressure (40 mmHg).
- Element used in a device that records body temperature and also in a device that records blood pressure.
- Fever; temperature values greater than 37.0°C or 98.6°F.
- Heartbeat at a rate greater than 100 beats/minute.
- Inflatable component of a sphygmomanometer that wraps around the patient's arm during recording of a blood pressure.
- Listening for sounds produced within the body.
- The lower number in a recorded blood pressure fraction; marks the pressure at the last distinct tap heard on the sphygmomanometer.
- Lower-than-normal body temperature; values below 96.0°F.
- Normal tension or tone; pertaining to having normal blood pressure.
- Noted along with volume and strength when counting the pulse rate.
- Oxygen deficiency.
- Pulse taken using fingertips placed at the wrist.
- The site used to find the pulse for an infant.
- Sounds originating within the blood passing through the vessel or produced by vibratory motion of the arterial wall.
- A systolic blood pressure of 140 mmHg or greater and diastolic blood pressure of 90 mmHg or greater.
- Temporary cessation of spontaneous respirations.
- A type of thermometer that is gently inserted into the ear canal.
- Unusually slow heartbeat and pulse; below 50 beats/minute.

12

Extraoral and Intraoral Examination

LEARNING OBJECTIVES

Upon successful completion of these exercises, you will be able to:

1. Identify and define key terms and concepts related to providing an intraoral and extraoral patient examination.
2. List and describe the objectives for examination of the oral cavity and adjacent structures by the dental hygienist.
3. List and describe the steps for a thorough, systematic examination.
4. Accurately describe conditions and lesions found during an oral examination.
5. List the warning signs of oral cancer and discuss the follow-up procedure for a suspicious lesion.

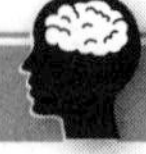

KNOWLEDGE EXERCISES

Write your answers for each question in the space provided.

1. In your own words, explain the purpose of performing an intraoral and extraoral examination for each patient.

___

___

2. Before you get ready to perform an examination for your patient, you first need to:

Review:

___

___

Examine:

___

___

Explain:

___

___

3. In your own words, explain the advantages of using a systematic sequence for the patient examination.

___

___

___

4. List and briefly describe the types of intraoral/ extraoral examinations.

____

____

____

____

____

____

____

____

5. Identify the anatomical landmarks shown in Figures 12-1, 12-2, and 12-3 by writing the appropriate term on each line.

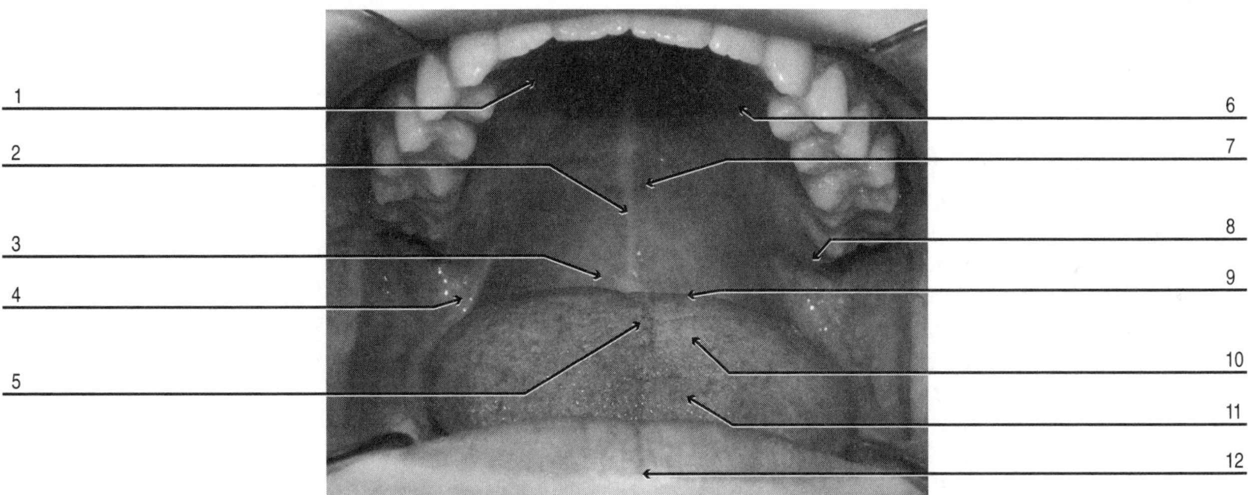

Figure 12-1

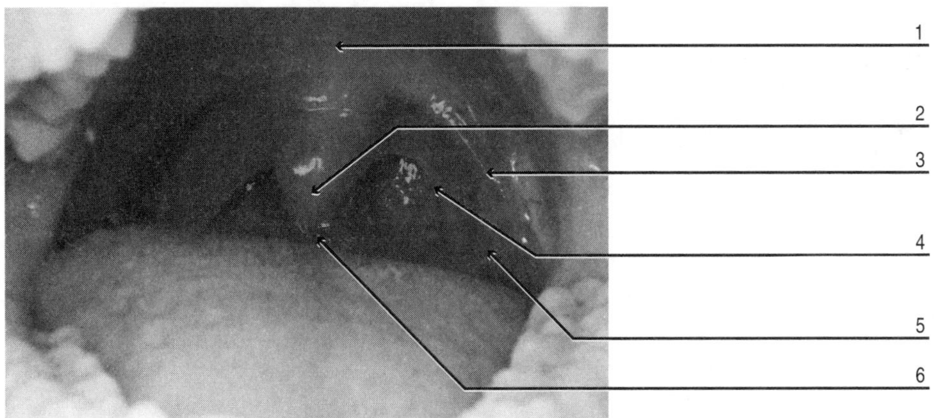

Figure 12-2

6. List the methods used to accomplish the extraoral and intraoral examinations:

____

____

____

____

____

____

7. What is auscultation?

____

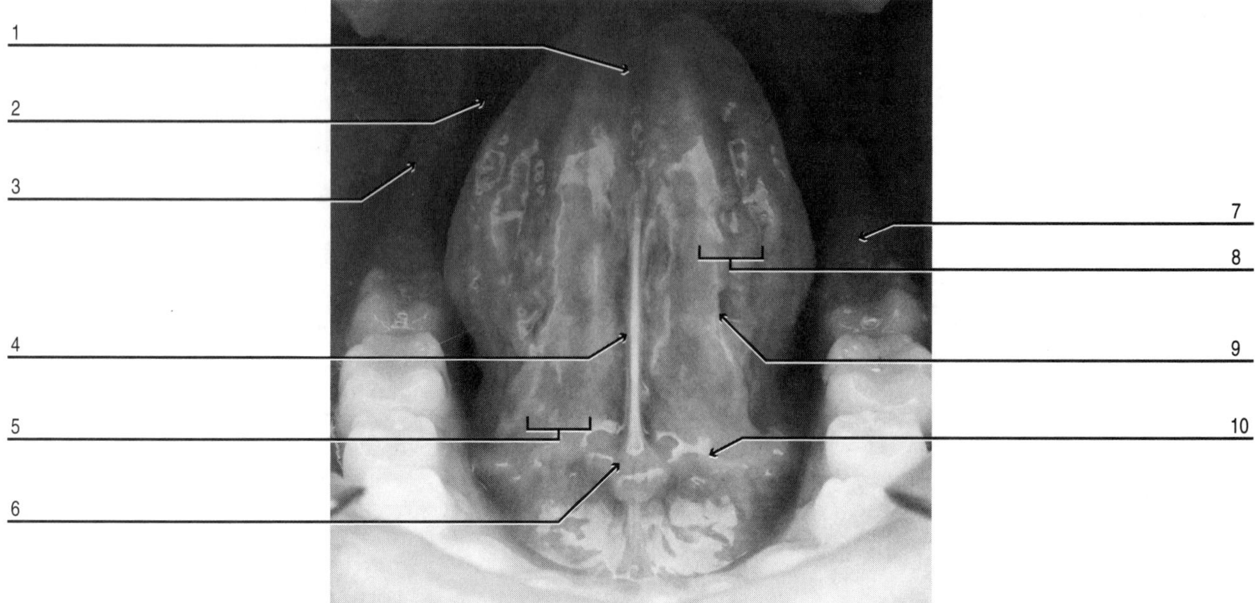

Figure 12-3

8. Match the types of palpation with the appropriate definition and description. There are two answers for each type of palpation.

Types of Palpation	Definition/Description
Digital: ____ and ____	A. Use of finger or fingers and thumb from each hand applied simultaneously in coordination
Bimanual: ____ and ____	B. Use of a finger C. Two hands used at the same time to examine corresponding structures on opposite sides of the body
Bilateral: ____ and ____	D. Use of finger and thumb of the same hand E. Palpation of the lips
Bidigital: ____ and ____	F. Index finger applied to the inner border of the mandible beneath the canine–premolar area to determine the presence of a torus mandibularis G. Index finger of one hand palpates the floor of the mouth inside, while a finger or fingers from the other hand press on the same area from under the chin externally H. Fingers placed beneath the chin to palpate the submandibular lymph nodes

9. In your own words, explain where lymph nodes in the cervical chain are located.

10. Describe the difference in the location of the submental and submandibular lymph nodes.

11. In your own words, define the following types of documentation recorded for each oral lesion.

History:

Location and extent:

Physical characteristics:

12. Identify the characteristics you would expect to observe for each of the following types of oral lesions.

Indurated:

Blisterform:

Pustule:

Plaque:

Ulcer:

Erythema:

Torus:

Papillary:

13. Early oral cancer takes many forms. Write a brief description of the characteristics you might observe for each of the five basic forms listed below.

White areas:

Red areas:

Ulcers:

Masses:

Pigmentation:

14. What characteristics indicate that a lesion should be biopsied?

15. When is a cytologic smear technique used to evaluate an oral lesion?

____

____

16. List the methods for examining cells in a suspicious lesion.

____

____

____

17. Briefly describe exfoliative cytology in your own words.

____

____

____

____

18. Match each laboratory report category with its description.

Laboratory Report Category	Description
___ Class I	A. Normal
___ Unsatisfactory	B. Uncertain (possible for cancer)
___ Class V	C. Slide is inadequate for diagnosis
___ Class II	D. Probable for cancer
___ Class IV	E. Atypical, but not suggestive of malignant cells
___ Class III	F. Positive for cancer

19. Using the information in Box 12-2 and Table 12-1 in the textbook, imagine that your patient presents with the conditions listed in Infomap 12-1 in the workbook. Complete the infomap by identifying the indications and influences on the appointment associated with each observation.

INFOMAP 12-1

OBSERVATION		INDICATION AND INFLUENCES ON THE APPOINTMENT
Overall appraisal of patient	Labored breathing	
Face	Evidence of fear or apprehension	
Skin	Multiple light brown macules	
Eyes	Eyeglasses (corrective)	
Nodes—submental; submandibular	Lymphadenopathy; induration	
Temporomandibular joint	Tenderness; sensitivity; noises (clicking, popping, grating)	
Lips	Blisters, ulcers	
Breath odor	Cigarette odor	
Labial and buccal mucosa	Multiple red nodules on left buccal mucosa	
Tongue	Coating	
Floor of mouth	Limitation or freedom of movement of tongue	
Saliva	Evidences of dry mouth; lip wetting	
Hard palate	Tori	
Soft palate, uvula	Large uvula	
Tonsillar region, throat	Large tonsils	

COMPETENCY EXERCISES

Apply information from the chapter and use critical thinking skills to complete the competency exercises. Write responses on paper or create electronic documents to submit your answers.

1. In your own words, explain the importance of careful description and documentation of any abnormality discovered during an intraoral and extraoral examination.

2. In your own words, describe the sequence of steps you will follow to provide a systematic and comprehensive extraoral and intraoral examination for your patient.

3. Your patient, Kurt Bachleim, age 23 years, presents with localized, coalescing multiple lesions on the right buccal mucosa. Mr. Bachleim also has an exostosis extending from tooth 12 to tooth 15 and trismus. Describe what you would expect to see and any possible adaptations you will need to make for the appointment.

4. Your patient, Yoon Chang, presents with a tiny (about 1 mm) bluish-black lesion on the top right half of her tongue. She said that it wasn't bothering her at all. You palpate the lesion, but do not feel anything unusual. Ms. Chang reports that the same thing had come up on her palate a few weeks ago. As you continue to question her, she mentions that she has had a broken blood vessel or two on her fingers in the past. She had actually forgotten about it until you started asking questions. Dr. Pine is not in the office today, so you document the lesion in the patient record in order to discuss it with him tomorrow and decide appropriate follow-up procedures.

   Use your institution's guidelines for writing in the patient record and the information in Chapter 12 to describe the lesion on Ms. Chang's tongue.

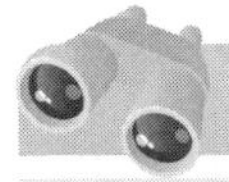

BOX 12-1 MeSH TERMS

Use a combination of MeSH terms and other key words to develop an effective and efficient PubMed literature search strategy.

Diagnosis, oral	Auscultation
Anatomic landmarks	Self-examination
Mouth	Lymph nodes
Palpation	Oral ulcer

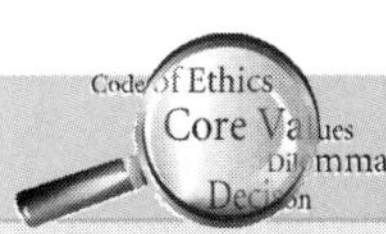

EVERYDAY ETHICS

Before completing the learning exercises below, reread and reflect on the Everyday Ethics Scenario and Questions for Consideration in this chapter of the textbook. It may also be useful to review the Dental Hygiene Ethics discussion in Chapter 1, the Ethical Applications in the introduction pages for each section in the textbook, as well as the Codes of Ethics in textbook Appendices I–IV.

Collaborative Learning Activity

NOTE: The Everyday Ethics Scenario in this chapter contains two different ethical components for the dental hygienist: providing information for her patient and approaching her coworkers to change office policies. Work with a group of students to provide alternate approaches for each of the two ethical concerns in the scenario.

Work with a small group to develop a 2- to 5-minute role-play that introduces the Everyday Ethics Scenario described in the chapter (a great idea is to video record your role-play activity). Then develop separate 2-minute role-play scenarios that provide at least two alternative approaches/solutions to resolving the situation. Ask classmates to view the solutions, ask questions, and discuss the ethical approach used in each. Ask for a vote on which solution classmates determine to be the "best."

Factors to Teach the Patient

This scenario is related to the following factors listed in this chapter of the textbook:

- ▷ The reasons for a careful extraoral and intraoral examination at each maintenance appointment.
- ▷ A method for self-examination. (The examination should include the face, neck, lips, gingiva, cheeks, tongue, palate, and throat. Any changes should be reported to the dentist and the dental hygienist.)
- ▷ The warning signs of oral cancer.

Aishia Williams presents with an oral lesion that may be malignant. She has previously been treated for a precancerous oral lesion and is at risk for recurrence. She has not been reevaluated for 18 months.

Use the motivational interviewing approach (Appendix D in this workbook) as a guide to write a statement explaining the need for careful follow-up and frequent evaluation by a dental professional as well as the need for Ms. Williams to perform a regular oral self-examination and to be aware of the warning signs of oral cancer.

Use the conversation you create to role-play this situation with a fellow student. If you are the patient in the role-play, be sure to ask questions. If you are the dental hygienist, try to anticipate questions and answer them in your explanation.

13

Dental Radiographic Imaging

LEARNING OBJECTIVES

Upon successful completion of these exercises, you will be able to:

1. Identify and define key terms, abbreviations, and concepts related to exposing and processing dental radiographs.
2. Describe procedures for producing and processing radiographic films and digital radiographic images.
3. Identify measures to protect yourself and your patient from ionizing radiation.
4. Select image receptor size and type, image receptor–holding devices, and clinical radiographic techniques for patient surveys.
5. Describe the positioning of individual intraoral image receptors based on area of the mouth and clinical technique.
6. Use guidelines to determine the indication for exposure of dental radiographs.
7. Identify probable causes of common radiographic inadequacies.

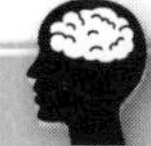

KNOWLEDGE EXERCISES

Write your answers for each question in the space provided.

Exposing and Processing Radiographs

1. In your own words, state two important objectives of dental radiology.

____

____

____

____

____

____

2. Using the diagrams and descriptions in the textbook as a reference, describe in your own words how X-rays are produced after the power switch on the X-ray machine is activated.

____

____

____

____

____

____

____

____

____

3. Collimation refers to:

4. How does a change in mA affect the final radiographic image?

5. Identify how increasing the kilovoltage affects the image density.

6. How is image contrast affected by increasing the kilovoltage?

7. List two advantages of high kVp.

8. List three advantages of lengthening the target-to-image receptor distance during exposure of patient radiographs.

9. How is the target-to-image receptor distance lengthened on an individual X-ray unit?

10. Identify three components to consider when selecting dental radiograph film.

11. What are the advantages of using digital radiography?

12. Correctly sequence the following steps in producing an *indirect* digital radiograph, numbering them from 1 to 5 (1 = first step; 5 = final step).
    _____ Electronic charge activates the sensor
    _____ Image is scanned using a laser scanner
    _____ Image stored on the PSP plate
    _____ Sensor placed in patient's mouth
    _____ Image displayed on computer

13. What type of digital imaging uses a sensor with a cord attached?

14. List the four types of image receptors.

Radiation Safety

1. Identify three factors that influence the biologic effects of radiation on cells.

2. List human tissues and organs that are highly radiosensitive.

3. List three ways to protect yourself from primary and leakage radiation while making patient radiographs.

4. Relative to your patient's head, where can you best stand to protect yourself from secondary radiation?

5. List the ways you can protect your patient during exposure of dental radiographs.

Clinical Techniques

1. Describe a complete dental radiographic survey.

2. When a rectangular PID is used for beam collimation while exposing dental radiographs, how do you adjust the X-ray machine to accommodate both horizontal and vertical film/sensor positioning?

3. Match the area of the mouth or teeth listed below with the radiographic film or sensor size most frequently used.

Intraoral Area	Film/Sensor Size
____ Overlapping anterior teeth	A. Size no. 0
____ Permanent dentition bitewings	B. Size no. 1
____ Primary teeth	C. Size no. 2
____ Adult posterior (periapical view)	
____ Child maxillary (occlusal view)	

4. When exposing a periapical image receptor of tooth 12, directing the central ray with too much vertical angle will produce an image of the tooth with roots that appear to be very ____________.

5. Identify three reasons why the paralleling technique usually produces better images with increased patient safety compared to the bisecting-angle technique.

6. When positioning the film inside the patient's mouth, the stippled or colored side of the film packet is placed:

7. To maintain a visually open contact on a bitewing radiograph, the horizontal angle of the central beam is directed:

8. How do you position the patient's head when you are making an occlusal survey image of the mandibular teeth?

9. If the patient's head is tilted to the side or the occlusal plane is not parallel with the floor, the angle

of the PID must be altered to adapt the central ray to the patient's position. List two conditions that must be met when you are using the paralleling technique to expose periapical radiographs.

____

____

____

____

10. List the reasons why images of oral structures on a panoramic radiograph may have poor detail or be distorted even if you are very careful to use proper techniques when exposing the radiograph.

____

____

____

____

11. Identify one reason a panoramic image may be ordered instead of or in addition to periapical images for an individual patient.

____

____

In and Out of the Darkroom

1. Exposure to radiation changes the silver halide crystals coating traditional X-ray film to ____________ and ____________ ions.

2. After developing the film, only the amount of ______________ corresponding to radiolucency and radiopacity remains.

3. The fixer solution removes the ______________ crystals that were not exposed to radiation.

4. Correct processing temperature and time for optimal manual processing are _____°F and _____ minutes.

5. If the temperature of the solutions is higher than the optimal, the amount of time that the film remains in the developer should be ____________.

6. What kind of safelight filter is used in a darkroom when processing both intraoral and extraoral films?

____

____

7. Match the image inadequacy commonly found on dental radiographs (first column) with the most probable cause of the problem (second column).

Image Inadequacy	Probable Cause
_____ Dark lines across film	A. Extreme increase in vertical angle
_____ Double image	B. Film exposed twice
_____ Foreshortening	C. Bent film
_____ Large dark stain on one end of the film safelight	D. Unsafe safelight
_____ Light image with a pattern overlaying the image	E. Sudden temperature change in processing solutions
_____ Puckered surface	F. Static electricity
_____ Stretched appearance of images	G. Film placed backward in mouth
_____ Whole film too dark	H. Overlap of film in developer

8. List anatomic landmarks (besides the teeth) you might observe on a radiograph of your patient's mandibular incisor area.

____

____

____

9. Name a mandibular structure that could appear on a maxillary third molar radiograph.

____

____

____

10. Identify the factors that will enhance interpretation of images on patient radiographs.

____

____

____

____

____

____

____

____

____

____

COMPETENCY EXERCISES

Apply information from the chapter and use critical thinking skills to complete the competency exercises. Write responses on paper or create electronic documents to submit your answers.

1. In your own words, explain the relationship between the tooth, the image receptor, and the central beam of radiation when using the paralleling technique. (*Hint*: Use your hands as a three-dimensional way to "draw" the images so you can visualize them as you try to explain.)

2. Mrs. Honey Davis, age 42, presents in your clinic for her initial appointment. She states she has come because she needs her teeth cleaned and because a tooth on the upper left side of her mouth has been bothering her. She has not been to visit a dentist for 2 years. She states that she had a lot of X-rays taken when she was last examined by her previous dentist just before she moved to your town but that she did not bring them with her today.

   When collecting your initial assessment data, you identify no positive clinical signs/symptoms of periodontal disease and no clinical evidence of active dental caries. She has six small amalgam restorations in her posterior teeth; only tooth 19 has a restoration on a proximal surface. However, Mrs. Davis reports intermittent use of mint candy to combat a feeling of dry mouth caused by a medication she takes. You also note an accumulation of biofilm on proximal tooth surfaces.

   You are planning to ask Dr. Gray, your employer, to examine Mrs. Davis. You know that he will probably order some X-rays. Using Tables 13-4, 13-5, and 13-6 in the textbook, determine which X-rays would be recommended for Mrs. Davis and why.

3. You plan to expose a periapical radiograph of Mrs. Davis's tooth 15 using the paralleling technique. Explain the following:

   Where the front edge of the image receptor should be positioned.

   How the image receptor is placed relative to the long axis of tooth 15 and the mesial/distal line of that tooth.

   How the central beam of radiation is directed relative to the long axis of tooth 15.

   Where the lingual cusp of tooth 15 should rest in a disposable styrofoam film/sensor holder.

4. After you take all of the images prescribed for Mrs. Davis and place the films in a paper cup, you will go into the darkroom to process the films. Write out a step-by step procedure for infection control and processing the films. For comparison, describe the infection control procedures for processing an indirect digital image.

5. In spite of your attempts to reassure him of the appropriateness and safety of the bitewing X-rays prescribed by the dentist, your patient, Jeff Darlington, has refused to have any X-rays taken at his recall appointment. Using your institution's guidelines for writing in patient records, document that he has refused the recommended exposures.

6. Gather a variety of dental radiographs taken in your clinic that are currently not being used for patient care. Place them in X-ray mounts for easy viewing. Evaluate the radiographs using Table 13-8, in the textbook.

   Identify any errors in technique or processing and describe possible causes and corrections you can make to eliminate the problem. Compare your evaluation of the images with those made by one or two of your student colleagues. Discuss any differences in the way you each evaluated the same image or the corrective measure you described for an error.

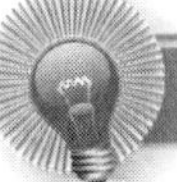

DISCOVERY EXERCISE

Gather a variety of dental radiographs taken in your clinic and identify as many anatomical landmarks as you can. What additional resources will help you to identify the landmarks visible on each film?

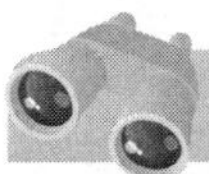

BOX 13-1 MeSH TERMS

Use a combination of MeSH terms and other key words to develop an effective and efficient PubMed literature search strategy.

Radiography, dental	Tomography scanners, X-ray Computed
Radiography, dental, digital	Radiation, ionizing
Radiography, panoramic	Scattering, radiation
Radiography, bitewing	Electromagnetic radiation
X-ray film	Film dosimetry
X-ray intensifying screens	Gamma rays
Radiation equipment and supplies	

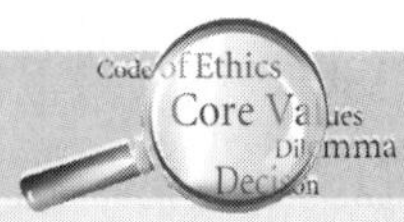

EVERYDAY ETHICS

Before completing the learning exercises below, reread and reflect on the Everyday Ethics Scenario and Questions for Consideration in this chapter of the textbook. It may also be useful to review the Dental Hygiene Ethics discussion in Chapter 1, the Ethical Applications in the introduction pages for each section in the textbook, as well as the Codes of Ethics in textbook Appendices I - IV.

Individual Learning Activity

Imagine that you are the dental hygienist in this scenario. Answer each of the questions for consideration at the end of the scenario.

Discovery Activity

Ask a friend or relative who is not involved in health care to read the scenario and discuss it with you from the perspective of a "patient" who receives services within the healthcare system. Discuss what you learned from the concerns, insights, or difference in perspective that person expressed.

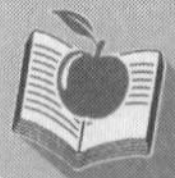

Factors To Teach The Patient

This scenario is related to the following factors listed in this chapter of the textbook:

▷ When the patient asks about the safety of radiation

As you talk with Mr. Glazier, you realize that not only is he concerned about why additional X-rays are necessary, but he is also extremely concerned about the safety and negative effects of the additional dose of radiation he will receive. Using the examples of patient conversations from Appendix D in this workbook as a guide, write a statement explaining all of the safety factors in place in your clinic to protect him from excessive exposure to radiation.

Use the conversation you create to role-play this situation with a fellow student. If you are the patient in the role-play, be sure to ask questions. If you are the dental hygienist, try to anticipate questions and answer them in your explanation.

Crossword Puzzle

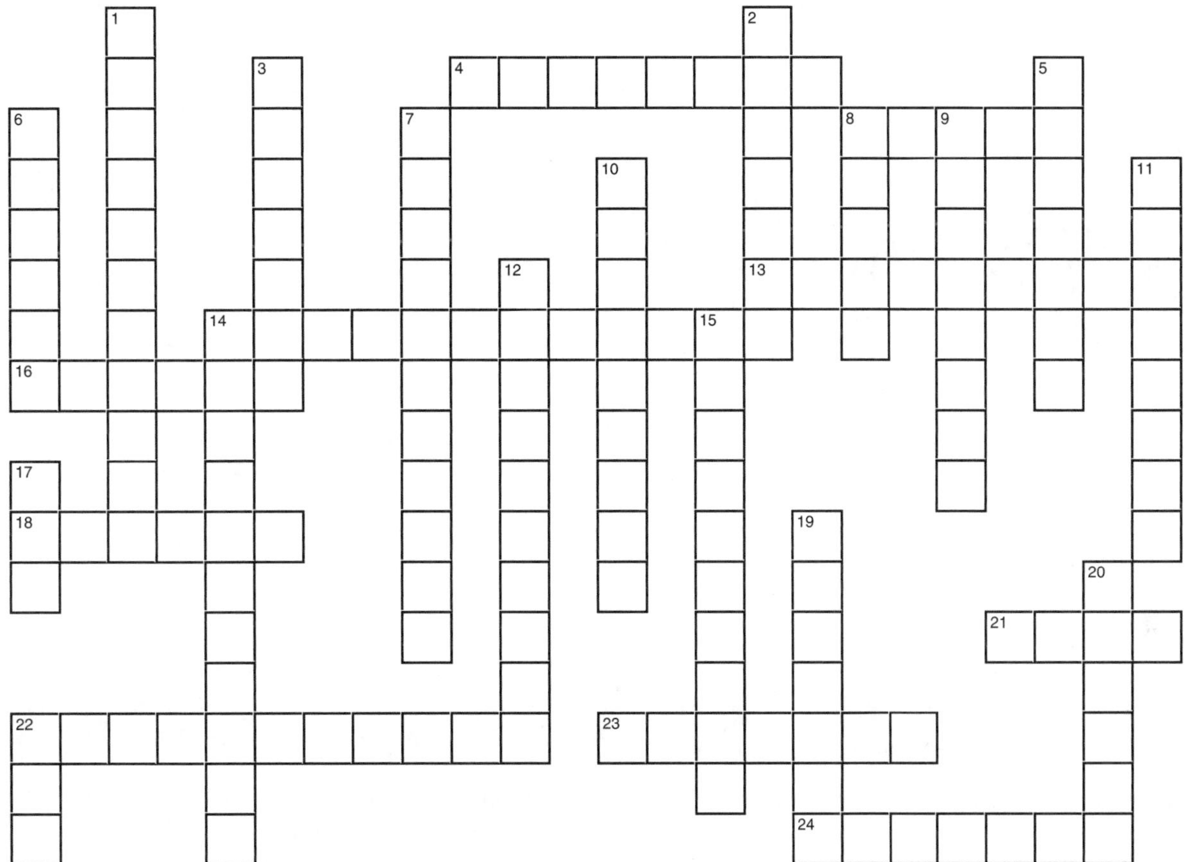

Puzzle Clues

Across

4. Secondary shadow that surrounds the periphery of the primary shadow; a blurred margin.
8. As low as reasonably achievable.
13. Branch of science that deals with the use of radiation in diagnosis and treatment of disease.
14. Appearance of dark images on a radiograph as a result of the greater amount of radiation that penetrates low-density objects.
16. Dose of radiation that is, or could be, sufficient to cause death.
18. Small intraoral detector that captures a digital radiographic image.
21. Dose of radiation absorbed when the central beam passes through body tissue.
22. Maximum dose of radiation a person can receive and not expect significantly harmful results.
23. Radiation that has been deviated from its primary direction during passage through a substance.
24. An error of technique that results when the beam of radiation does not completely cover the sensor. (two words).

Down

1. Technique used for controlling the size and shape of the primary radiation beam.
2. Beam of X-ray photons that bounces in all directions from anode of an x-ray machine.
3. Filmless radiography system that stores images on a computer
5. Tungsten filament, which is a coiled wire heated to generate a cloud of electrons; has a negative charge.
6. Beam of primary radiation that comes off the anode to exit the x-ray machine directly through the position indicating device.
7. The art and science of making radiographs.
8. A tungsten target embedded in a copper stem, positioned at an angle to the electron beam; has a positive charge
9. Dose of radiation imparted at a specific exposure point.
10. Minimum dose that produces any detectable effect on body tissues.
11. Appearance of redness on human skin that can be caused by a high does of radiation.
12. Dose that results from repeated exposure to radiation.
14. The appearance of light (white) images on a radiograph; result of the amount of radiation absorbed by dense objects.
15. Beam of radiation directed at right angles to the film or sensor when using the paralleling technique (two words)
17. The type of image receptor that is read by a laser scanner (acronym).
19. Body cells; with the exclusion of germ cells.
20. Digital imaging system that uses a charged-coupled device or complementary-metal-oxide semiconductor.
22. Acronym that refers to the collimator cone of the x-ray machine.

14

Study Models

LEARNING OBJECTIVES

Upon successful completion of these exercises, you will be able to:

1. Identify and define key terms and concepts related to making oral study models.
2. List and discuss the purposes and uses of study models.
3. Identify the supplies, steps, and procedures involved in taking an impression.
4. List the supplies, steps, and procedures involved in making a study model.

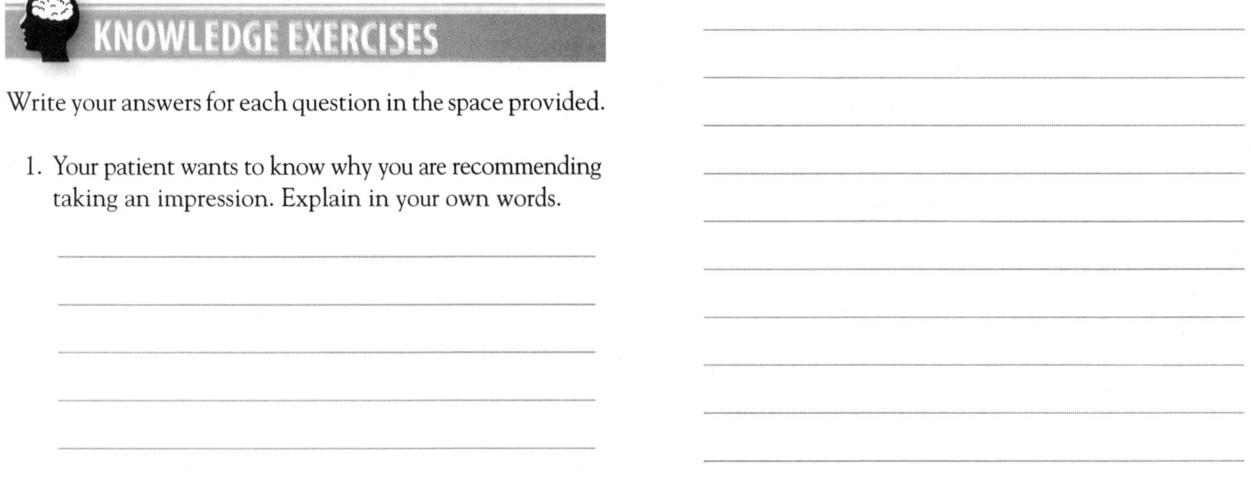

KNOWLEDGE EXERCISES

Write your answers for each question in the space provided.

1. Your patient wants to know why you are recommending taking an impression. Explain in your own words.

2. You are asked to order all the supplies you will need for taking patient impressions and pouring study models. List the supplies you will order.

____
____
____
____
____
____
____
____
____
____
____
____
____
____
____
____
____
____

3. You have tried in the impression tray for your patient. In checking the width of the tray, you allowed for an adequate thickness of impression material on the facial and lingual surfaces of each tooth to provide _______________ to the impression.
Your patient has a tooth in prominent linguoversion, so you allowed for a minimum thickness of _______________ in.
As you checked the length of the tray, you made sure to allow coverage of the _______________ area of the mandible and the _______________ of the maxilla.

4. The steps involved in taking a maxillary impression are listed below. You have already tried in and prepared the tray. Number the list in the correct order (1 = first step; 6 = last step).
_____ Seat the tray from posterior to anterior.
_____ Maintain equal pressure on each side of the tray.
_____ Rinse under cool running water and proceed with disinfection for maxillary model.
_____ Insert the tray with a rotary motion.
_____ Elevate the cheek over the edge of the impression to break the seal, and remove the impression with a sudden jerk.
_____ Ask the patient to form a tight O with the lips to mold the impression material.

5. The impression tray is seated with a slight _______________ motion.

6. Seat the _______________ portion of the tray in the patient's mouth before seating the _______________ portion.

7. A _______________ around the borders of the tray can help prevent discomfort.

8. The front border of a maxillary study model is trimmed to a _______________, and the front border of the mandibular model is _______________.

9. Each of the following statements **is** *not correct*. Write a *corrected statement* in the space provided.

9a. A removable oral prosthesis is left in the patient's mouth while the impression is taken.

____
____

9b. Spatulating the impression material for 2 minutes will allow the chemical reactions to proceed uniformly.

____
____

9c. Ideal gelation time for impression material is between 7 and 9 minutes when the room temperature is 20–21°C (68–70°F).

____
____

9d. The patient is positioned in a supine position when you take an impression.

____
____

9e. The teeth are wet with the air/water syringe before the impression is taken.

____
____

9f. You can wait until you have a break in your schedule before you pour the alginate impression.

____
____

9g. When taking an impression, vestibular areas, occlusal surfaces, and undercut areas inside the patient's mouth can be precoated with wax.

____
____

10. Dental stone is sensitive to changes in the relative humidity of the atmosphere. List some strategies that protect the stone.

____

____

____

11. The steps involved in mixing dental stone are given below. First complete the sentences, and then number the list in the correct order (1 = first step; 6 = last step).

_____ Sift in the powder gradually to__________ and to allow each particle to become _________.

_____ Measure the water and powder according to the manufacturer's specifications. (The ratio of water to powder is 30 to 40 mL water for ________ g of stone.)

_____ Wait briefly until all powder is wet, then vibrate to __________________.

_____ Place measured water (which is at __________ temperature) in a clean, dry mixing bowl.

_____ The result is a______________ consistency.

_____ Use a vacuum mixer.

12. Water added to the stone when mixing controls the strength, rigidity, and hardness of the model.

Increasing the water to dental stone ratio ____________ the strength of the model.

Temperature affects the setting time of the dental stone: ____________ water increases it, and ____________ water decreases it.

13. Complete the following sentences to describe the process of pouring the anatomic portion of the model.

Shake any______ ______ out of the impression.

Start at the most posterior tooth and allow the mix to flow through the impression. Use ____________ amounts and vibrate continually. ____________ the impression so the material passes into the tooth indentions and flows slowly down the side, and across the ____________ surface or the ____________ edge.

Air is trapped when the process is hurried or _______ ____________________________.

When all tooth indentations are covered, add larger amounts of mix to slightly ________________ the impressions, then vibrate.

14. The base of the study model can be made using a number of techniques. In your own words, briefly describe each of the following techniques.

Rubber model base former

____

____

____

____

____

____

____

____

____

____

____

____

Two-step or double pour

____

____

____

____

____

____

____

____

Boxing technique

____

____

____

____

____

____

____

____

____

____

15. The exact proportions of the study models and the steps required to accomplish the trimming and finishing depend on several factors. List these factors.

____

____

____

16. In your own words, describe the proportions and planes of an acceptable finished study model. Use the figures in Chapter 14 of the textbook to help you visualize your descriptions.

____

____

____

____

____

____

____

____

____

____

17. Complete the following sentences related to finishing and polishing the completed model.
Allow models to dry thoroughly for ______________.
Smooth the art portion with ______________.
Soak in heated soap solution for ______________.
Rub with a ______________.
______________ may be used to help polish the model.

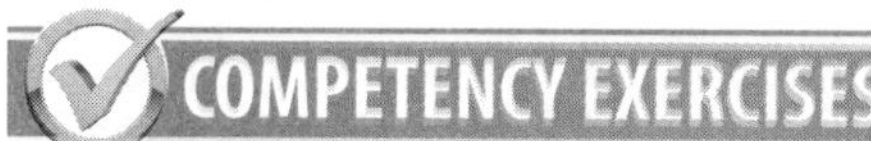

COMPETENCY EXERCISES

Apply information from the chapter and use critical thinking skills to complete the competency exercises. Write responses on paper or create electronic documents to submit your answers.

Privesh Doshi is a dental assistant at the dental clinic in which you are practicing. Dr. Pecharo has asked you to teach Privesh how to take an impression (assume that you are in a state or province where it is legal for dental assistants to make impressions). You decide the best way to teach is to make a checklist so Privesh can follow it every time he is taking an impression.

1. Create the checklist.
2. Privesh is concerned about making the patient gag. Give him some suggestions on how to prevent this.
3. Privesh is concerned about taking the impressions. He needs more information on how to mix the alginate material and wants to know how much time he has to insert the material into the patient's mouth. Explain these procedures.
4. The alginate impression that Privesh took this morning has been sitting on the counter in the laboratory for 4 hours. What are your concerns?

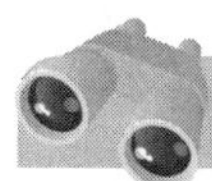

BOX 14-1 MeSH TERMS

Use a combination of MeSH terms and other key words to develop an effective and efficient PubMed literature search strategy.

Dental impression materials

Dental impression technique

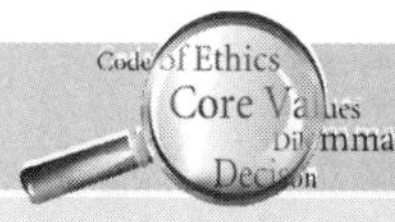

EVERYDAY ETHICS

Before completing the learning exercises below, reread and reflect on the Everyday Ethics Scenario and Questions for Consideration in this chapter of the textbook. It may also be useful to review the Dental Hygiene Ethics discussion in Chapter 1, the Ethical Applications in the introduction pages for each section in the textbook, as well as the Codes of Ethics in textbook Appendices I–IV.

Discovery Activities

Ask a dental hygienist who has been practicing for a year or more to read the scenario. Provide them with a copy of the Code of Ethics as well. Share the responses you have made to answer each question and ask that person to discuss the situation with you. What insights did you have or what did you learn during this discussion?

Ask a friend or relative who is not involved in health care to read the scenario and discuss it with you from the perspective of a "patient" who receives services within the healthcare system. Discuss what you learned from the concerns, insights, or difference in perspective that person expressed.

Factors To Teach The Patient

This scenario is related to the following factors listed in this chapter of the textbook:

- ▷ Importance and purposes of study models; reasons for comparative models after treatment or at a later date.
- ▷ Use of the models of other patients to show effects of treatment or what can happen if the prescribed treatment is not carried out.

You have just seated your patient, Mrs. Lorna Patel. Refer to Appendix C in the workbook to review her care plan. Before this appointment, Mrs. Patel was unaware of the generalized moderate attrition in her mouth.

Using the motivational interviewing approach outlined in Appendix D of the workbook as a guide, write a statement explaining to Mrs. Patel the need to take the alginate impression to make study models so you can document her condition. Be sure to discuss the need to fabricate a night guard and why study models will help you do that. Compare your conversation with one developed by a student colleague to identify any missing information.

15

Dental Biofilm and Other Soft Deposits

LEARNING OBJECTIVES

Upon successful completion of these exercises, you will be able to:

1. Identify and define key terms and concepts related to oral soft deposits.
2. Differentiate dental biofilm from pellicle, materia alba, and food debris in terms of composition, significance, and detection.
3. Discuss the implications of dental biofilm in terms of periodontal disease and caries.
4. Describe the essentials for dental caries as well as other contributing factors.

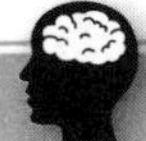

KNOWLEDGE EXERCISES

Write your answers for each question in the space provided.

1. In your own words, describe each of the four types of nonmineralized tooth deposits listed below

Acquired pellicle:

Dental biofilm:

Materia alba:

Food debris:

2. Why is acquired pellicle significant?

____
____
____
____
____
____

3. Acquired pellicle is composed primarily of

____
____
____
____

4. ________________ pellicle can become embedded in the tooth structure, particularly where the tooth surface is partially demineralized.

5. Make a drawing of the shape of each of these types of bacteria.

Bacillus
Staphylococci
Streptococci
Spirella
Vibrios

6. Label the left side of Figure 15-1 to identify the microorganisms present in biofilm. To the right of the figure, indicate the timeframe for the development of the observed changes in the bacteria over time when the teeth are not cleaned.

7. How does the dental hygienist detect biofilm during patient assessment?

____
____
____

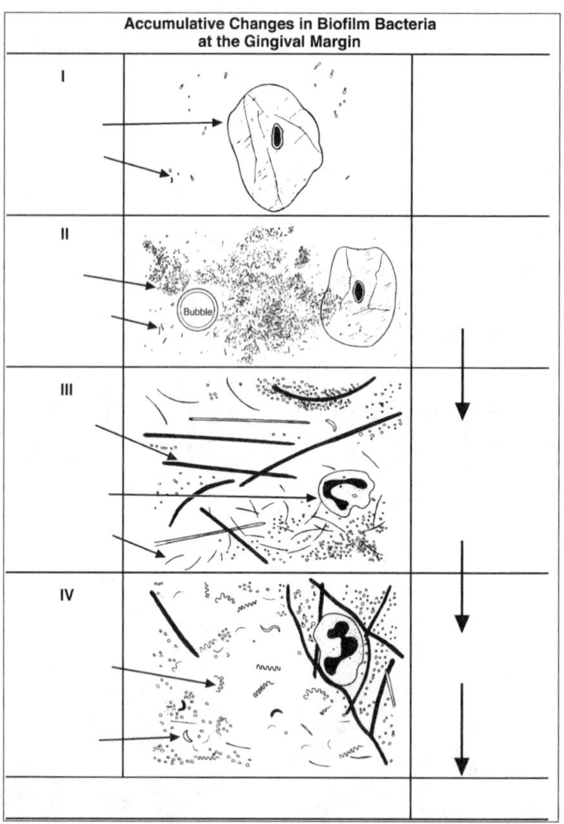

Figure 15-1

8. The interactions involved in the formation of biofilm are listed below. Number the list in the correct order (1 = first interaction; 5 = last interaction).
______ Secretion of extracellular matrix
______ Bacteria adhere to pellicle
______ Biofilm growth
______ Bacteria multiply and colonize
______ Release of cells to spread and colonize other areas

9. Gingivitis is clinically evident within ____________ when biofilm is left undisturbed on tooth surfaces.

10. Match the following descriptions of biofilm with the correct type. Each type is used more than once.

Type of Biofilm	Description
A. Supragingival biofilm	______ Shape and size are affected by the friction of tongue, cheeks, and lips
	______ The main source of nutrients for bacterial proliferation is gingival crevicular fluid
	______ Coronal to the margin of the free gingiva
	______ May become thicker as the diseased pocket wall becomes less tight
B. Subgingival biofilm	______ Heaviest collection on areas not cleaned daily by patient
	______ Found most often on the cervical third, especially facial surfaces, the lingual mandibular molars, and proximal surfaces
	______ Down growth of bacteria from supragingival biofilm
	______ Diseased pocket; primarily gram-negative, motile, spirochetes, rods
	______ Sources of nutrients for bacterial proliferation are saliva and ingested food
	______ Made up of three layers
	______ The structure is an adherent, densely packed microbial layer over pellicle on the tooth surface

11. Describe the microbial structure for each of the following types of subgingival biofilm

Unattached biofilm:

Tooth-attached biofilm:

Epithelium-attached biofilm:

12. List the microorganisms in each layer of subgingival biofilm.

Initial layer:

Intermediate layer:

Top layer:

13. What three minerals are more concentrated in biofilm than in saliva?

14. List the patient self-care interventions that can increase the amount of fluoride in dental biofilm.

15. Carbohydrate intake can contribute to the ____________ of biofilm microorganisms to each other and the teeth.

16. Explain the significance of the two types of cariogenic microorganisms in biofilm.

17. What is the typical pH level in dental biofilm prior to eating?

18. What happens to the pH level of dental biofilm immediately following the intake of sucrose?

19. Explain the significance of the change in pH level of biofilm following intake of sucrose.

20. When thinking about prevention of dental caries, the quantity (amount) of dietary carbohydrate consumption is less critical than the ______________ of sucrose intake.

COMPETENCY EXERCISES

Apply information from the chapter and use critical thinking skills to complete the competency exercises. Write responses on paper or create electronic documents to submit your answers.

1. Your patient, Daron Horwitz, is curious about how to remove the soft deposits in his mouth. He presents with biofilm, materia alba, and food debris. Discuss patient instructions for the removal of all three deposits.

2. As you evaluate Mrs. Eltheia Shore, you note that she presents with a significant amount of supragingival, subgingival, gingival, and fissure biofilm. Educate her about the factors that can contribute to biofilm accumulation and the surfaces most commonly affected. Describe the strategies used for detection of biofilm.

3. You are providing patient education for Alison Alverez and her 10-year-old son, Juan. Juan has multiple carious lesions, and his mother is very interested in preventing more from occurring. Juan drinks soda daily. He purchases a 32-oz. bottle on his way to school and sips the soda every chance he gets. Juan's mother remembers hearing something about acids in the mouth and wants to know more about this. Describe your patient education approach.

4. Your patient is Nguyen Tho Phan, a 58-year-old research microbiologist. Her area of research is disease prevention, and she wants to understand the major pathogens that are identified in destructive periodontal disease and caries. If Nguyen presents with mutans streptococci, what disease is she most at risk for? Her brother has periodontal disease, and Nguyen want to know if he would have the same bacteria in his mouth. What is your response?

5. Specific microorganisms, a susceptible tooth surface, and a diet high in cariogenic foods are essential for caries to develop. List some recommendations you can provide for an adult patient for prevention of dental caries.

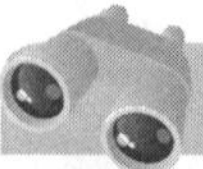

BOX 15-1 MeSH TERMS

Use a combination of MeSH terms and other key words to develop an effective and efficient PubMed literature search strategy.

Biofilms	Dental pellicle
Bacterial processes	Biofilms
Dental deposits	Gram-positive bacteria
Dental plaque	Gram-negative bacteria

EVERYDAY ETHICS

Before completing the learning exercises below, reread and reflect on the Everyday Ethics Scenario and Questions for Consideration in this chapter of the textbook. It may also be useful to review the Dental Hygiene Ethics discussion in Chapter 1, the Ethical Applications in the introduction pages for each section in the textbook, as well as the Codes of Ethics in textbook Appendices I - IV.

Individual Learning Activity

Imagine that you have observed what happened in the scenario, but are not one of the main characters involved in the situation. Write a reflective journal entry that:

describes how you might have reacted (as an observer—not as a participant),

expresses your personal feelings about what happened,

or

identifies personal values that affect your reaction to the situation.

Collaborative Learning Activity

Work with another student colleague to role-play the scenario. The goal of this exercise is for you and your colleague to work though the alternative actions in order to come to consensus on a solution or response that is acceptable to both of you.

Factors To Teach The Patient

This scenario is related to the following factors listed in this chapter of the textbook:

- ▷ Location, composition, and properties of dental biofilm with emphasis on its role in dental caries and periodontal infections.
- ▷ Effects of personal oral care procedures in the prevention of dental biofilm.
- ▷ Biofilm control procedures with special adaptations for individual needs.

You have just seated your patient, Mrs. Lorna Patel. Refer to her completed care plan in Appendix C to review the assessment findings, concentrating on her dental history and dental findings.

Use the motivational interviewing approach (see Appendix D) to write a patient education conversation explaining to Mrs. Patel the appearance of acute gingivitis and the impact of effective brushing and flossing after a specified period of time. You may also want to refer to the figure in Knowledge Exercise 6 in this chapter when writing your statement. Compare your conversation with a student colleague to identify any missing information.

Crossword Puzzle

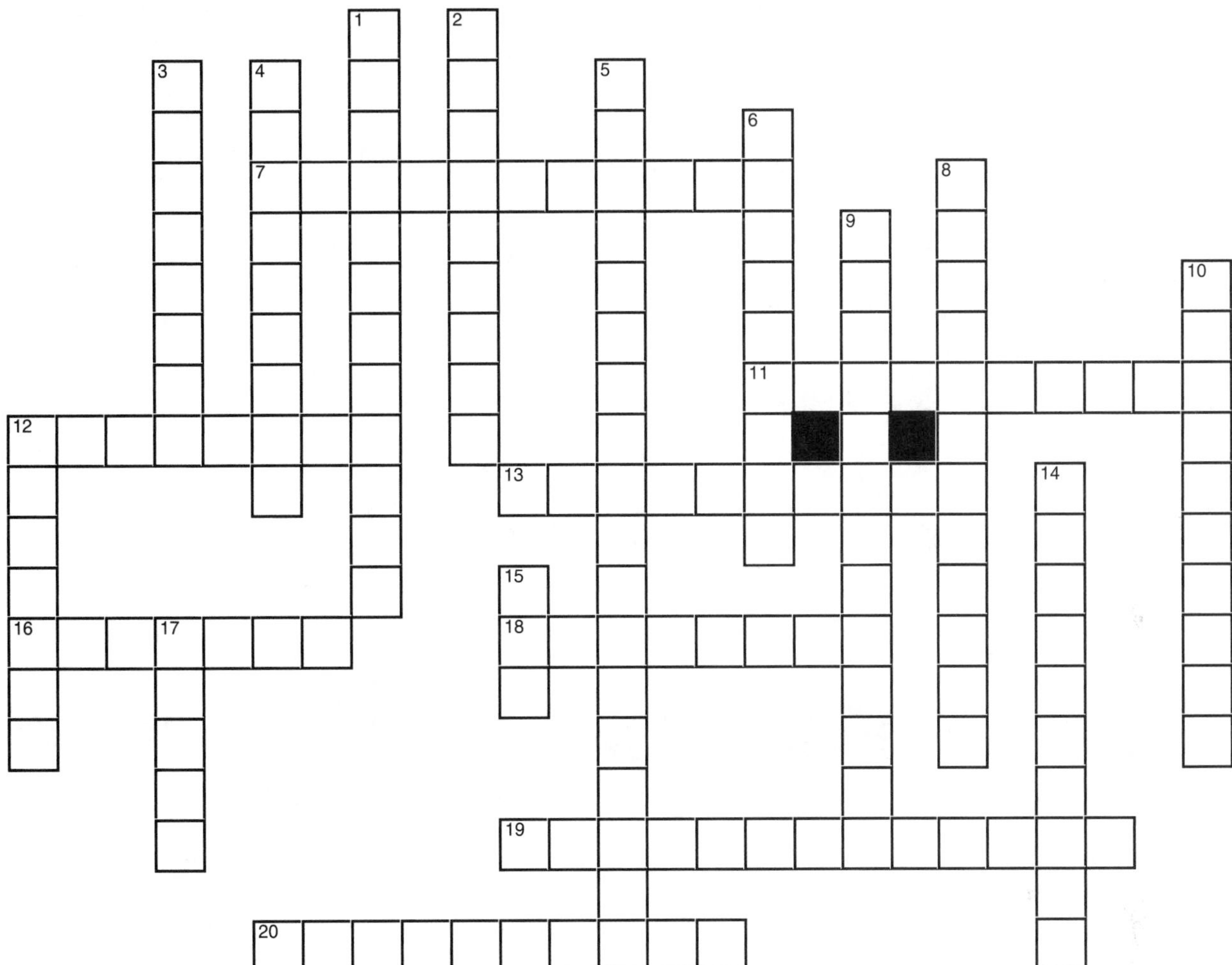

Puzzle Clues

Across

7. Organism that is able to live under more than one specific set of environmental conditions.
11. Conducive to the initiation or development of dental caries.
12. Heterotrophic microorganism that lives and grows in complete (or almost complete) absence of oxygen.
13. When combined with frequent fermentable carbohydrate exposure, promotes the growth of dental biofilm.
16. Any matrix-enclosed bacterial populations adherent to each other and/or to surfaces or interfaces.
18. Disease-producing agent or microorganism.
19. Minute living organism.
20. The action of a substance in attracting and holding other materials or particles on its surface.

Down

1. Dental biofilm conducive to the formation of dental calculus.
2. Not made up of or containing cells.
3. Ability to survive only in a particular environment
4. Invasion and multiplication of a microorganism in body tissues.
5. Initiates the caries process (two words).
6. White blood corpuscle that functions to protect the body against infection and disease.
8. Contributes to the progression of a carious lesion.
9. A cell-to-cell communication process activated between bacterial cells during the growth stage of biofilm development.
10. The microscopic living organisms of a region.
12. Microorganisms that live and grow in the presence of free oxygen.
14. Pleomorphic, gram-negative bacteria that lack cell walls.
15. Substance secreted to form a matrix as bacteria multiply within dental biofilm (acronym).
17. The collective organisms of a given locale.

16

The Teeth

LEARNING OBJECTIVES

Upon successful completion of these exercises, you will be able to:

1. Identify and define key terms and concepts related to the teeth.
2. Discuss various types of dental caries in terms of classification, development, and detection.
3. Describe noncarious dental lesions, their causes and their appearance.
4. Describe a clinical examination of the teeth.
5. Detail the development and eruption of permanent teeth.
6. Identify various strategies for the recognition of carious lesions and describe tests for vitality.

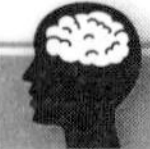

KNOWLEDGE EXERCISES

Write your answers for each question in the space provided.

1. List the three divisions of the human dentition.

2. List five factors that may contribute to enamel hypoplasia during tooth development.

3. In your own words, describe the appearance of various types of hypoplasia.

4. List the teeth most frequently affected by enamel hypoplasia and explain why these particular teeth are affected first?

____

____

____

____

____

5. Describe the appearance of an initial attrition lesion.

____

____

6. What might one see on a radiograph of a tooth that presents with attrition?

____

____

____

7. Match the term to the correct definition.

Term	Definition
___ Abrasion	A. Loss of tooth substance by a chemical process that does not involve bacterial action
___ Attrition	B. Condition in which a tooth is forced into the alveolar bone through trauma
___ Avulsion	C. Dislocation of a tooth
___ Erosion	D. Partial displacement of a tooth from its socket
___ Extrusion	E. Mechanical wearing away of tooth substance by forces other than mastication
___ Intrusion	F. Complete displacement of a tooth from its socket
___ Luxation	G. Wearing away of a tooth as a result of tooth-to-tooth contact

8. Complete Infomap 16-1 to help you differentiate among attrition, erosion, and abrasion.

9. Match the description of types of dental caries with the correct term. Each term may be used more than once.

Terminology	Description
A. Simple	_____ Involves more than two tooth surfaces
B. Compound	_____ & _____ Caries on the occlusal surface of a molar
C. Complex	_____ Covering two surfaces
D. Pit and fissure	_____ Closure of the enamel plates is imperfect
E. Smooth surface	_____ Occurs in proximal tooth surfaces
	_____ Mesio-occlusal caries, for example

10. Match the description of types of dental caries with the correct term. Each term may be used more than once or not be used at all.

Terminology	Description
A. Simple	_____ Involves one tooth surface
B. Compound	_____ & _____ The buccal groove of a mandibular molar, for example
C. Complex	_____ Distal-occlusal caries
D. Pit and fissure	_____ Irregularity occurs where three or more lobes of the developing tooth join
E. Smooth surface	_____ Caries in an area where there is no pit, groove, or other fault

11. Match the description with the correct Dr. G.V. Black classification. Each classification may be used more than once.

G.V. Black Classifications	Descriptions
A. Class I	_____ Pits or fissures on occlusal surfaces of premolars or molars
B. Class II	_____ Lingual surfaces of maxillary incisors
C. Class III	_____ Proximal surfaces of premolars
	_____ Transillumination useful for detection
	_____ & _____ Early caries can be detected using radiographs
	_____ Proximal surfaces of incisors and canines that do not involve the incisal angle

12. Match the description with the correct Dr. G.V. Black classification. Each classification may be used more than once.

G.V. Black Classifications	Descriptions
A. Class IV	_____ Cervical third of facial or lingual surfaces (not pit or fissure)
B. Class V	_____ Proximal surfaces of incisors or canines that involve the incisal angle
C. Class VI	_____ Transillumination is useful for detection
	_____ Incisal edges of anterior teeth and cusp tips of posterior teeth

13. What clinical signs denote an untreated **incipient** carious lesion?

____

____

____

____

____

INFOMAP 16-1

CONDITION	DEFINITION	OCCURRENCE	ETIOLOGY	PREDISPOSING FACTORS	APPEARANCE
Attrition					
Erosion					
Abrasion					

14. List two causes of early childhood caries.

____

____

15. List the relevant findings for each response during an electric pulp test.

Result of Vitality Test	Finding
No response	
Lingering pain after removal of stimulus	
Pain subsides promptly	

16. List and describe the types of thermal tests used to determine pulpal vitality.

____

____

____

____

17. List the factors that can influence response or reaction to the thermal tests.

____

____

____

____

____

18. Using the numbers 1 - 5, order the phases of the self-cleansing mechanism of the teeth during mastication.
    _______ Food particles brought back by the tongue to the occlusal surfaces for additional chewing.
    _______ Food is forced out by the pressure of the bite.
    _______ Food enters the mouth.
    _______ Food particles remaining on the teeth are removed.
    _______ The teeth are brought together for chewing.

COMPETENCY EXERCISES

Apply information from the chapter and use critical thinking skills to complete the Competency exercises. Write responses on paper or create electronic documents to submit your answers.

1. Your patient presents with both Class II and V dental caries. Describe how you detected each of these lesions.

2. Your patient, Oliver Summerlin, uses a hard toothbrush and an abrasive nonfluoride-containing dentifrice. He wears a partial denture on the mandible and takes a medication that causes xerostomia. You note abrasion in all four quadrants and root caries on the facial surfaces of teeth 27–30. Differentiate abrasion from root caries, and discuss the prevention of both root caries and abrasion.

3. Your patient at 3:00 is Paulo Jacoby. He is 16 years old, is an avid basketball player, and never wears a mouthguard. Describe potential oral injuries.

4. Clive Williams is 10 years old. He wants to know if he will get "more grown-up teeth." Explain to him the formative stages that his remaining teeth are in and the age at which most children can expect more permanent teeth to erupt.

5. Clive's cousin Jamal is 5 years old. He and Clive have a bet as to who still has the most teeth to erupt. Who will win the bet and why?

6. Jamal's sister wants to get in on the bet. She is 15 years old and says she will not have any more teeth erupt because all of her teeth are in and she is a grown-up. She has never had any teeth extracted. Who will win the bet and why?

DISCOVERY EXERCISE

Review the data collection forms that are used in your dental hygiene program. What form will you use to document each of the examination features that are listed in Table 16-2 in the textbook?

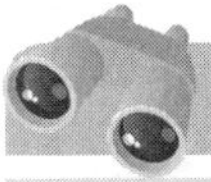

BOX 16-1 MeSH TERMS

Use a combination of MeSH terms and other key words to develop an effective and efficient PubMed literature search strategy.

Dentition, mixed	Tooth abrasion
Dentition, permanent	Tooth attrition
Dentition, primary	Tooth erosion
Dental caries	Tooth exfoliation
Tooth demineralization	Tooth abnormalities

EVERYDAY ETHICS

Before completing the learning exercises below, reread and reflect on the Everyday Ethics Scenario and Questions for Consideration in this chapter of the textbook. It may also be useful to review the Dental Hygiene Ethics discussion in Chapter 1, the Ethical Applications in the introduction pages for each section in the textbook, as well as the Codes of Ethics in textbook Appendices I–IV.

Individual Learning Activity

Imagine that you are the dental hygienist in this scenario. Answer each of the questions for consideration at the end of the scenario.

Discovery Activity

Ask a friend or relative who is not involved in health care to read the scenario and discuss it with you from the perspective of a "patient" who receives services within the health-care system. Discuss what you learned from the concerns, insights, or difference in perspective that person expressed.

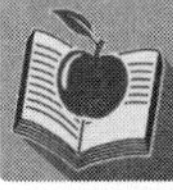

Factors To Teach The Patient

This scenario is related to the following factors listed in this chapter of the textbook:

- ▷ The cause and process of enamel or root caries formation and development for the patients at risk.
- ▷ Methods for prevention of dental caries, such as fluorides, biofilm prevention and control, and control of cariogenic foods in the diet.
- ▷ Methods for prevention of early childhood caries. (Nothing but plain water should be used in bedtime or nap-time nursing bottles. Avoid the use of a sweetener on a pacifier. Use of a cup for milk or juice by the baby's first birthday.)

Andrea Carfagno has arrived in the reception area of the clinic. She is holding her 26-month-old daughter, Nicole, and her 9-month-old twin boys are in a stroller. Nicole is your patient today. The girl is holding a baby bottle filled with fruit juice. She is a happy, attentive youngster who is anxious to please.

Use the principles of motivational interviewing (Appendix D) as a guide to write a dialogue explaining the need to have Nicole switch from a bottle to a cup. Be sure to address the use of fruit juices in a bottle and to explain early childhood caries. These issues pertain to both Nicole and her brothers.

Use the conversation you create to role play this situation with a fellow student. If you are the patient in the role play, be sure to ask questions. If you are the dental hygienist, try to anticipate questions and answer them in your explanation.

Crossword Puzzle

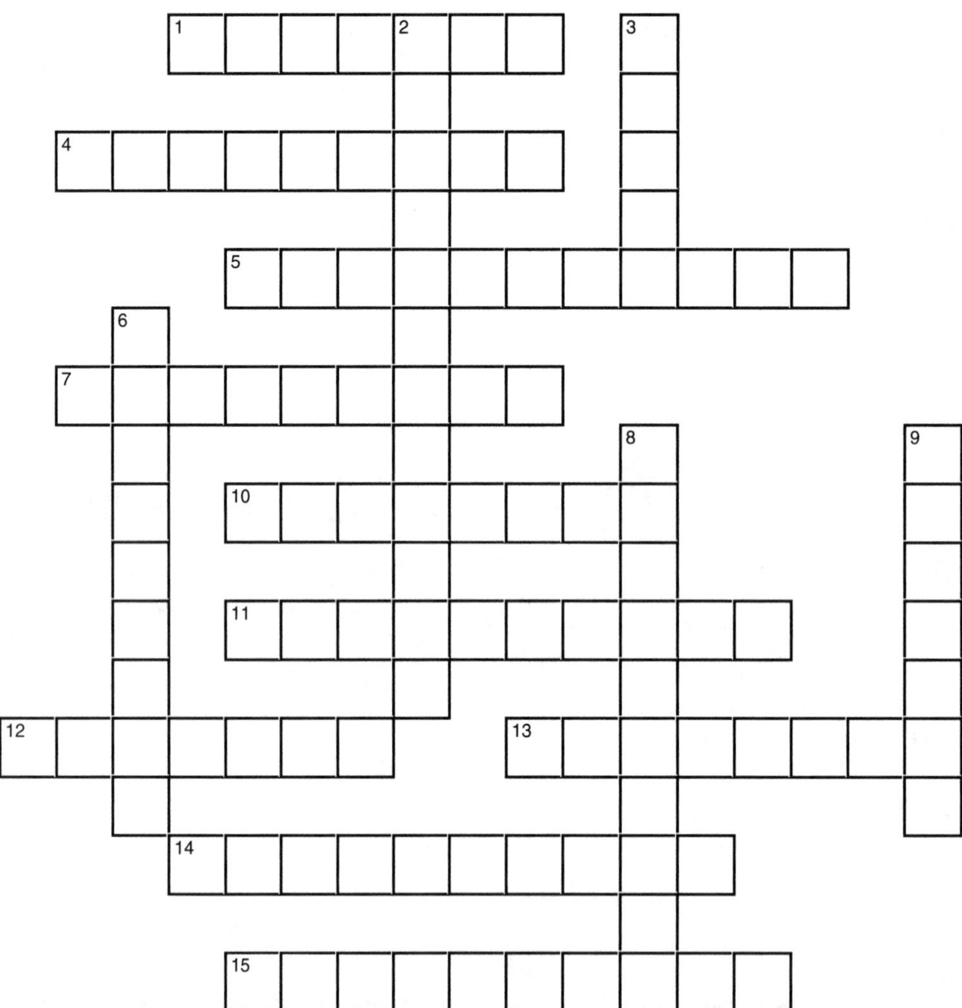

Puzzle Clues

Across

1. A term used to refer to the first teeth.
4. Very early carious lesion.
5. Natural loss of primary teeth following physiologic resorption of root structure.
7. Dental caries that occur on a surface adjacent to a restoration.
10. Carious lesion that has not progressed.
11. Any substance that promotes dental caries.
12. An oral habit of grinding, clenching, or clamping the teeth.
13. Traumatic separation of a tooth from the alveolus.
14. Gradual dissolution of a mineralized tissue.
15. Incomplete or defective formation of the enamel.

Down

2. Production and development of enamel.
3. A small, flattened surface on a tooth that results from attrition or repeated parafunctional contact.
6. A term that refers to primary teeth.
8. Without teeth.
9. The widespread formation of dental caries.

17

The Occlusion

LEARNING OBJECTIVES

Upon successful completion of these exercises, you will be able to:

1. Identify and define key terms and concepts related to occlusion.
2. Classify malocclusions for both adult and child patients.
3. Discuss functional occlusion in terms of occlusal and proximal contacts.
4. Identify the types of trauma from occlusion, including clinical and radiographic findings.

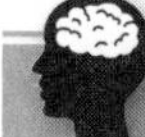

KNOWLEDGE EXERCISES

Write your answers for each question in the space provided.

1. Fill in the blanks in the following statements concerning facial profiles.

   Your patient presents with a prominent maxilla and a mandible posterior to its normal relationship. This is known as a convex, or ______________ profile.

   This patient's cousin has slightly protruded jaws, which give the facial outline a relatively flat appearance. This is known as a straight, or ______________profile.

   The father of your patient is waiting in the reception area. He has a prominent, protruded mandible and a normal maxilla. This is known as a concave, or ______________ profile.

2. Match the following definitions with the correct term from the list.

Definitions	Terms
____ Consists of all contacts during chewing, swallowing, or other normal action	A. Centric relation
____ Maximum intercuspation or contact of the teeth of the opposing arches; also called habitual occlusion	B. Centric occlusion
____ Any contact of opposing teeth that occurs before the desirable intercuspation	C. Static occlusion
____ Seen when jaws are closed in centric relation	D. Normal occlusion
____ Most unstrained, retruded physiologic relation of the mandible to the maxilla from which lateral movements can be made	E. Functional occlusion
____ Abnormal or deviated function	F. Malocclusion
____ Any deviation from the physiologically acceptable relationship of the maxillary arch and/or teeth to the mandibular arch and/or teeth	G. Occlusal prematurity
____ All teeth in the maxillary arch are in maximum contact with all teeth in mandibular arch in a definite pattern; maxillary teeth slightly overlap the mandibular teeth on the facial surfaces	H. Parafunctional

3. Match the following definitions with the correct term from the list.

Definitions	Terms
____ Rigid fixation of a tooth to the surrounding alveolus as a result of ossification of the periodontal ligament; prevents eruption and orthodontic movement	A. Ankylosis
____ Diastema, or gap, in the tooth row occasionally observed in the human primary dentition	B. Dental ankylosis
____ Tooth movement that occurs when disease is present	C. Primate space
____ Infantile pattern of suckle/swallow movement in which the tongue is placed between the incisor teeth or alveolar ridges	D. Diastema
____ Space between two adjacent teeth in the same arch	E. Drifting
____ Union or consolidation of two similar or dissimilar hard tissues previously adjacent but not attached	F. Pathologic migration
____ Migration with a healthy periodontium	G. Facet
____ Shiny, flat, worn spot on the surface of a tooth, frequently on the side of a cusp	H. Tongue thrust

4. Match the following definitions with the correct term from the list.

Definitions	Terms
____ Head-holding instrument used to obtain cephalometric radiographs	A. Orthopedics
____ Orienting device for positioning the head for radiographic examination and measurement	B. Orthodontic and dentofacial orthopedics
____ Specialty area of dentistry concerned with the diagnosis, supervision, guidance, and treatment of the growing and mature dentofacial structures	C. Cephalostat
____ Process of evaluating dental and skeletal relationships by way of measurements obtained directly from the head or from cephalometric radiographs and tracings made from the radiographs	D. Cephalometer
____ Correction of abnormal form or relationship of bone structures	E. Cephalometric analysis
____ Removable dental appliance usually made of plastic that covers a dental arch and is designed to minimize the damaging effects of bruxism and other oral habits	F. Occlusal guard

5. Label each of the following figures (Figures 17-1–17-15) with the condition illustrated by the figure; then write a short description of your observations about each condition.

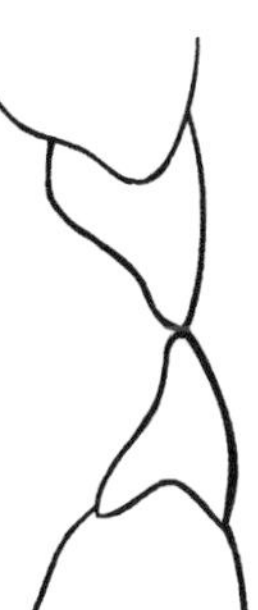
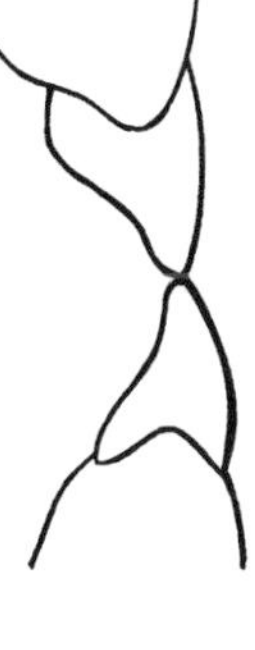

Figure 17-1

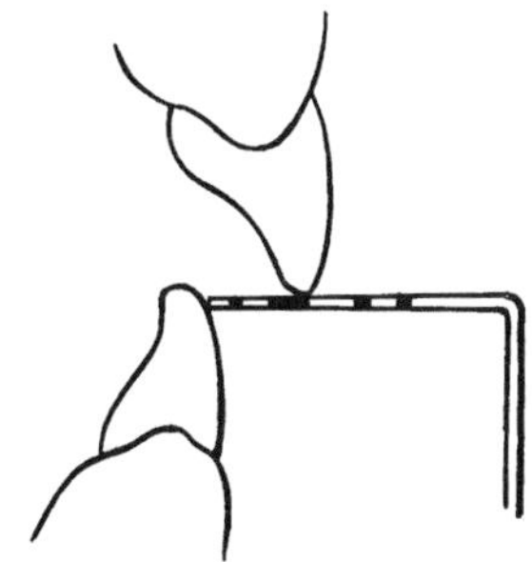

Figure 17-2

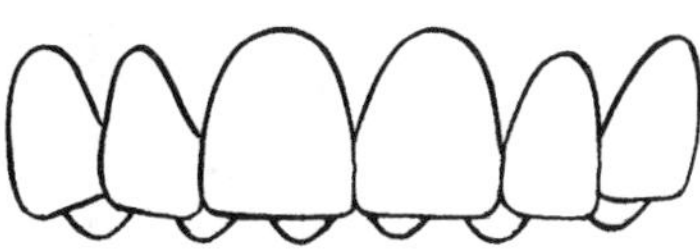

Figure 17-3

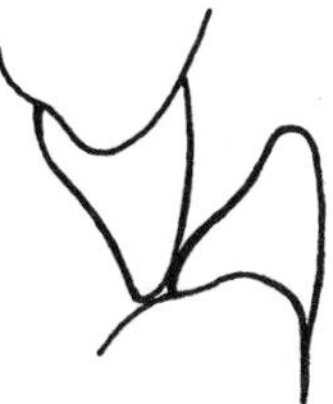

Figure 17-4

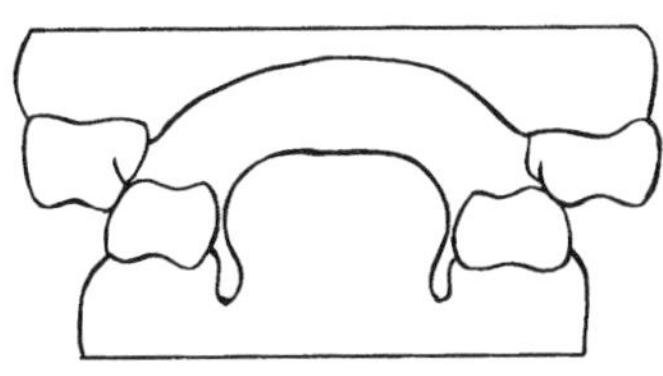

Figure 17-5

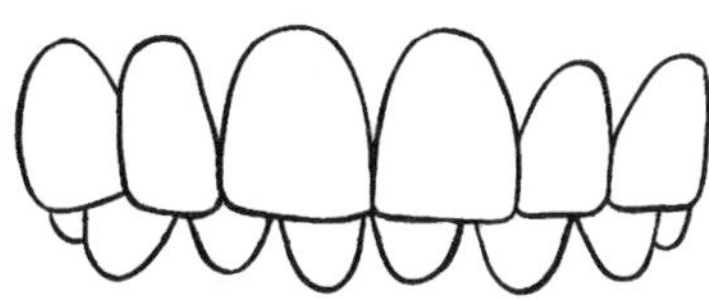

Figure 17-6

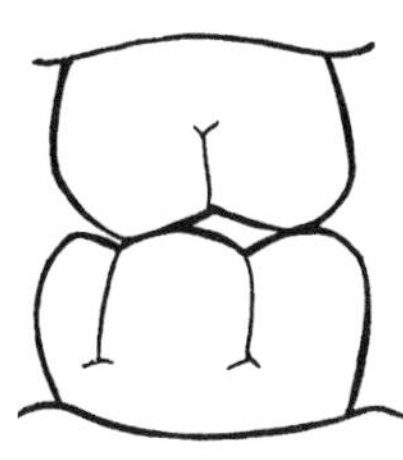

Figure 17-7

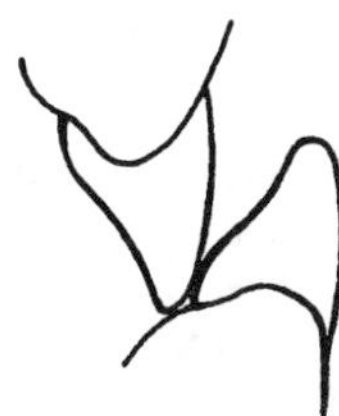

Figure 17-8

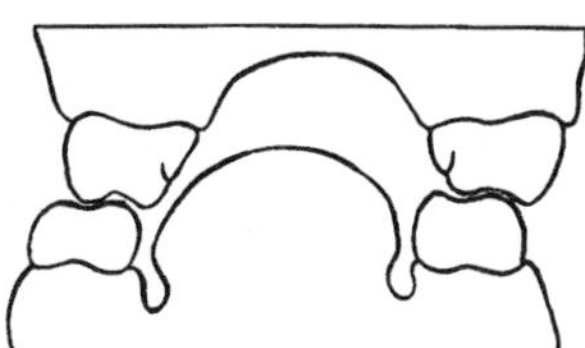

Figure 17-9

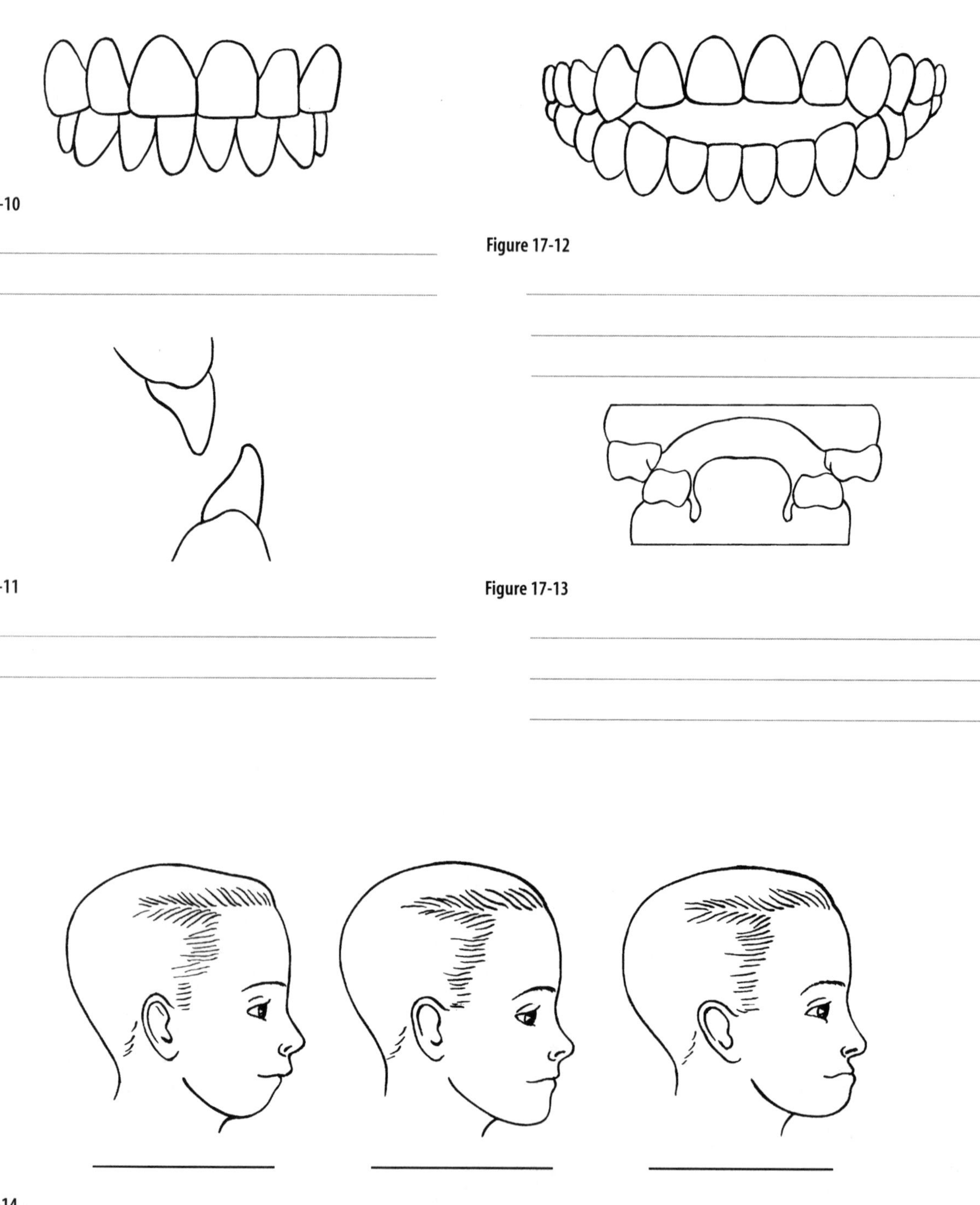

Figure 17-10

Figure 17-12

Figure 17-11

Figure 17-13

Figure 17-14

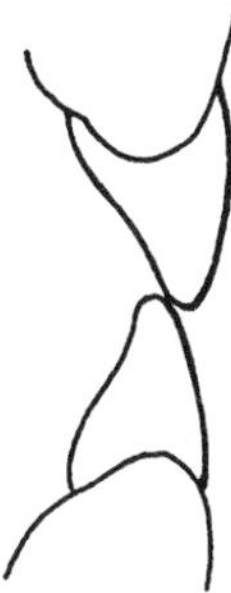

Figure 17-15

____

____

6. Fill in the blanks as you think about the occlusion of the primary teeth.

   The primary canine relation is ______________the permanent dentition.

   When a patient has primate spaces in the ______________ arch, you see these between the canine and first molar.

   In the ______________ arch, you see primate spaces between the lateral incisor and canine.

   You can expect the second primary molar relation to appear as the ______________cusp of the maxillary second primary molar occluding with the ____________ groove of the mandibular second primary molar.

   There can be variations in distal surfaces relationships, called terminal steps. An example is when the ____________ surface of the mandibular primary molar is ____________to that of the maxillary, thereby forming a mesial step.

   Although there can be morphologic variation in molar size, maxillary and mandibular primary molars are approximately the same in ______________width.

   When a patient has a terminal step, the first permanent molar erupts directly into ______________ occlusion.

   A terminal plane occurs when the ______________ surfaces of the maxillary and mandibular primary molars are on same vertical plane.

   The maxillary molar is ______________ mesiodistally than the mandibular molar.

   When a patient has a terminal plane, the first permanent molars erupt ____________to ____________.

   Primate spaces affect the eruption of the ______________.

7. Functional occlusion consists of all contacts during chewing, swallowing, and other normal action. Functional occlusion is associated with performance. List some reasons why normal functional occlusion benefits the patient.

   ____

   ____

   ____

   ____

   ____

   ____

   ____

   ____

   ____

   ____

8. Match each definition with the correct term. Each term is used more than once.

Terms	Definitions
A. Functional contact	_____ Made outside the normal range of function
B. Parafunctional contact	_____ When contact is lost, teeth can drift into spaces created by unreplaced missing teeth
C. Proximal contact	_____ This results from occlusal habits and neuroses
	_____ Normal contact that is made between the maxillary teeth and the mandibular teeth during chewing and swallowing
	_____ This is potentially injurious to the periodontal supporting structures, but only in the presence of bacterial plaque and inflammatory factors
	_____ Attrition or wear of the teeth occurs at this type of contact
	_____ This creates wear facets and attrition on the teeth
	_____ Each contact is momentary, so the total contact time is only a few minutes each day
	_____ Tooth-to-tooth contact; bruxism, clenching, tapping
	_____ This serves to stabilize the position of teeth in the dental arches and to prevent food impaction between the teeth
	_____ Tooth-to-hard-object contact; nail biting, occupational use (tacks or pins), use of smoking equipment (pipestem or hard cigarette holder)
	_____ Tooth-to-oral-tissues contact; lip or cheek biting
	_____ Pathologic migration

9. Refer to Figure 17-16 when answering the following questions.

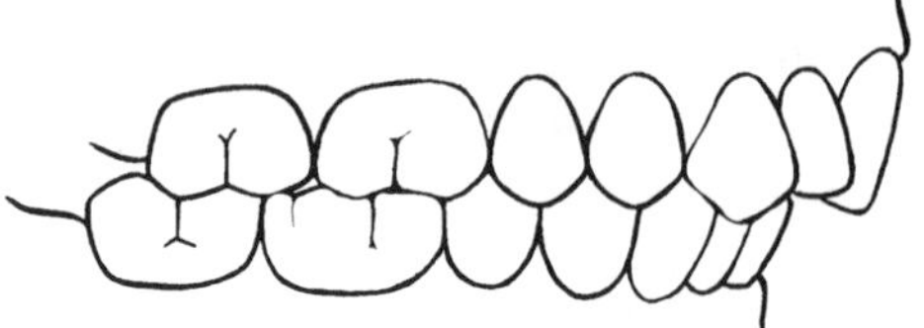

Figure 17-16

Using a red pencil, mark the teeth you will evaluate to determine this patient's classification of occlusion.

Describe the tooth relationships that will influence your decision about the patient's classification of occlusion.

What is this patient's classification of occlusion?

10. Refer to Figure 17-17 when answering the following questions.

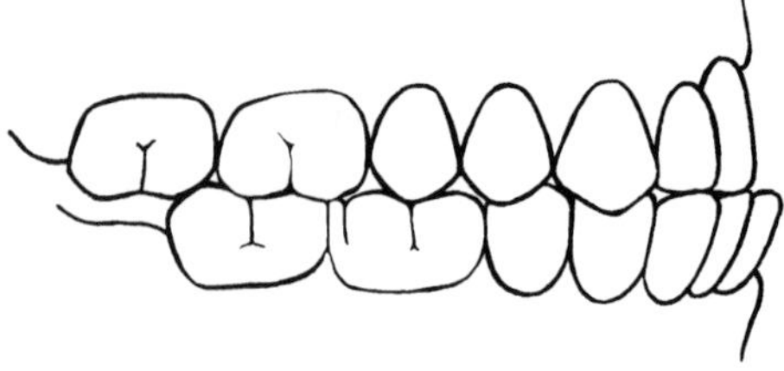

Figure 17-17

Using a red pencil, mark the teeth you will evaluate to determine this patient's classification of occlusion.

Describe the tooth relationships that will influence your decision about the patient's classification of occlusion.

What is this patient's classification of occlusion?

11. Refer to Figure 17-18 when answering the following questions.

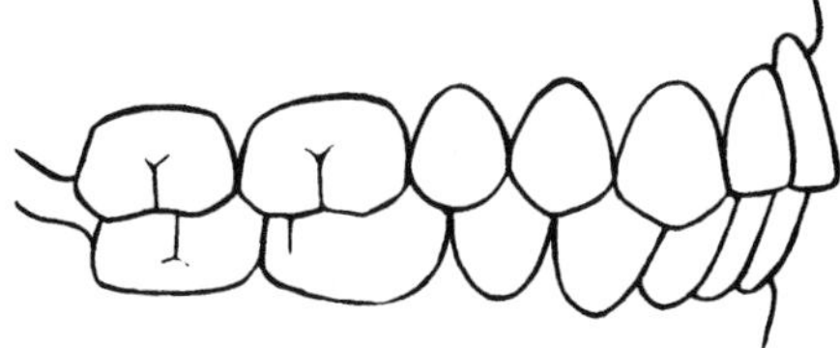

Figure 17-18

Using a red pencil, mark the teeth you will evaluate to determine this patient's classification of occlusion.

Describe the tooth relationships that will influence your decision about the patient's classification of occlusion.

What is this patient's classification of occlusion?

12. Refer to Figure 17-19 when answering the following questions.

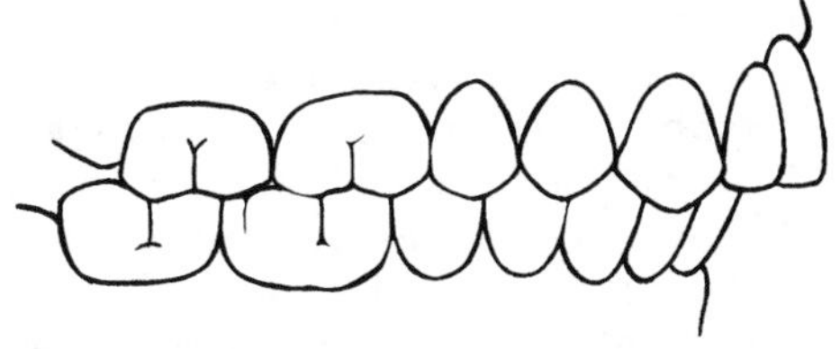

Figure 17-19

Using a red pencil, mark the teeth you will evaluate to determine this patient's classification of occlusion.

Describe the tooth relationships that will influence your decision about the patient's classification of occlusion.

What is this patient's classification of occlusion?

COMPLETENCY EXERCISES

Apply information from the chapter and use critical thinking skills to complete the competency exercises. Write responses on paper or create electronic documents to submit your answers.

1. You are performing an examination to determine whether your patient has an overbite. Describe the strategies you will use and how you will describe your findings. Which figures located in this workbook chapter will help you explain an overbite to your patient?

2. You are asked to explain an overjet. Which figure from this chapter of the workbook will help you do this? Describe the procedure for evaluating an

overjet, and then go back to the figure you selected and determine the approximate overjet reading for this patient.

3. Your patient, Song Yee, presents with chronic, generalized, moderate periodontal disease. Song just had new restorations placed on teeth 30 and 3. You are concerned about her occlusion because you have seen evidence of both primary and secondary trauma in her mouth. She wants to understand the term you used and to understand these concepts by being given an example of what you saw in her mouth. Explain to Song the clinical and radiographic findings that you have evaluated in order to determine that her occlusion is a factor in her periodontal disease.

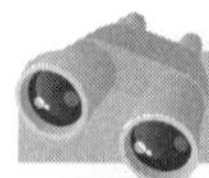

BOX 17-1 MeSH TERMS

Use a combination of MeSH terms and other key words to develop an effective and efficient PubMed literature search strategy.

Orthodontics	Malocclusion
Dental occlusion	Malocclusion, angle Class I
Dental occlusion, balanced	Malocclusion, angle Class II
Dental occlusion, centric	Malocclusion, angle Class III
Dental occlusion, traumatic	

EVERYDAY ETHICS

Before completing the learning exercises below, reread and reflect on the Everyday Ethics Scenario and Questions for Consideration in this chapter of the textbook. It may also be useful to review the Dental Hygiene Ethics discussion in Chapter 1, the Ethical Applications in the introduction pages for each section in the textbook, as well as the Codes of Ethics in textbook Appendices I–IV.

Collaborative learning Activity

Work with another student colleague to role-play the scenario. The goal of this exercise is for you and your colleague to work through the alternative actions in order to come to consensus on a solution or response that is acceptable to both of you.

Discovery Activity

Summarize this scenario for faculty member at your school and ask them to consider the questions that are included. Is their perspective different than yours or similar? Explain.

Factors To Teach The Patient

This scenario is related to the following factors listed in this chapter of the textbook:

- ▷ Interpretation of the general purposes of orthodontic care (function and aesthetics) to patients referred by the dentist to an orthodontist.
- ▷ Dependence of masticatory efficiency on the occlusion of the teeth.
- ▷ Influence of masticatory efficiency on food selection in the diet.
- ▷ Influence of masticatory efficiency and diet on the nutritional status of the body and oral health.

Your patient, Placido Perez, is a 35-year-old insurance salesman. He is overweight and reports that he can eat only soft foods because of the way he bites. Although Placido admires that famous late-night talk show host that everyone tells him he looks like, he is unhappy with his appearance. He presents with a class III malocclusion.

Use the motivational interviewing approach (see Appendix D) and the figures in this chapter of the workbook as a guide to help you write a statement explaining to Placido what you see in his mouth and what ideal occlusion looks like. Explain why referral to an orthodontist may be recommended.

Use the conversation you create to role-play this situation with a fellow student. If you are the patient in the role-play, be sure to ask questions. If you are the dental hygienist, try to anticipate questions and answer them in your explanation.

18

The Periodontium

LEARNING OBJECTIVES

Upon successful completion of these exercises, you will be able to:

1. Identify and define key terms and concepts related to the gingiva.
2. Identify the clinical features of the periodontal tissues that must be examined for a complete assessment.
3. List the markers for periodontal infection and classify them by type, degree of severity, and causative factors.
4. Identify gingival landmarks and discuss their significance.

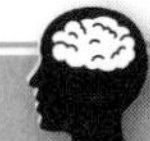

KNOWLEDGE EXERCISES

Write your answers for each question in the space provided.

1. Use the following terms to label the following figure with each of the components of the gingiva and periodontium.
   - *Alveolar bone*
   - *Alveolar mucosa*
   - *Attached gingiva*
   - *Cementoenamel junction*
   - *Enamel*
   - *Free gingiva*
   - *Free gingival groove*
   - *Gingival margin*
   - *Gingival sulcus*
   - *Junctional epithelium*
   - *Mucogingival junction*

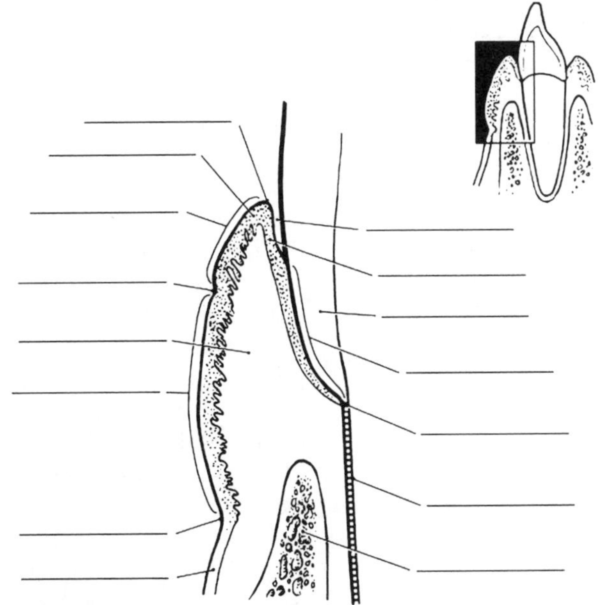

2. Draw the following gingival fibers in their correct position on the following figure. Use colored pencils to help differentiate.
   - *Alveologingival fibers*
   - *Circumferential fibers*
   - *Dentogingival fibers*
   - *Dentoperiosteal fibers*

3. Draw and label the periodontal ligament in the correct position on the same diagram.

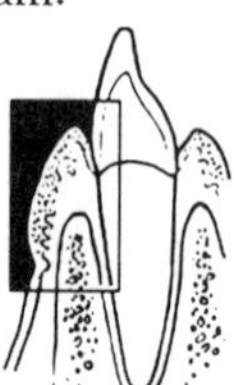

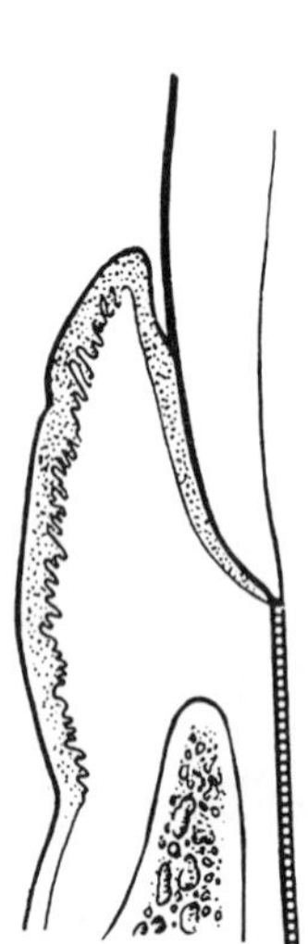

4. Match each term with the appropriate definition.

Terms Related to the Gingiva	Definition
_____ Generalized _____ Marginal _____ Clinical crown _____ Papillary _____ Anatomic root _____ Diffuse _____ Anatomic crown _____ Localized _____ Clinical root	A. A change that is confined to the free or marginal gingiva B. The gingiva is involved about all or nearly all of the teeth throughout the mouth C. A change that involves a papilla but not the rest of the free gingiva around a tooth D. Spread out, dispersed; affects the gingival margin, attached gingiva, and interdental papillae; may extend into alveolar mucosa E. Indicates the gingiva around a single tooth or a specific group of teeth F. The part of the tooth above the attached periodontal tissues; can be considered the part of the tooth where clinical treatment procedures are applied G. The part of the tooth below the base of the gingival sulcus or periodontal pocket; the part of the root to which periodontal fibers are attached H. The part of the tooth covered by enamel I. The part of the tooth covered by cementum

5. Define the following terms in your own words. (*Hint:* You may want to think about location as you define each term.)

Masticatory mucosa

____

____

Lining mucosa

____

____

____

____

Cementum

____

____

____

____

Alveolar bone

____

____

____

____

Free gingival groove

____

____

Gingival sulcus (crevice)

____

____

____

____

____

Interdental gingiva

____

____

Col

____

____

____

6. Use the following terms to label the following diagram of teeth and gingiva.
   - *Alveolar mucosa*
   - *Attached gingiva*
   - *Free gingiva*
   - *Interdental papilla*
   - *Mandibular labial frenum*
   - *Maxillary labial frenum*
   - *Mucogingival junction*

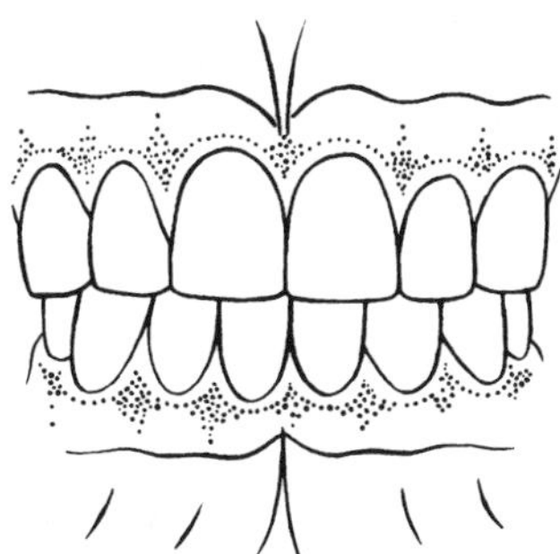

7. Match the gingival fiber group with the correct location and purpose.

Gingival Fiber Group	Location and Purpose
_____ Dentogingival fibers	A. From the cervical area of one tooth across to an adjacent tooth (on the mesial or distal side only) to provide resistance to separation of teeth
_____ Transseptal fibers	B. From the cementum in the cervical region into the free gingiva to give support to the gingiva
_____ Dentoperiosteal fibers	C. From the root apex to adjacent surrounding bone to resist vertical forces
_____ Apical fibers	D. From the root above the apical fibers obliquely toward the occlusal to resist vertical and unexpected strong forces
_____ Interradicular fibers	E. From the alveolar crest into the free and attached gingiva to provide support
_____ Circumferential fibers	F. From the cervical cementum over the alveolar crest to blend with fibers of the periosteum of the bone
_____ Oblique fibers	G. From the cementum in the middle of each root to the adjacent alveolar bone to resist tipping of the tooth
_____ Alveolar crest fibers	H. From the alveolar crest to the cementum just below the cementoenamel junction to resist intrusive forces
_____ Alveologingival fibers	I. Continuous around the neck of the tooth to help maintain the tooth in position
_____ Horizontal fibers	J. From the cementum between the roots of multirooted teeth to the adjacent bone to resist vertical and lateral forces

8. To complete this exercise using the following figure, you will need red, blue, and green pencils.
   - On the left-hand side of the diagram, color the interdental papilla in both the maxillary and mandibular arch in red.
   - On the right-hand side of the drawing, color the free gingiva in blue.
   - On the right-hand side of the drawing, color the attached gingiva in green.

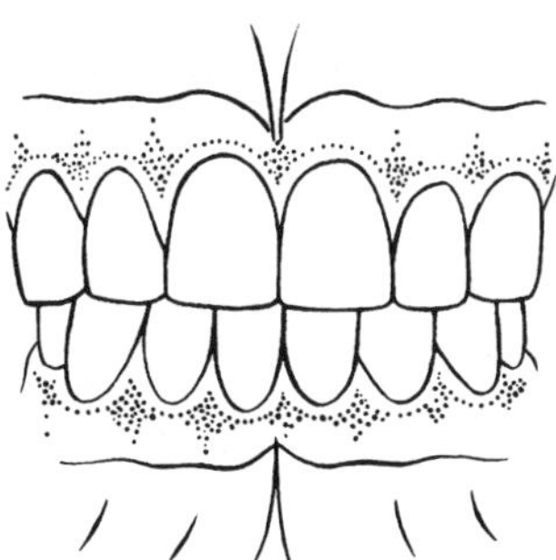

9. You are getting ready to do an examination of Patrice Davis, who is a professional ice skater and is curious about everything. She wants to know exactly how you are going to check her "gum tissues," and she does not want you to "skate over anything." She really wants to have a nice smile for the competitions! Explain the purpose of the examination to Patrice and list the markers you will use to describe the appearance of her oral tissues.

____

____

____

____

____

____

____

____

____

____

____

____

____

____

____

COMPETENCY EXERCISES

Apply information from the chapter and use critical thinking skills to complete the competency exercises. Write responses on paper or create electronic documents to submit your answers.

1. Your patient, Tucker McLeimgreen, presents with clinically normal-appearing gingiva. Describe in your own words what you expect to observe as you examine Tucker's gingival tissues both visually and with a probe.

2. Your patient, Xin Singer, is very concerned about the areas of localized, wide, shallow recession she has on teeth 6 and 7 and the narrow, deep (with missing attached gingiva) recession she has on teeth 24 and 25. Using the figures in the textbook chapter as a guide, draw a sketch of the recession that is described here. Then identify the points you will discuss with Xin.

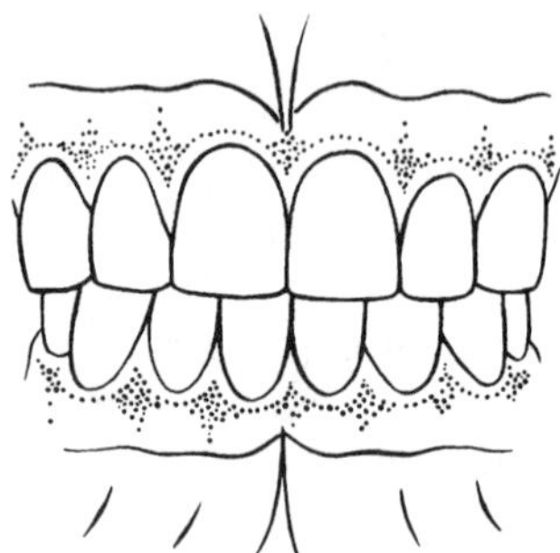

3. Your patient, Frank Catty, presents with gingiva that looks like the tissue pictured in Figure 18-12B in the textbook. On the basis of your understanding of this condition, describe Frank's gingival tissue using the following markers: color, size, shape, consistency, surface texture, position of the gingival margin, and bleeding.

4. You are providing care for Kathleen Gallagher. She is a research scientist particularly interested in inflammation. You have just completed the gingival examination and are planning to discuss the information you have gathered and the causes for the oral changes you have documented. Kathleen has not received dental care for 5 years, and she is worried about her "bleeding gums" and wants to know exactly why these changes are occurring. Refer to Table 18-1 in the textbook to help you collect your thoughts and then explain the *reasons* for each change listed below.
   - *Color: bright red*
   - *Size: enlarged*
   - *Shape: bulbous papillae*
   - *Consistency: soft, spongy (dents readily when pressed with probe)*
   - *Surface texture: smooth, shiny gingiva*
   - *Position of gingival margin: enlarged; higher on the tooth, above normal; pocket deepened*
   - *Position of junctional epithelium: probing is within normal limits*
   - *Bleeding: spontaneous*
   - *Exudate: none on pressure*

5. For some types of patient records, you will need to describe a patient's condition in sentence form. In the space provided, document a brief gingival description that you will include in Kathleen Gallagher's record.

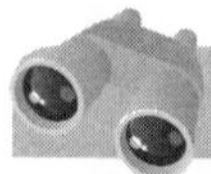

BOX 18-1 MeSH TERMS

Use a combination of MeSH terms and other key words to develop an effective and efficient PubMed literature search strategy.

Periodontium	Gingiva
Alveolar process	Periapical tissue
Dental cementum	Periodontal ligament
Epithelial attachment	Hemidesmosomes

EVERYDAY ETHICS

Before completing the learning exercises below, reread and reflect on the Everyday Ethics Scenario and Questions for Consideration in this chapter of the textbook. It may also be useful to review the Dental Hygiene Ethics discussion in Chapter 1, the Ethical Applications in the introduction pages for each section in the textbook, as well as the Codes of Ethics in textbook Appendices I–IV.

Individual Learning Activities

Identify a situation you have experienced that presents a similar ethical dilemma. Write about what you would do differently now than you did at the time the incident happened—support your discussion with concepts from the dental hygiene codes of ethics.

Discovery Activity

Summarize this scenario for faculty member at your school and ask them to consider the questions that are included. Is their perspective different than yours or similar? Explain.

Factors To Teach The Patient

This scenario is related to the following factors:

- ▷ Characteristics of normal healthy gingiva.
- ▷ The significance of bleeding; healthy tissue does not bleed.
- ▷ Relationship of findings during a gingival examination to the personal daily care procedures for infection control.

You have just seen Kathleen Gallagher, the patient described in Competency Exercise 4. She is very anxious now that you have told her about all the implications of your findings from the gingival examination.

Working with the data you have collected and the causative factors you have identified, and using the principles of motivational interviewing in Appendix D as a guide, write a dialogue explaining what type of tissue changes you would like to see at Kathleen's next appointment.

Use the conversation you create to role-play this situation with a fellow student. If you are the patient in the role-play, be sure to ask questions. If you are the dental hygienist, try to anticipate questions and answer them in your explanation.

Crossword Puzzle

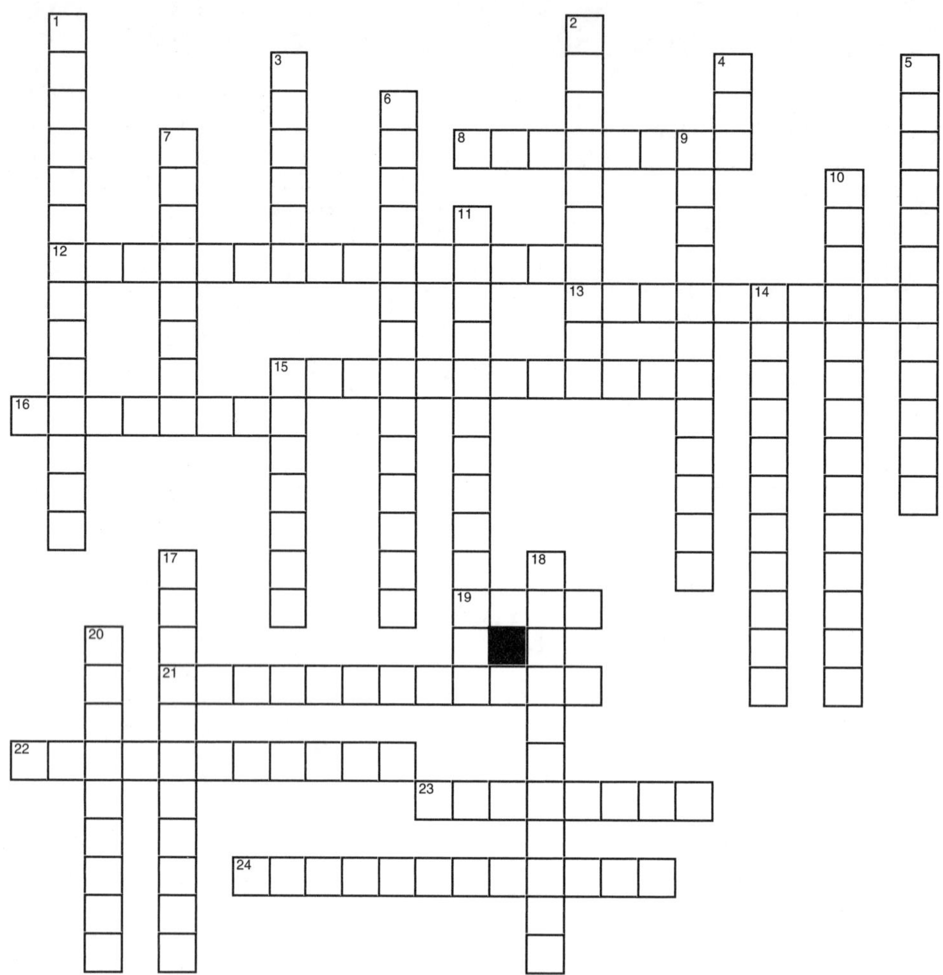

Puzzle Clues

Across

8. A fibrous change of the mucous membrane as a result of chronic inflammation.
12. Measured from the CEJ to the base of the sulcus or pocket (two words).
13. Base of the sulcus; formed by cementum, periodontal ligament, and the alveolar bone.
15. Tissue that surround and support the teeth.
16. A space between two natural teeth.
19. The type of epithelial tissue that serves as a liner for the intraoral mucosal surfaces.
21. The distance from the gingival margin to periodontal attachment at the base of the pocket (two words).
22. Increase in size of tissue or organ caused by an increase in size of its constituent cells.
23. The type of epithelium that is composed of a layer of flat, scalelike cells; or may be stratified.
24. Junction between the attached gingiva and the alveolar mucosa.

Down

1. The type of mucosal lining in which the stratified squamous epithelial cells retain their nuclei and cytoplasm.
2. Fiber-producing cell of the connective tissue.
3. Narrow fold of mucous membrane that passes from a more fixed to a more movable area of the oral mucosa.
4. Contains leukocytes, degenerated tissue elements, tissue fluids, and microorganisms.
5. Variation in gingival color related to complexion or race.
6. The development of a horny layer of flattened epithelial cells.
7. Fibrous connective tissue that surrounds and attaches the roots of teeth to the alveolar bone.
9. Characterized by increased blood flow, increased permeability of capillaries, and increased collection of defense cells and tissue fluid/usually produces alterations in color, size, shape, and consistency of tissue.
10. Abnormal thickening of the keratin layer (stratum corneum) of the epithelium.
11. One of two structures that together create a cell junction and form an attachment between junctional epithelial cells and the tooth surface.
14. Abnormal increase in volume of a tissue or organ caused by formation and growth of new normal cells.
15. Fills the interproximal area between two teeth.
17. Formation of pus.
18. The act of chewing.
20. The pitted, orange-peel appearance frequently seen on the surface of the attached gingiva.

19

Periodontal Disease Development

LEARNING OBJECTIVES

Upon successful completion of these exercises, you will be able to:

1. Identify and define key terms and concepts related to the development of periodontal disease.
2. Classify and describe periodontal diseases and conditions.
3. Discuss the development of gingival and periodontal infections.
4. Identify risk factors for development of periodontal disease.

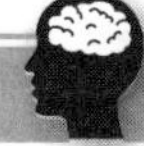

KNOWLEDGE EXERCISES

Write your answers for each question in the space provided.

1. Using the information in Table 19-1, describe each of the four types of biofilm-induced *gingival diseases*.

____
____
____
____
____
____
____
____
____
____

2. Match the gingival disease with its origin.

Gingival Disease	Origin
______ Generalized gingival candidosis	A. Bacterial
______ Phemphigoid	B. Viral
______ Varicella zoster infections	C. Fungal
______ Lupus erythematous	D. Systemic condition/ mucocutaneous disorder
______ *Neisseria gonorrhea*–associated lesions	
______ Linear gingival erythema	
______ Recurrent oral herpes	
______ Lichen planus	
______ *Treponema pallidum*–associated lesions	
______ Histoplasmosis	
______ Erythema multiforma	

3. List one example of a gingival lesion of genetic origin.

____

4. Identify three dental restorative materials that could cause an allergic reaction in the form of a gingival lesion.

____

____

____

5. List two terms that describe the locations of chronic and aggressive periodontitis.

____

____

6. Periodontitis as a manifestation of systemic disease can be associated with hematologic disorders. Name some conditions in which you may find this association.

____

____

7. Periodontitis can be associated with genetic disorders. Name some conditions in which you may find this association.

____

____

____

____

____

____

____

____

____

____

8. Name the necrotizing periodontal diseases.

____

____

9. List three types of abscesses of the periodontium.

____

____

____

10. List the term used to describe lesions associated with endodontic lesions.

____

11. List localized tooth-related factors that modify or predispose the area to biofilm-induced gingival diseases/periodontitis.

____

____

____

____

12. List mucogingival deformities and conditions around the teeth that are manifestations of systemic disease.

____

____

____

____

____

13. Match each descriptive statement with the appropriate stage of development of gingivitis and periodontal disease. Each answer may be used more than once.

Developmental Stage	Description
A. Initial lesion	______ Inflammatory response to biofilm occurs within 2–4 days
B. Early lesion	______ Biofilm becomes older and thicker (7–14 days; time reflects individual differences)
	______ Migration and infiltration of white blood cells into the junctional epithelium and gingival sulcus
	______ Signs of gingivitis become apparent with slight gingival enlargement
	______ No clinical evidence of change
	______ Infiltration of fluid, lymphocytes, and neutrophils with a few plasma cells into the connective tissue
	______ The gingivitis is reversible when biofilm is controlled and inflammation is reduced; healthy tissue may be restored
	______ Increased flow of gingival sulcus fluid

14. Match each descriptive statement with the appropriate stage of development of gingivitis and periodontal disease. Each answer may be used more than once.

Developmental Stage	Description
C. Established lesion	______ Inflammation spreads through the bone marrow and out into the periodontal ligament
D. Advanced lesion	______ Fluid and leukocyte migration into tissues and sulcus increase; plasma cells are related to areas of chronic inflammation
	______ Exposed cementum where Sharpey fibers were attached becomes altered by inflammatory products of bacteria and the sulcus fluid
	______ Clear evidence of inflammation is present, with marginal redness, bleeding on probing, and spongy marginal gingiva; later, chronic fibrosis develops
	______ Proliferation of the junctional and sulcular epithelium continues in an attempt to wall out the inflammation
	______ Inflammation spreads through the loose connective tissue along (beside) the blood vessels to the alveolar bone
	______ Connective tissue fibers below the junctional epithelium are destroyed; the epithelium migrates along the root surface
	______ Bacteria from supragingival biofilm enter the sulcus and provide the source for subgingival biofilm
	______ Diseased cementum contains a thin superficial layer of endotoxins from the bacterial breakdown
	______ Formation of pocket epithelium

15. In your own words, define and describe a periodontal pocket. Include the following in your description:
    - *What distinguishes a pocket from a sulcus?*
    - *Describe the walls and the base of a pocket.*
    - *Compare the histology of a healthy pocket and the histopathology of a diseased pocket.*

16. Use the following terms to label Figure 19-1, which illustrates types of periodontal pockets.
    - *Normal relationship*
    - *Gingival pocket*
    - *Periodontal pocket*
    - *Suprabony*
    - *Intrabony*
    - *Cementoenamel junction*
    - *Alveolar bone*
    - *Gingival tissue*
    - *Calculus*

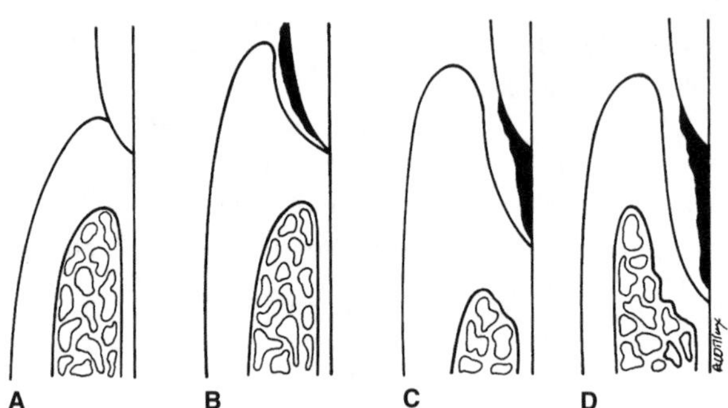

A. ______________________________

B. ______________________________

C. ______________________________

D. ______________________________

17. In your own words, describe a pseudopocket.

____

____

____

____

____

____

____

____

18. When a pocket is identified as an infrabony pocket, where is the base of the pocket?

____

____

19. Match each of the following definitions with the correct term.

Factor	Definition
A. Etiologic factor	_____ A factor that lends assistance to, supplements, or adds to a condition or disease
B. Predisposing factor	_____ A factor that results from or is influenced by a general physical or mental disease or condition
C. Risk factor	_____ A factor that is the actual cause of a disease or condition
D. Contributing factor	_____ A factor in the immediate environment of the oral cavity or specifically in the environment of the teeth or periodontium
E. Local factor	_____ A factor that renders a person susceptible to a disease or condition
F. Systemic factor	_____ An exposure that increases the probability that disease will occur

20. List the types of information/data collected during a basic periodontal examination.

____

____

____

____

____

____

21. List the symptoms of periodontal disease that a patient may notice or feel.

____

____

____

____

____

22. Match the term to the description of periodontal disease.

Term	Description
____ severity	A. More than 30% of the gingiva is involved
____ marginal	B. Spread out, dispersed, affects multiple tissues
____ papillary	C. Change confined to free gingiva
____ generalized	D. Involvement around a single tooth or specific group of teeth
____ diffuse	E. Quantity of clinical attachment loss
____ localized	F. The tissue change does not involve the free gingiva

COMPETENCY EXERCISES

Apply information from the chapter and use critical thinking skills to complete the competency exercises. Write responses on paper or create electronic documents to submit your answers.

1. After probing, you determine that disease is limited to the gingiva. Discuss the care planning objectives and some questions you may have for your patient.
2. Your next patient presents with apical positioning of the periodontal attachment, with alveolar bone loss and other indications of periodontitis. Identify some questions, concerns, and general guidelines you will consider as you start to plan treatment for this patient.
3. As you assess your patient Chu His, you observe that clear evidence of inflammation is present, with marginal redness, bleeding on probing, and spongy marginal gingival. He has a history of diabetes, candidiasis infections, and an allergy to dental restorative materials. Describe the disease classification you would use for this patient.
4. You detect a Class II furcation on tooth 30 and a Class III furcation involvement on tooth 31 as you collect data for your 10:00 patient, Woody Green. Woody asks many questions and wants to understand what these terms mean. Explain the terms to him, and use drawings of the teeth to help describe the conditions.
5. You are asked to develop patient education materials for the practice you are in. You decide to focus on local contributing factors in disease development. Develop a checklist that can be filled out during a patient education session to identify specific factors relevant for each individual patient.

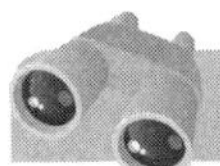

BOX 19-1 MeSH TERMS

Use a combination of MeSH terms and other key words to develop an effective and efficient PubMed literature search strategy.

Periodontal diseases	Gingivitis
Periodontitis	Gingival pocket
Periodontal pocket	Gingival recession
Gingival diseases	Gingival hyperplasia

EVERYDAY ETHICS

Before completing the learning exercises below, reread and reflect on the Everyday Ethics Scenario and Questions for Consideration in this chapter of the textbook. It may also be useful to review the Dental Hygiene Ethics discussion in Chapter 1, the Ethical Applications in the introduction pages for each section in the textbook, as well as the Codes of Ethics in textbook Appendices I–IV.

Discovery Activity

Ask a dental hygienist who has been practicing for a year or more to read the scenario. Provide a copy of the Code of Ethics as well. Share the responses you have made to answer each question and ask that person to discuss the situation with you. What insights did you have or what did you learn during this discussion?

Collaborative Learning Activity

Work with a small group to develop a 2- to 5-minute role-play that introduces the everyday ethics scenario described in the chapter (a great idea is to video record your role-play activity). Then develop separate 2-minute role-play scenarios that provide at least two alternative approaches/solutions to resolving the situation. Ask classmates to view the solutions, ask questions, and discuss the ethical approach used in each. Ask for a vote on which solution classmates determine to be the "best."

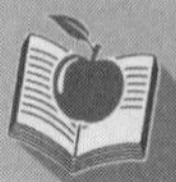

Factors To Teach The Patient

This scenario is related to the following factors listed in this chapter of the textbook:

- ▷ Factors that contribute to disease development and progression.
- ▷ What a risk factor is and the importance of planning personal and professional care to include risk factor problems.

During data collection for your patient, Maria Manuela Rodriguez, you note the following information:

- She smokes two packs of cigarettes per day.
- She takes 10 mg Fosamax (alendronate) per day to prevent/control osteoporosis.
- There is a family history of diabetes.
- She is overweight.
- She takes 10 mg Procardia three times per day to treat her high blood pressure and ventricular arrhythmia (this is nifedipine, which is a calcium channel blocker).
- She tends to have a soft diet.

Use the principles of motivational interviewing as a guide to write a dialogue explaining Maria's risk factors for periodontal disease. Use the ideas from this written dialogue to role-play a counseling session with a student colleague.

Word Search

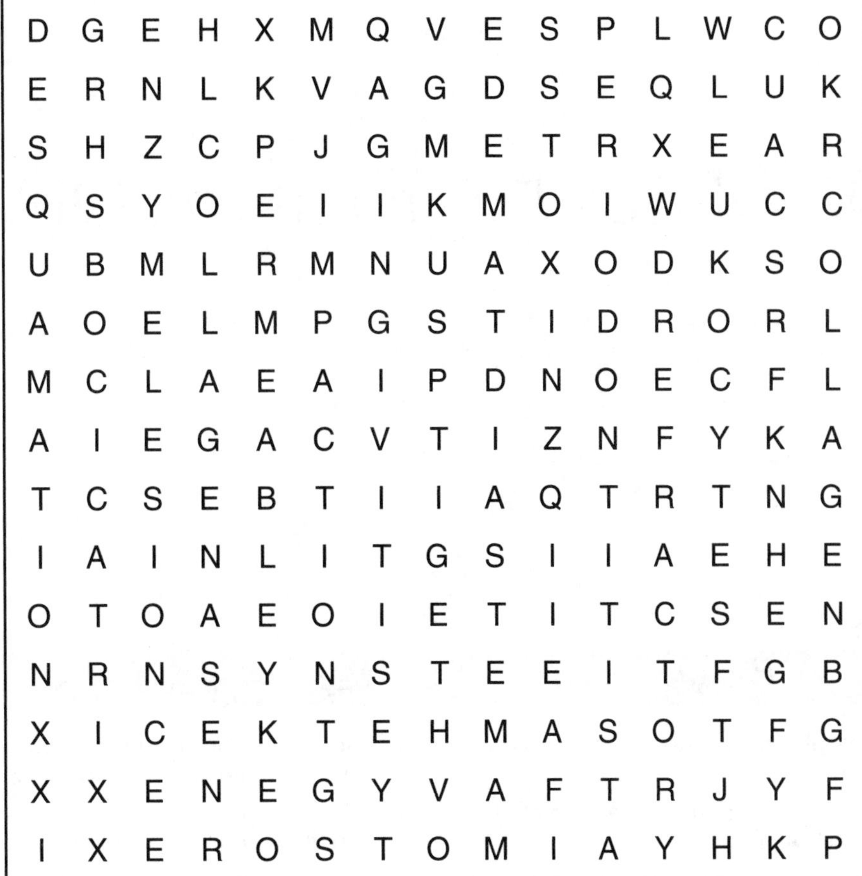

Word Search Clues

- Refers to wounds, sores, ulcers, tumors, or any other tissue damage.
- The numbers of these increase inside the diseased pocket as inflammation increases.
- White fibers of the connective tissue.
- Poison; protein produced by certain animals, higher plants, and pathogenic bacteria.
- Shedding of the outer epithelial layer of the stratified squamous epithelium of skin or mucosa.
- Accumulation of excessive fluid in cells or tissues.
- Not readily responsive to treatment.
- Forceful wedging of food into the periodontium by occlusal forces.
- Inflammation of the gingiva.
- A space or abnormal opening; in dentistry, a space between two adjacent teeth in the same dental arch.
- Enzyme that contributes to the hydrolysis of collagen.
- Inflammation of the periodontium.
- Protein secreted by body cells that acts as a catalyst to induce chemical changes in other substances.
- Permitting passage of a fluid.
- Dryness of the mouth from a lack of normal secretions.
- Fibrous tissue left after the healing of a wound.

20

Periodontal Examination

LEARNING OBJECTIVES

Upon successful completion of these exercises, you will be able to:

1. Identify and define key terms and concepts related to oral examination procedures.
2. Describe the purpose and procedure for the use of each instrument in a basic examination setup.
3. Discuss the implications of various oral findings identified during the examination.

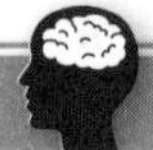

KNOWLEDGE EXERCISES

Write your answers for each question in the space provided.

1. List the basic instruments used for the periodontal examination.

2. Describe the types of mirror surfaces in your own words.

3. Describe the purposes and uses of mouth mirrors.

4. Match each term with the correct definition.

Examination Procedures Term	Definition
_____ Horizontal bone loss	A. A slender instrument, usually round in diameter with a rounded tip, designed for examination of the teeth and soft tissues
_____ Clinical attachment level	B. Probing depth as measured from the cementoenamel junction (or other fixed point) to the location of the probe tip at the coronal level of attached periodontal tissues
_____ Explorer	C. Determination of the accuracy of an instrument by measurement of its variation from a standard
_____ Bifurcation	D. The distance from the gingival margin to the location of the periodontal probe tip at the coronal border of attached periodontal tissues
_____ Fremitus	E. A slender stainless-steel instrument with a fine, flexible, sharp point used for examination of the surfaces of the teeth to detect irregularities
_____ Tactile	F. A vibration perceptible by palpation
_____ Explorer tip	G. Pertaining to touch
_____ Calibration	H. The ability to distinguish relative degrees of roughness and smoothness
_____ Probe	I. Two roots
_____ Probing depth	J. Slender, wirelike, circular in cross section, and tapering to a fine, sharp point
_____ Tactile discrimination	K. When the crest of the bone is parallel with a line between the cementoenamel junctions of two adjacent teeth

5. How does the application of air improve assessment procedures?

6. List the purposes of using an explorer.

7. List the parts of an explorer.

8. List five characteristics of an explorer that contribute to increased tactile sensitivity.

9. List two sensory stimuli engaged through use of an explorer.

10. What operator techniques will contribute to increased tactile sensitivity?

11. What information is learned by the dental hygienist through auditory stimuli when using an explorer?

12. Why is it important to not remove the explorer from the pocket after each stroke?

13. What action will prevent damage to the tissue by the tip and point of the explorer during subgingival exploring?

14. What are the purposes of using a periodontal probe?

15. When is a plastic periodontal probe used?

16. Describe the purpose and use of a probe with a curved working end.

17. What is the difference between a sulcus and a periodontal pocket?

18. What is measured during periodontal probing?

19. In addition to measuring the depth of a pocket/sulcus, what additional information can be identified with a probe?

20. List factors that influence the accuracy of the probing measurements.

21. List five sources of error in periodontal probing.

22. List three factors that interfere with probing.

23. The probe reading in part A of Figure 20-1 is ________. The probe reading in part B of the figure is ________.

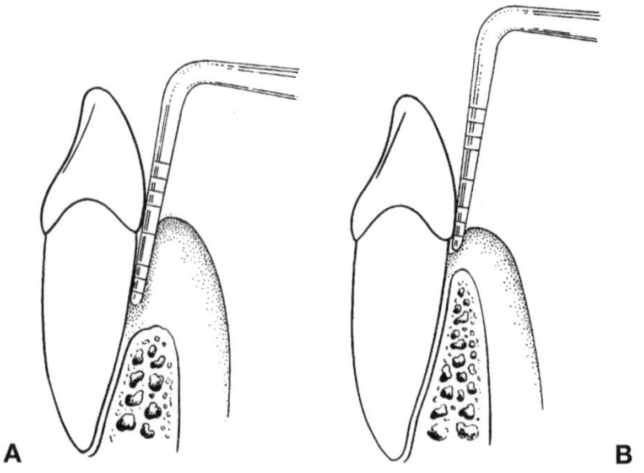

A B

FIGURE 20-1

24. Match the health status of the periodontium with the appropriate location of the probe tip.

Periodontal Status	Location of Probe Tip
_____ Gingivitis and early periodontitis	A. At the base of the sulcus or crevice, at the coronal end of the junctional epithelium
_____ Normal healthy tissue	B. Penetrates through the junctional epithelium to reach attached connective tissue fibers
_____ Advanced periodontitis	C. Within the junctional epithelium

25. What types of preliminary assessments should be done prior to the periodontal examination?

26. When probing a **sulcus**, which tooth structure is touched by the probe?

27. When probing a **pocket**, which tooth structures are touched by the probe?

28. Describe why it is important to keep the probe as parallel to the long axis of the tooth as possible.

29. The probe is adapted to individual teeth and surfaces. In your own words, describe how to adapt the probe for each of the following structures.

- *Molars and premolars*

- *Anterior teeth*

- *Proximal surfaces*

30. Identify the six measurements recorded for each tooth in the periodontal probing record.

31. Describe what you would do if you encountered a significant calculus deposit during probing.

32. What is meant by the term, "walking stroke?"

33. Describe CAL.

34. Explain the significance of clinical attachment loss?

35. List two fixed points that can be used during the calculation of CAL.

36. List the steps for determining CAL in the presence of visible gingival recession.

37. List the steps for determining CAL when the CEJ is covered by gingiva.

38. True or false (circle one). Provide a reason for your answer. The probing depth equals the clinical attachment level when the free gingival margin is level with the cementoenamel junction.

39. True or false (circle one). Provide a reason for your answer. When there is visible recession, the probing depth is greater than the clinical attachment loss.

40. List three reasons to conduct a mucogingival examination.

41. Describe one method to make the facial mucogingival margin become visible.

42. Describe how to measure the width of the attached gingiva.

43. Describe why it is important to use two single-ended metal instruments with wide blunt ends to measure mobility.

44. Match the level of mobility to its descriptor.

Miller Index of Tooth Mobility	Description
N	____ Slight mobility, greater than normal
1	____ Vertical as well as horizontal movement
2	____ Physiologic mobility
3	____ Greater than 1 mm displacement

45. What is fremitus?

____

____

46. Why are only maxillary teeth used to determine fremitus?

____

____

47. Briefly describe how to conduct the examination for fremitus.

____

____

____

____

____

____

____

____

____

____

48. Describe the clinical findings of each stage of furcation involvement.

Glickman Furcation Grade	Description
I	
II	
III	
IV	

49. Match each tooth with the appropriate anatomic features. There are two answers for each type of tooth.

Type of Tooth	Anatomic Features
_____ and _____ Mandibular molars	A. Furcation area is accessible from the mesial and distal aspects, under the contact area
_____ and _____ Maxillary molars	B. Palatal root and two buccal roots (mesiobuccal and distobuccal); access for probing is from the mesial, buccal, and distal surfaces
_____ and _____ Maxillary first premolars	C. Bifurcation
_____ and _____ Maxillary primary molars	D. Widespread roots
_____ and _____ Mandibular primary molars	E. Furcation area is accessible from the facial and lingual surfaces
	F. Trifurcation

50. Match the tooth surface irregularities with the correct tactile sensation. Each answer is used more than once.

Tooth Surface Irregularity	Tactile Sensation
_____ Enamel pearl	A. Normal
_____ Smooth surface of enamel	B. Irregular: increases or elevations in tooth surface
_____ Carious lesion	C. Irregular: depressions, grooves
_____ Anatomic configurations, such as cingula, furcations	
_____ Abrasion	
_____ Root surface that has been planed	
_____ Calculus	
_____ Erosion	
_____ Irregular margins (overhang)	
_____ Pits such as those caused by enamel hypoplasia	
_____ Areas of cemental resorption on the root surface	
_____ Unusually pronounced cementoenamel junction	
_____ Deficient margins	
_____ Overcontoured restoration	
_____ Rough surface of a restoration	

51. Radiographic evidence of periodontal disease includes changes in:

____

____

____

52. Describe how normal bone level appears in a dental radiograph.

____

____

53. What is vertical bone loss?

54. Describe horizontal bone loss.

55. How does the periodontal ligament appear in a dental radiograph?

COMPETENCY EXERCISES

Apply information from the chapter and use critical thinking skills to complete the competency exercises. Write responses on paper or create electronic documents to submit your answers.

1. Your employer, Dr. Harriet Golden, asks you put together instrument kits for the office and label them "basic assessment setup." Identify the instruments you have placed in the kit and discuss why you have included each one.

2. Whenever you are using air, you should take care to avoid some very specific situations that may hurt or startle the patient. List some of these situations and describe how you would avoid them.

3. When your instructor verifies your probing, many differences are found. You are having difficulty and need to look at the factors that affect probe determinations and probing procedures. Knowing the right question to ask yourself is a great way to solve a problem. Develop questions that will help you look at these factors and allow you to self-evaluate your own performance.

4. Identify the number on the handle of each explorer in your student kit. Describe the design of the working end, shank, handle, and construction of each one and specify its use.

5. Your patient Tony Wade presents with both mobility (III on teeth 22–27) and fremitus (+ on teeth 6–11). You note generalized bleeding and probe readings of 5–8 mm. The radiographs show horizontal bone loss in all posterior and anterior areas and vertical bone loss on the distal side of tooth 29. The crestal lamina dura is indistinct, irregular, and radiolucent throughout Tony's mouth. There are furcation involvements on teeth 30 and 31. The periodontal ligament spaces are thickened on teeth 28 and 29. Describe how the pocket depth, mobility, and fremitus findings were determined.

6. Label Tony's radiograph in Figure 20-2 with the following findings.

Findings

- *Horizontal bone loss*
- *Vertical bone loss*
- *Change in crestal lamina dura*
- *Furcation involvement*
- *Changes in the periodontal ligament*

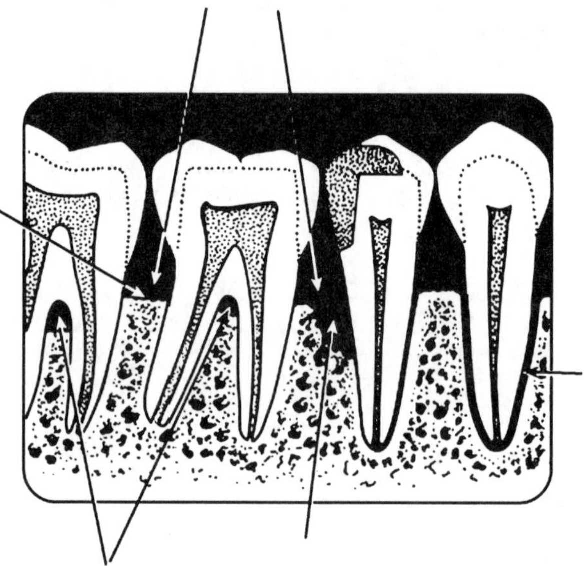

FIGURE 20-2

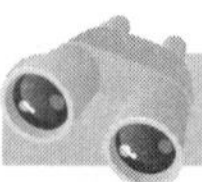

BOX 20-1 MeSH TERMS

Use a combination of MeSH terms and other key words to develop an effective and efficient PubMed literature search strategy.

Periodontium	Gingival pocket
Periodontal pocket	Gingival recession
Periodontal ligament	Periodontal attachment Loss
Epithelial attachment	Alveolar bone loss
Gingiva	Tooth mobility

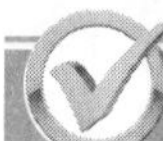

COMPETENCY EXERCISE

Apply information from the chapter and use critical thinking skills to complete the competency exercises. Write responses on paper or create electronic documents to submit your answers.

1. Compare and contrast the distribution of supragingival and subgingival calculus. Discuss how the distribution affects your detection strategies.

2. Your patient, John Weston, is wondering about calculus formation. He is trying to understand the exact time frame of the process. Help him understand calculus formation by defining pellicle, biofilm, and calculus and discussing the influencing factors. Make a list or draw a picture that describes calculus formation in terms of minutes, hours, and days.

3. Explain the impact of the formation of calculus on John Weston's oral health.

4. While scaling in the mandibular right quadrant, you are having varying degrees of difficulty detecting and removing the calculus. Describe the three modes of calculus attachment. Explain how each mode affects detection and removal.

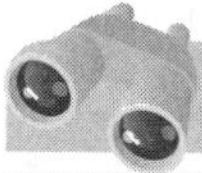

BOX 21-1 MeSH TERMS

Use a combination of MeSH terms and other key words to develop an effective and efficient PubMed literature search strategy.

Biofilms	Dental pellicle
Dental calculus	Dental scaling
Dental plaque	Minerals

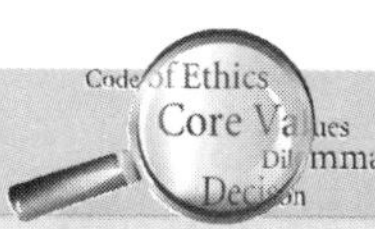

EVERYDAY ETHICS

Before completing the learning exercises below, reread and reflect on the Everyday Ethics Scenario and Questions for Consideration in this chapter of the textbook. It may also be useful to review the Dental Hygiene Ethics discussion in Chapter 1, the Ethical Applications in the introduction pages for each section in the textbook, as well as the Codes of Ethics in textbook Appendices I–IV.

Individual Lea Activity

Imagine that you a. dental hygienist in this scenario. Answer each of the q ns for consideration at the end of the scenario.

Discovery Activity

Summarize this scenario fo. y member at your school and ask them to consider th tions that are included. Is their perspective different th urs or similar? Explain.

Factors To Teach The Patient

This scenario is related to the following factors:

- ▷ That good oral hygiene and frequent professional care for complete scaling are consistent with low levels of supragingival and subgingival calculus.
- ▷ The effect of calculus on the health of the periodontal tissues and, therefore, on the general health of the oral cavity.
- ▷ What to expect from use of an anticalculus dentifrice.
- ▷ The importance of selecting products with an ADA Seal of Approval.

Louisa Gregory, a 53-year-old first-grade teacher, is busy with her two daughters, aged 12 and 14. She does not take time for herself and has come to the dental hygiene clinic after a 5-year absence. She uses any type of toothpaste that is on sale, and her current dentifrice is in a decorative dispenser; she does not know anything else about i. pt that it matches her bathroom perfectly! As you exa ouisa's mouth, you see generalized heavy supragingival bgingival calculus. She wants to know what to do ab his hard stuff" on her teeth.

Use a motivational interviewing approach (see App)) to create a conversation to educate Louisa about the i. of good oral hygiene and frequent professional care for c plete scaling on the levels of supragingival and subging calculus. Be sure to address product selection criteria and th need for the use of an anticalculus toothpaste.

Use the conversation you create to role-play this situation with a fellow student. If you are the patient in the role-play, be sure to ask questions. If you are the dental hygienist, try to anticipate questions and answer them in your explanation.

22

Dental Stains and Discolorations

LEARNING OBJECTIVES

Upon successful completion of these exercises, you will be able to:

1. Identify and define key terms and concepts related to dental stains and discolorations.
2. Classify various stains as to their location and source.

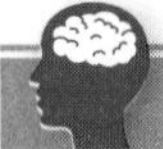

KNOWLEDGE EXERCISES

Write your answers for each question in the space provided.

1. Match the following terms with the correct definition.

Term	Definition
A. Chlorophyll	_______ Incomplete development or underdevelopment of an organ or a tissue
B. Endogenous	_______ Producing color or pigment
C. Chronologic	_______ Imperfect formation of enamel; hereditary condition in which the ameloblasts fail to lay down the enamel matrix properly or at all
D. Chromogenic	_______ Originating outside or caused by factors outside
E. Dentinogenesis imperfecta	_______ Hereditary disorder of dentin formation in which the odontoblasts lay down an abnormal matrix; can occur in both primary and permanent dentitions
F. Amelogenesis imperfecta	_______ Produced within or caused by factors within
G. Hypoplasia	_______ Situated entirely within
H. Intrinsic	_______ Green plant pigment essential to photosynthesis
I. Exogenous	_______ Arranged in order of time
J. Extrinsic	_______ Derived from or situated on the outside; external

2. Stains are classified by location and source.
   - *List examples of extrinsic exogenous stains.*

   ____
   ____
   ____
   ____
   ____
   ____

   - *List examples of intrinsic endogenous stains.*

   ____
   ____
   ____
   ____
   ____
   ____

   - *List examples of intrinsic exogenous stains.*

   ____
   ____
   ____
   ____
   ____
   ____

3. Your patient presents with a stained pulpless tooth. Describe the clinical appearance of the stain and explain how it was formed. The patient is scheduled for endodontic treatment on another tooth and wants to know if that tooth will also stain. What would you tell this patient?

   ____
   ____
   ____
   ____
   ____
   ____
   ____
   ____
   ____
   ____
   ____
   ____

4. Clinically you observe enamel that is partially or completely missing because of a generalized disturbance of the ameloblasts. Teeth are yellowish-brown or gray-brown. What is this condition is called?

   ____

5. Your patient was born with erythroblastosis fetalis (Rh incompatibility). This condition may a leave the teeth with a ______________________ hue.

6. Complete Infomap 21-1 to help you organize information about extrinsic stains.

INFOMAP 22-1

TYPE OF STAIN	APPEARANCE	DISTRIBUTION	OCCURRENCE	CAUSE/ORIGIN	CLINICAL ISSUES
Yellow					
Green					
Other green					
Black line					
Tobacco					
Other brown					
Orange and red					
Metallic-industrial					
Metallic-drugs					

COMPETENCY EXERCISES

Apply information from the chapter and use critical thinking skills to complete the competency exercises. Write responses on paper or create electronic documents to submit your answers.

1. Your 1:30 patient, Fawez Sadarage, 47 years old, presents with a stain on all the second and third molars caused by tetracycline. Describe the stain that you might see and list some follow-up questions you will ask Mr. Sadarage. Indicate why you would ask the questions.

2. The patient in the scenario posed in Question 1 presented with generalized gray-brown stain on second and third molars. Why weren't all teeth affected?

3. At what age do you think the patient took the antibiotic?

4. Several strategies will help you recognize and identify stains that you observe during assessment of the oral cavity. Explain the types of stains (color and cause) that can be identified using each of the strategies listed below.
   - *Medical history*
   - *Questions about industrial occupation*
   - *Questions about dietary habits*
   - *Dental history*
   - *Dental charting (e.g., endodontic therapy, restorative materials)*

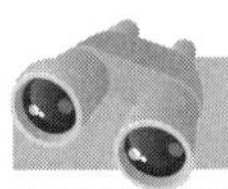

BOX 21-1 MeSH TERMS

Use a combination of MeSH terms and other key words to develop an effective and efficient PubMed literature search strategy.

Dental polishing	Amelogenesis imperfecta
Dental prophylaxis	Dental enamel hypoplasia
Tooth bleaching	Dentin dysplasia
Tetracyclines	Dentinogenesis imperfecta
Fluorosis, dental	Odontodysplasia

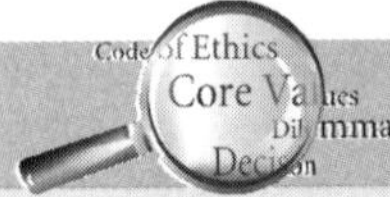

EVERYDAY ETHICS

Before completing the learning exercises below, reread and reflect on the Everyday Ethics Scenario and Questions for Consideration in this chapter of the textbook. It may also be useful to review the Dental Hygiene Ethics discussion in Chapter 1, the Ethical Applications in the introduction pages for each section in the textbook, as well as the Codes of Ethics in textbook Appendices I–IV.

Collaborative Learning Activity

Answer each of the questions for consideration at the end of the scenario in the textbook. Compare what you wrote with answers developed by another classmate and discuss differences/similarities.

Discovery Activity

Summarize this scenario for faculty member at your school and ask them to consider the questions that are included. Is their perspective different than yours or similar? Explain.

Factors To Teach The Patient

This scenario is related to the following factors listed in this chapter of the textbook:

- ▷ Predisposing factors that contribute to stain accumulation.
- ▷ Personal care procedures that can aid in the prevention or reduction of stains.
- ▷ Advantages of starting a smoking-cessation program.
- ▷ Reasons for not using an abrasive dentifrice with vigorous brushing strokes to lessen or remove stain accumulation.
- ▷ The need to avoid tobacco, coffee, tea, and other beverages or foodstuffs that can stain to prevent discoloration of new restorations.

Your patient, Shaneeka Harris, is a 21-year-old college student. She has recently started to smoke cigarettes and marijuana and drinks a lot of coffee and tea. Her last blood test showed that she was anemic, and her physician has prescribed daily oral doses of iron. Shaneeka is finding college overwhelming and very stressful. The reason she made an appointment in the dental hygiene clinic is because she has noticed that her teeth have a brown and gray-green stain, and she is really unhappy with how they look. She does not remember having all these stains before.

Use a motivational interviewing approach (see Appendix D) as a guide to develop a dialogue you might use to help Shaneeka understand the factors affecting stain accumulation and the removal and prevention strategies.

Use the conversation you create to role-play this situation with a fellow student. If you are the patient in the role-play, be sure to ask questions. If you are the dental hygienist, try to anticipate questions and answer them in your explanation.

23

Indices and Scoring Methods

LEARNING OBJECTIVES

Upon successful completion of these exercises, you will be able to:

1. Identify and define key terms and concepts related to dental indices and scoring methods.
2. Identify the purpose, criteria for measurement, scoring methods, range of scores, and reference or interpretation scales for a variety of dental indices.
3. Select and calculate dental indices for use in a specific patient or community situation.

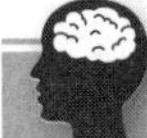

KNOWLEDGE EXERCISES

Write your answers for each question in the space provided.

Dental Indices Infomaps

Infomaps are tables that place related information about different factors of one topic on a single page. This method of organizing not only allows you to learn information as you transfer key points from the textbook but also provides a study guide that lets you visually compare and contrast the different dental indices easily and effectively.

Transfer enough basic information about each index from the textbook to the appropriate infomap so that you can use the collected data to complete the competency exercises for this chapter. The blank Infomaps 23-1–23-5 are found on the next few pages.

INFOMAP 23-1 ORAL HYGIENE STATUS INDICES

INDEX	WHAT IS MEASURED?	TEETH AND/OR SURFACES SCORED	CRITERIA USED FOR MEASUREMENT	SCORING/CALCULATION OF INDEX	REFERENCE SCALES, RANGE OF SCORES, AND ADDITIONAL INFORMATION
Biofilm index					
Biofilm control record					
Biofilm-free score					
PHP					
OHI-S					

INFOMAP 23-2 GINGIVAL HEALTH INDICES

INDEX	WHAT IS MEASURED?	TEETH AND/OR SURFACES SCORED	CRITERIA USED FOR MEASUREMENT	SCORING/CALCULATION OF INDEX	REFERENCE SCALES, RANGE OF SCORES, AND ADDITIONAL INFORMATION
SBI					
GBI					
EIBI					
GI					

INFOMAP 23-3 INDIVIDUAL AND COMMUNITY PERIODONTAL INDICES

INDEX	WHAT IS MEASURED?	TEETH AND/OR SURFACES SCORED	CRITERIA USED FOR MEASUREMENT	SCORING/CALCULATION OF INDEX	REFERENCE SCALES, RANGE OF SCORES, AND ADDITIONAL INFORMATION
PSR					
CPI					

INFOMAP 23-4 DENTAL CARIES INDICES

INDEX (AND AUTHOR)	WHAT IS MEASURED?	TEETH AND/OR SURFACES SCORED	CRITERIA USED FOR MEASUREMENT	SCORING/CALCULATION OF INDEX	REFERENCE SCALES, RANGE OF SCORES, AND ADDITIONAL INFORMATION
DMFT					
DMFS					
dft and dfs					
deft and defs					
dmft and dmfs					
ECC and S-ECC					
RCI					

INFOMAP 23-5 FLUOROSIS INDICES

INDEX	WHAT IS MEASURED?	TEETH AND/OR SURFACES SCORED	CRITERIA USED FOR MEASUREMENT	SCORING/CALCULATION OF INDEX	ADDITIONAL INFORMATION
Dean's fluorosis index					
TSIF					

COMPETENCY EXERCISES

Apply information from the chapter and use critical thinking skills to complete the competency exercises. Write responses on paper or create electronic documents to submit your answers.

Community Case Scenario #1: Answer the following questions based on this community case scenario.

You and your classmates conducted an oral health screening of 100 residents at the Mountain View Nursing Home using the ASTDD Basic Screening Survey for Older Adults as part of a statewide initiative to identify the oral health needs of this population. This statewide survey is being conducted because the Department of Community Health received a grant and is planning to set up a mobile clinic to provide dental services for nursing home residents in your city. There is not enough money to offer all possible services for this group of people, but the health department is hoping to provide enough care to meet most of the people's needs.

The screening revealed that 50 residents had both upper and lower dentures, no one presented with root fragments, 25 had untreated decay, and 25 demonstrated need for periodontal care. There were nine residents with suspicious lesions and 14 residents needing care within the next week.

Use the rough data in the scenario to answer the following questions.

1. How many residents participated in the basic screening survey?

____

2. What percentage of the residents have untreated decay?

____

3. What percentage of the residents require evaluation of suspicious lesions?

____

4. What percentage of the residents have an urgent need for care?

____

5. What percentage of the residents need periodontal care?

____

Community Case Scenario #2: Answer the following questions based on this community case scenario.

You, several student colleagues, and some of the faculty members at your school are asked to be part of a statewide, community-based oral health surveillance project conducted by your local Department of Community Health. The project requires that you collect data during the local Toothtown Activity Center Health Fair for young adults aged 17–25.

You are excited to be participating in calibration exercises, collecting data with other members of your school team, and then actually calculating and interpreting the results of your own data collection. What a great way to learn about the dental indices you have just been studying!

6. The Department of Community Health has decided to use the DMFT index to collect data about the caries experience of the group of individuals at the activity center. Discuss the advantages and disadvantages of using this index instead of the DMFS index for community screening.

7. After participating in the screening day at the Toothtown Activity Center, you feel quite confident about using the DMFT index and OHI-S to score individuals as well as the GI that your team decided to use. Now it is time to calculate the results and practice interpreting your findings.

Using the information in Table 23-1, calculate the individual DMFs, the total group DMF, and the group average DMF.

8. Using the data in Table 23-1, calculate the percentage of DMF teeth in this group that currently have decay.

TABLE 23-1 CALCULATING DMF DATA

INDIVIDUAL	D	M	F	INDIVIDUAL DMF
Abbe	12	0	14	
Bill	0	0	6	
Charlie	4	2	0	
David	1	0	6	
Edwin	3	0	0	
Frank	0	1	1	
Grace	4	0	6	
Harry	6	0	7	
Ida	18	2	0	
Joe	2	0	5	
Total				
Group average DMF				

9. Using the data in Table 23-1, calculate the percentage of DMF teeth that have been restored.

10. Using the data in Table 23-1, calculate the percentage of individuals in this group who have at least one decayed tooth.

11. Using the data in Table 23-1, calculate the percentage of individuals in this group who have treatment needs.

12. Use Tables 23-2 and 23-3 to calculate a GI score for Grace and an average GI score for all the individuals in the group.

13. What does Grace's GI score mean?

TABLE 23-2 CALCULATING GI DATA: AREA SCORES FOR GRACE

TOOTH	D	M	F	L
3 (16)	2	0	2	0
9 (21)	0	0	0	0
12 (24)	1	0	1	0
19 (36)	2	0	2	0
25 (41)	0	0	0	0
28 (44)	1	0	1	0
Total				
GI score				

TABLE 23-3 CALCULATING THE GROUP AVERAGE GI SCORE

NAME	GI SCORE
Charlie	2.9
Harry	1.0
Ida	1.7
Joe	2.6
Grace	?________
Total	
Group average GI	

14. What is your interpretation of the average gingival health of the group?

15. Imagine that you have calculated GI scores for more than 150 individuals who were screened at the Activity Center Health Fair. You calculate that this group's average score is 2.78. How can you use this group average score as baseline data to evaluate the effect of oral hygiene presentations that you and your students will provide at a later time? In other words, explain how you might use this baseline average GI score to determine whether the people in this community were motivated to better oral health because of your education project.

16. Use Table 23-4 to calculate a DI score, a CI score, and an OHI-S score for Bill.

17. Use Table 23- 5 to calculate a group OHI-S score. Make sure to include Bill's score.

TABLE 23-4 OHI-S DATA FOR BILL

TOOTH	DI	CI
3 (16)	3	0
8 (11)	3	0
14 (26)	3	2
19 (36)	3	0
24 (31)	3	0
30 (46)	2	0
Total		
Scores		
OHI-S score		

TABLE 23-5 CALCULATING GROUP OHI-S DATA

INDIVIDUAL	OHI-S SCORE
Abbe	4.33
Bill	?________
Charlie	1.20
David	1.03
Edwin	1.00
Group OHI-S	

18. What does each individual person's OHI-S score indicate about his or her oral cleanliness? What does the average group score indicate?

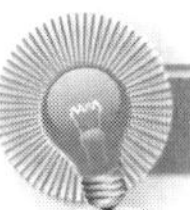

DISCOVERY EXERCISE

Explore the Association of State and Territorial Dental Directors website (http://www.astdd.org) to locate information about the *Basic Screening Surveys: An Approach to Monitoring Community Oral Health* community data collection system. Many states in the United States use this system to gather oral health surveillance data. Download and study all of the components that are available on the website to help you learn about how this oral health surveillance system works. Consider purchasing the training videotape so you and your classmates can be trained to use the system in a future community screening.

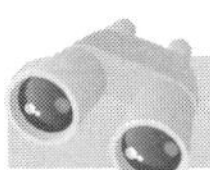

BOX 23-1 MeSH TERMS

Use a combination of MeSH terms and other key words to develop an effective and efficient PubMed literature search strategy.

Data collection	Population surveillance
Dental health surveys	Public health surveillance
Dental plaque index	Incidence
DMF index	Prevalence
Oral hygiene index	World Health Organization
Periodontal index	

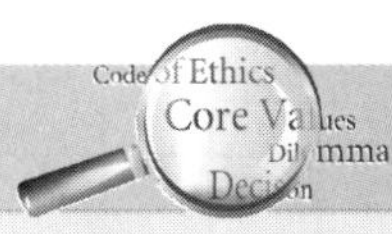

EVERYDAY ETHICS

Before completing the learning exercises below, reread and reflect on the Everyday Ethics Scenario and Questions for Consideration in this chapter of the textbook. It may also be useful to review the Dental Hygiene Ethics discussion in Chapter 1, the Ethical Applications in the introduction pages for each section in the textbook, as well as the Codes of Ethics in textbook Appendices I–IV.

Individual Learning Activity

Identify a situation you have experienced that presents a similar ethical dilemma. Write about you would do differently now than you did at the time the incident happened—support your discussion with concepts from the dental hygiene codes of ethics.

Collaborative Learning Activity

Answer each of the questions for consideration at the end of the scenario in the textbook. Compare what you wrote with answers developed by another classmate and discuss differences/similarities.

Factors To Teach The Patient

This scenario is related to the following factors listed in this chapter of the textbook:

- ▷ How an index is used and calculated and what the scores mean.
- ▷ Correlation of index scores with current oral health practices and procedures.
- ▷ Procedures to follow to improve index scores and bring the oral tissues to health.

As you are marking the areas of biofilm on the patient form, Mrs. Combs asks why dental hygienists always bother to do all that "extra work" just to provide oral hygiene instructions. Apparently no one had ever explained it to her before.

Using a motivational interviewing approach (see Appendix D), develop an imaginary dialogue explaining these dental indices to your patient.

Use the conversation you create to role-play this situation with a fellow student. If you are the patient in the role-play, be sure to ask questions. If you are the dental hygienist, try to anticipate questions and answer them in your explanation.

Crossword Puzzle

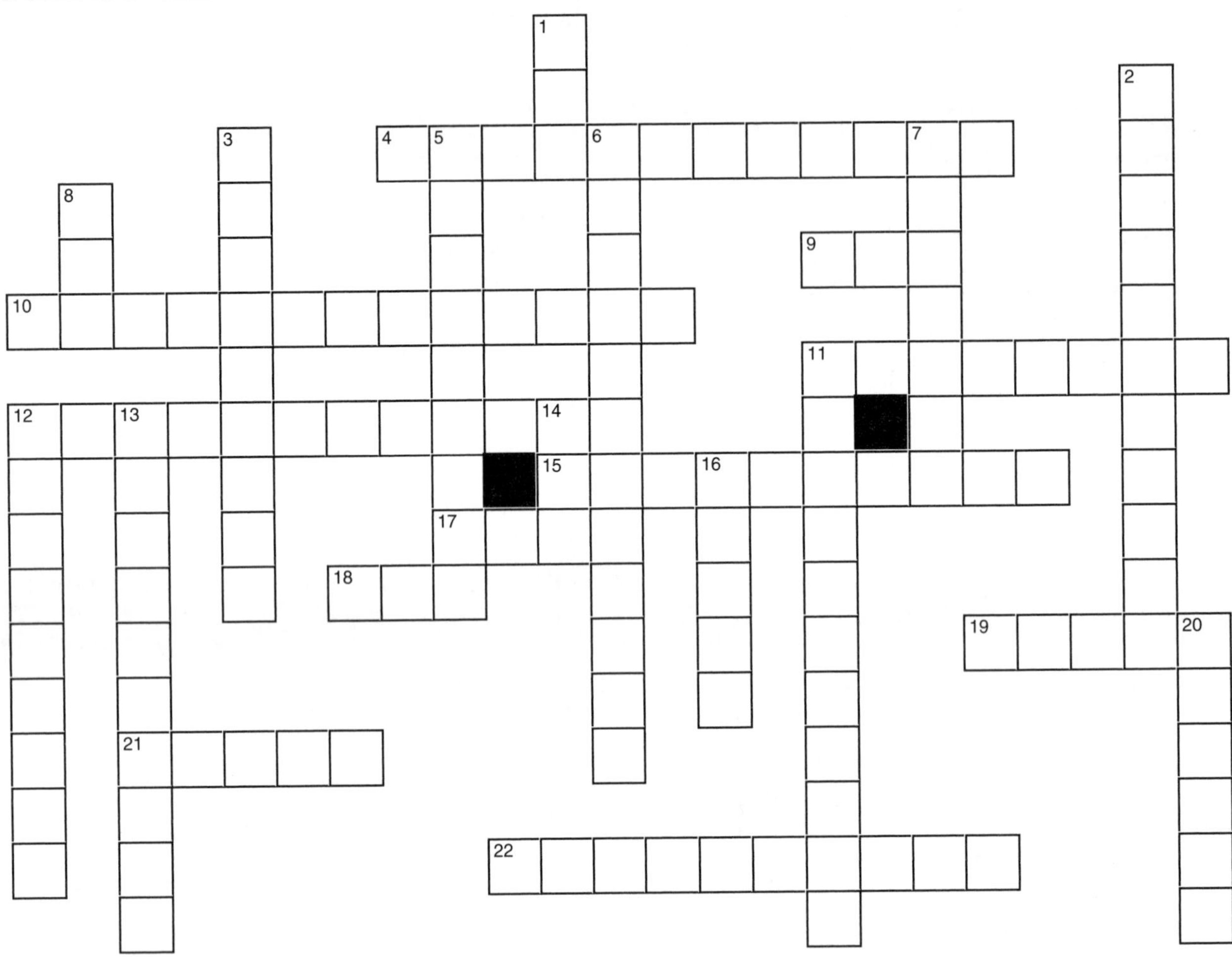

Puzzle Clues

Across

4. Index that is used to assesses thickness of dental biofilm at the gingival area (two words).
9. A community screening index designed for use by dental and nondental screeners.
10. A sweeping motion of the dental probe determines bleeding evaluation when this index is used (two words).
11. Refers to index teeth numbers 3, 9, 12, 19, 25, and 28; teeth used for classic epidemiological studies of periodontal disease.
12. The systematic collection of oral health data for use in planning public health programs.
15. The total number of cases of some disease or condition in a given population.
17. An index that combines a debris score and a calculus score using specific surfaces of six teeth.
18. Index similar to the community periodontal index used to screen individual patients in a private practice setting.
19. Index that measures fluorosis using six categories.
21. An expression of clinical observations in numerical values.
22. A type of index that measures all the evidence of a condition, past and present.

Down

1. Index used to determine caries experience.
2. A determination of accuracy and consistency between examiners; affects the reliability of data collection.
3. Refers to the number of new cases of a disease that occur during a certain period of time.
5. A factor that is measured and analyzed to describe health status.
6. An index that measures conditions that are not able to be changed; in other words, evidence of the condition will remain even after treatment; example is dental caries.
7. This index uses a triangular wooden interdental cleaner to identify areas of interproximal bleeding.
8. This index uses unwaxed dental floss to determine areas of interproximal gingival bleeding.
11. Consistency of measurement; enhanced by calibration of examiners.
12. Refers to a brief initial exam for an individual or an assessment of many individuals to determine a certain characteristic in a population.
13. Type of index which measures a condition that can be changed and no evidence of the condition will remain; example is dental biofilm.
14. Periodontal screening index used for community oral health surveillance that can be used in conjunction with a code related to loss of attachment.
16. Measures what it is intended to measure.
20. A category of indices that measures only the presence or absence of a condition.

SECTION IV Summary Exercises

Assessment

Chapters 10–23

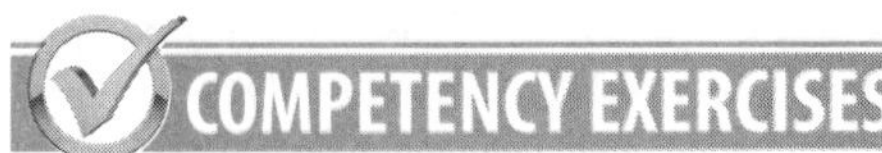

Apply information from the chapter and use critical thinking skills to complete the competency exercises. Write responses on paper or create electronic documents to submit your answers.

SECTION IV – PATIENT ASSESSMENT SUMMARY			
Patient Name: *Mrs. Lorna Patel*	Age: *49*	Gender: M F	☑ Initial Therapy ☐ Maintenance
Provider Name: *D.H. Student*	Date: *Today*		☐ Re-evaluation
Chief Complaint: *Gum tissues bleed when brushing and flossing. Mouth is dry all the time.*			
Assessment Findings			
Health History • *History of high blood pressure managed by medication* • *Cholesterol managed by medication* • *Mitral valve prolapse* • *Allergy to penicillin* • *Zocar 20 mg/1 per day* • *Caltrate 1 per day* • *Enapril 10 mg/hydrochlorothiazide 15 mg/1 per day* • *Multiple vitamin 1 per day* • *Clindamycin 20.0 g taken 1 hour before appointment* • *ASA Classification - II* • *ADL level - 0*	**At Risk For:**		
Social and Dental History • *1.5 years since last recall* • *Localized 4 – 5 mm probing depths* • *Flosses daily* • *Rinses with Listerine* • *Mouth dry all the time* • *Uses mints and candy for dry mouth* • *Uses bottled water with no fluoride content*	**At Risk For:**		

Dental Examination

- *Moderate dental biofilm along cervical margins and proximal surfaces*
- *Generalized supra- and subgingival calculus*
- *Light yellow stain*
- *Posterior gingiva red and bleeding on probing*
- *Generalized moderate attrition (evidence of bruxism)*
- *Numerous faulty MOD amalgam restorations*
- *Localized 4 – 5 mm maxillary and mandibular probing depths*

At Risk For:

Periodontal Diagnosis/Case Type and Status

Caries Management Risk Assessment (CAMBRA) Level:
☐ Low ☐ Moderate ☐ High ☐ Extreme

Read the Section IV Patient Assessment Summary to help you answer the following questions.

1. Identify follow-up questions to ask Mrs. Patel that will help you determine any additional information you need to complete this patient's dental hygiene care plan.

2. When you question her, Mrs. Patel states that she has been taking clindamycin, as prescribed by her physician, prior to each dental appointment for many years. Would you request a medical consultation with her physician prior to scheduling a scaling and root planing appointment for Mrs. Patel? Explain why or why not.

3. Use the assessment findings information you have for Mrs. Patel to complete the "At Risk For" sections of her Patient Assessment Summary.

4. Complete the Periodontal Diagnosis and CAMBRA sections of the Assessment Summary form. What assessment information was available on the form that helped you to make those decisions? What additional information would be helpful as you completed those sections of the Assessment Form?

DISCOVERY EXERCISES

1. Collect samples of the worksheets used for patient assessment record keeping from several dental practices in your community. Compare these systems with those used in your school clinic. Discuss the advantages and disadvantages of each system with your student colleagues.

2. Many patients you provide dental hygiene care for will not speak English (or the language that most people in your country speak) as their first language. Those patients can often have a more difficult time accurately completing health history information. Explore the Internet to discover health history forms that are translated into other languages. A fine place to start is at the MetDental.com website https://www.metdental.com/prov/execute/Content. This Web page includes a link leading you to a site where you can download and print health history forms in a variety of languages. Click on the resource center tab at the top of the page and then scroll down to find the link to Multilanguage Health History forms.

3. Look through the scientific literature to find periodontal disease studies that use some of the dental indices you learned about in Chapter 23 to collect data on periodontal disease status.

4. Explore the Internet to find oral health surveillance statistics for your community, state, or country. Analyze the statistics to describe the oral health status, and write a description of specific ways in which the oral health status of the population in your community might be improved by community-based dental hygiene interventions.

FOR YOUR PORTFOLIO

1. Include your personal written responses to the questions in the Everyday Ethics section from any of the chapters.

2. Complete patient assessment summaries for several patients who are scheduled with you in your clinic.

3. Demonstrate your interest and the development of your skills in providing culturally competent care by including any patient data collection or patient education materials that you discover for patients who are culturally different from yourself. Include a reflective journal entry describing ways that you can use these materials to enhance the quality of dental hygiene care you provide.

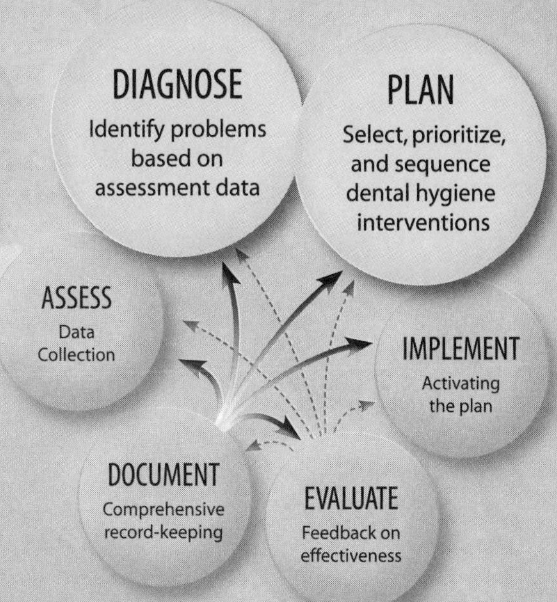

SECTION V

Dental Hygiene Diagnosis and Care Planning

Chapters 24-25

SECTION V LEARNING OBJECTIVES

Completing the exercises in this section of the workbook will prepare you to:

1. Use assessment data to write dental hygiene diagnostic statements.
2. Develop a formal dental hygiene care plan based on the dental hygiene diagnosis that sequences evidence-based dental hygiene interventions in order to address identified patient needs.
3. Identify and apply procedures for obtaining informed consent.
4. Document informed consent and the plan for patient care.

COMPETENCIES FOR THE DENTAL HYGIENIST (APPENDIX A)

Competencies supported by the learning in Section V

Core Competencies: C3, C4, C5, C7, C9, C10, C11, C12, C13

Health Promotion and Disease Prevention: HP1, HP2, HP3, HP4, HP5

Patient/Client Care: PC1, PC2, PC3, PC4, PC5, PC6, PC7, PC8, PC9, PC11, PC13

24

Planning for Dental Hygiene Care

LEARNING OBJECTIVES

Upon successful completion of these exercises, you will be able to:

1. Identify and define key terms and concepts related to planning dental hygiene care.
2. Identify and explain assessment findings and individual patient factors that affect patient care.
3. Identify additional factors that can influence planning for dental hygiene care.
4. Apply the evidence-based decision-making process to determine patient care recommendations.

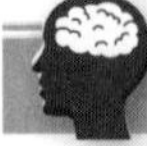

KNOWLEDGE EXERCISES

Write your answers for each question in the space provided.

1. Supply the term or concept that matches each of the following descriptions:
   A. Measure of ability to perform self-care.
   B. A measure that integrates a combination of physical and cognitive ability.
   C. Statements that identify a problem.
   D. An outcome that can be expressed as "excellent," "poor," or "guarded."
   E. Diagnostic model that uses the phrase "related to" to link identified patient problems with risk factors or etiology.
   F. Systemic conditions, behavioral factors, or environmental factors that can lead to increased probability of oral disease.
2. Identify factors from the patient assessment that are analyzed and considered when planning dental hygiene care.

3. Identify and briefly describe the issues indicated by the mnemonic OSCAR:

O

S

C

A

R

4. Briefly define each of the five ASA classification levels.

5. Define dental hygiene diagnosis in your own words.

6. List factors that determine prognosis after dental hygiene interventions.

7. In your own words, define anticipatory guidance.

8. What is the role of the patient in determining outcomes following dental hygiene care?

9. What is the purpose of preprocedural tissue conditioning with antimicrobials?

10. The need for anesthesia during dental hygiene procedures is determined by:

11. Your patient's clinical diagnosis, provided by the periodontist, is "Chronic Periodontitis." List the therapeutic goals of treatment for this patient.

COMPETENCY EXERCISES

Apply information from the chapter and use critical thinking skills to complete the competency exercises. Write responses on paper or create electronic documents to submit your answers.

1. At which ASA classification levels would you be most likely to consider contacting the patient's physician prior to planning for dental hygiene care? Provide a rationale for your answer.

2. Table 24-5 in the textbook contains a list of diagnostic models used in planning dental hygiene care along with a description of how diagnostic statements are constructed within the model. Which model seems closest to the approach your school clinic uses for planning individualized patient care? Explain.

3. For each of patient scenarios described below:

   Identify the OSCAR issue(s) that need to be evaluated.

   Determine the ASA classification you will assign when assessing the patient during planning of dental hygiene care.

   Write a justification for your selection.

   Scenario A: Mrs. Kujath is 90 years old and in very good physical and mental health. She has chronic arthritis, which is managed very well with daily pain medication, and only has minor problems with mobility, including sitting still for a long period of time. She doesn't really like the way her old denture looks, and she desires a new denture. She states that there is no problem about having the money to pay for the new denture.

   Scenario B: Mr. Diamond has type I diabetes. His blood sugar levels indicate that his diabetes is not well controlled. Mr. Diamond has numerous posterior teeth that present with significant bone loss, generalized mobility, and class II or III furcations. Moreover, he is not particularly compliant with your recommendations for self-care for those furcation areas.

   Scenario C: Mrs. Abdul must make a decision about treatment options for several teeth with severe periodontal involvement. Her health history indicates mild hypertension that is well controlled by medication. It has been many years since she has been to the dentist because of an extremely unpleasant dental experience she had as a child. She squirmed and protested when you measured her probing depths and, in general, had a very difficult time cooperating during the collection of assessment data. She says that she must talk with her son, as he will be bringing her for her appointments and also be paying for whatever treatment is decided upon.

   Scenario D: Ms. Anitha Jones has cerebral palsy. She arrives at the dental office in a wheelchair and is accompanied by an attendant. Because of extreme muscle spasticity caused by her condition, her arms and legs are in constant motion, sometimes lashing out unexpectedly, and she must have a variety of pads and restraints to maintain her position and safety in her wheelchair. You and her caregiver plan to transfer her from her wheelchair to the dental chair for treatment. Her health history indicates that she is *not* mentally disabled.

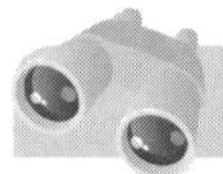

BOX 24-1 MeSH TERMS

Use a combination of MeSH terms and other key words to develop an effective and efficient PubMed literature search strategy.

Patient care planning	Prognosis
Risk factors	Activities of daily living
Periodontal diseases	Health education, dental
Diagnosis	

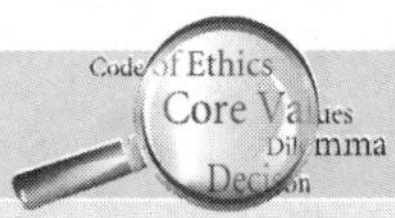

EVERYDAY ETHICS

Before completing the learning exercises below, reread and reflect on the Everyday Ethics Scenario and Questions for Consideration in this chapter of the textbook. It may also be useful to review the Dental Hygiene Ethics discussion in Chapter 1, the Ethical Applications in the introduction pages for each section in the textbook, as well as the Codes of Ethics in textbook Appendices I–IV.

Individual Learning Activity

Imagine that you have observed what happened in the scenario, but are not one of the main characters involved in the situation. Write a reflective journal entry that:

describes how you might have reacted (as an observer—not as a participant),

expresses your personal feelings about what happened,

or

identifies personal values that affect your reaction to the situation.

Discovery Activity

Ask a friend or relative who is not involved in health care to read the scenario and discuss it with you from the perspective of a "patient" who receives services within the healthcare system. Discuss what you learned from the concerns, insights, or difference in perspective that person expressed.

Factors To Teach The Patient

This scenario is related to the following factors listed in this chapter of the textbook:

- ▷ Why disease control measures are learned before and in conjunction with scaling.
- ▷ Facts of oral disease prevention and oral health promotion relevant to the patient's current level of healthcare knowledge and individual risk factors.

Your next patient, Jonathon Meyers, is a 26-year-old graduate student. He has not seen a dentist since he was a child. When his girlfriend told him about his bad breath, he decided to take advantage of the services offered at the dental clinic.

He presents with an aggressive periodontal condition in the lower anterior sextant of his mouth. Because he was not exposed to much dental education in his life, Jon has a low dental IQ and doesn't understand the cause and progression of dental disease. He smokes, demonstrates poor biofilm control, and states that he wants you to just "fix him up" with your treatments.

Using the Motivational Interviewing approach (see Appendix D), write a statement explaining why disease control measures must happen before and in conjunction with scaling. Explain his role in attaining and maintaining oral health.

Use the conversation you create to role-play this situation with a fellow student. If you are the patient in the role-play, be sure to ask questions. If you are the dental hygienist, try to anticipate questions and answer them in your explanation.

25

The Dental Hygiene Care Plan

LEARNING OBJECTIVES

Upon successful completion of these exercises, you will be able to:

1. Identify and define key terms and concepts related to the written dental hygiene care plan.
2. Identify the components of a dental hygiene care plan.
3. Write dental hygiene diagnostic statements based on assessment findings.
4. Prepare a written dental hygiene care plan.
5. Apply procedures for discussing a care plan with the dentist and the patient.
6. Identify and apply procedures for obtaining informed consent.

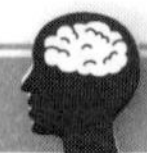

KNOWLEDGE EXERCISES

Write your answers for each question in the space provided.

1. Define the following terms in your own words.

   Dental hygiene intervention

   Informed consent

   Implied consent

   Informed refusal

2. Identify and define the three parts of a dental hygiene care plan.

3. List the 10 components of a written care plan.

4. List three individual patient requirements that can require significant adaptations in the written dental hygiene care plan.

5. Which of the following is a factor that might affect the *sequence* you select for quadrant scaling and root planing in a dental hygiene care plan? (Circle the correct answer.)
   A. Availability of a power-driven scaler
   B. Patient complaint of pain associated with a periodontal abscess
   C. The amount of calculus in the lower anterior sextant
   D. Chronic systemic disease

6. What is the purpose for explaining the entire treatment plan to the patient?

7. What are some important points to consider when explaining the dental hygiene care plan to the patient?

8. Identify five areas of information you will discuss with the patient when you are obtaining informed consent.

COMPETENCY EXERCISES

Apply information from the chapter and use critical thinking skills to complete the competency exercises. Write responses on paper or create electronic documents to submit your answers.

1. Explain the role of the patient in developing a plan for care that prioritizes the patient's needs.
2. Explain the relationship between the master treatment plan and the dental hygiene care plan.
3. Why are medical, personal, and clinical findings linked to actual or potential risk factors in the assessment findings section of a written dental hygiene care plan?
4. Using your institution's guidelines for writing in patient records, document that the dental hygiene care plan was presented to the supervising dentist prior to explaining the plan to the patient.
5. Use the following information from the case of Jonathon Meyers to answer the questions below. Jon has not seen a dentist since he was a child. When his girlfriend told him about his bad breath, he decided to take advantage of the services offered at the dental clinic in your school.

Jon presents with an aggressive periodontal condition in the lower anterior sextant of his mouth. He has a low dental IQ and doesn't understand the cause and progression of dental disease. He smokes, demonstrates poor biofilm control, and states that he wants you to just "fix him up" with your treatments.

A. Write at least one dental hygiene diagnosis statement related to the information provided about the patient in this scenario.
B. What interventions will you plan to target the problem(s) you identified?
C. Write a goal for each problem you identified. Include a time frame for meeting the goal. How will you measure whether or not Jon met the goal?

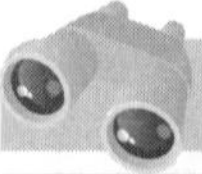

BOX 25-1 MeSH TERMS

Use a combination of MeSH terms and other key words to develop an effective and efficient PubMed literature search strategy.

Patient care planning	Treatment refusal
Comprehensive dental care	Patient-centered care
Informed consent	Health education, dental

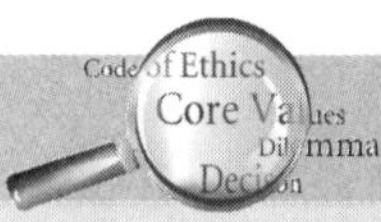

EVERYDAY ETHICS

Before completing the learning exercises below, reread and reflect on the Everyday Ethics Scenario and Questions for Consideration in this chapter of the textbook. It may also be useful to review the Dental Hygiene Ethics discussion in Chapter 1, the Ethical Applications in the introduction pages for each section in the textbook, as well as the Codes of Ethics in textbook Appendices I–IV.

Individual Learning Activity

Imagine that you have observed what happened in the scenario, but are not one of the main characters involved in the situation. Write a reflective journal entry that:

describes how you might have reacted (as an observer—not as a participant),

expresses your personal feelings about what happened,

or

identifies personal values that affect your reaction to the situation.

Discovery Activity

Ask a friend or relative who is not involved in health care to read the scenario and discuss it with you from the perspective of a "patient" who receives services within the healthcare system. Discuss what you learned from the concerns, insights, or difference in perspective that person expressed.

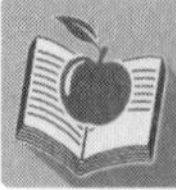

Factors To Teach The Patient

This scenario is related to the following factors listed in this chapter of the textbook:

- ▷ Why patient input into the final care plan is important.
- ▷ The patient's rights and responsibilities regarding informed consent.

Using the motivational interviewing approach (see Appendix D), write a statement explaining to Mrs. Kwan, the patient in the textbook everyday ethics scenario for this chapter, what informed consent means.

SECTION V Summary Exercises

Dental Hygiene Diagnosis and Care Planning

Chapters 24-25

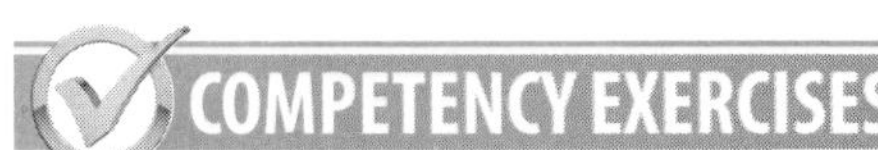

Apply information from the chapter and use critical thinking skills to complete the competency exercises. Write responses on paper or create electronic documents to submit your answers.

Read the Section V Patient Assessment Summaries to help you answer questions #1 and #2.

SECTION V – PATIENT ASSESSMENT SUMMARY #1			
Patient Name: *Mrs. Diane White*	Age: *27*	Gender: M [F]	☐ Initial Therapy ☑ Maintenance
Student (Clinician) Name: *D.H. Student*	Date: *Today*		☐ Re-evaluation

Chief Complaint:
Gum tissues bleed when brushing and flossing.
First trimester of pregnancy with nausea.

Assessment Findings	
Medical History • *First trimester of first pregnancy* • *Husband smokes cigarettes in house and car* • *ASA II and ADL level 0*	**At Risk For:** • *Embryo susceptible to injuries and malformations* • *Infant at risk for secondhand-smoke exposure*
Social and Dental History • *One year since last recall* • *Generalized 4-mm probing depths* • *Infrequent flossing* • *Several white spot lesions on cervical surfaces of posterior teeth* • *Uses bottled water with no fluoride content* • *Smell of fluoridated toothpaste makes her nauseated* • *Uses frequent, high-carbohydrate snacking to control nausea*	**At Risk For:** • *Increased incidence of dental caries* • *Increased risk of periodontal conditions*

Dental Examination	At Risk For:
• *Moderate dental biofilm along cervical margins and proximal surfaces* • *Posterior gingiva red and bleeding on probing* • *No radiographic bone changes*	• *Increased incidence of dental caries* • *Increased risk of periodontal conditions*
Periodontal Diagnosis/Case Type and Status: Biofilm-induced gingivitis	☐ Low ☐ Moderate ☐ High ☐ Extreme

SECTION V – PATIENT ASSESSMENT SUMMARY #2

Patient Name: *Melody Crane* Age: *15 months* Gender: M [F] ☑ Initial Therapy

☐ Maintenance

Student (Clinician) Name: *D.H. Student* Date: *Today* ☐ Re-evaluation

Chief Complaint:

Gum tissues bleed when mother brushes Melody's teeth.

Melody fights with mother when she brushes her teeth.

Assessment Findings

Medical History	At Risk For:
• *Frequent ear infections—three since birth* • *Liquid antibiotics—contain sweeteners*	• *Early childhood caries*
Social and Dental History	**At Risk For:**
• *Melody's initial dental visit* • *Teeth present at 6 months* • *Fluoridated water supply—but family drinks mostly bottled water* • *Fluoride toothpaste used 4× per week—unspecified amount of paste* • *Bottle fed two times daily at naptime and bedtime* • *At-will use of sippy cup for juice* • *Five-year-old brother with restorations on all primary molars and some anteriors* • *Parental lack of dental knowledge*	• *Early childhood caries* • *Fluorosis*
Dental Examination	**At Risk For:**
• *Moderate dental biofilm along cervical margins of maxillary incisors* • *White-spot lesions cervical of four maxillary incisors* • *Red maxillary anterior gingiva*	• *Early childhood caries* • *Gingivitis*
Periodontal Diagnosis/Case Type and Status: Gingivitis	**Caries Management Risk Assessment (CAMBRA) level:** ☐ Low ☐ Moderate ☐ High ☐ Extreme

1. Use a copy of the dental hygiene care-plan template in Appendix B, or use the care-plan format your school provides to write dental hygiene diagnosis statements for either of the patient summaries above.

2. Use the care-plan template or your school format to write a plan for clinical, education/counseling, and oral hygiene instruction/home care interventions for either Mrs. White or Melody Crane and her parents.

3. Use the care-plan template in Appendix B of the workbook, or the care-plan form used in your clinic to write a formal care plan from assessment data collected during an initial appointment of a patient you are providing care for in your school clinic.

4. Write an outline of important points to address when presenting the care plan to the patient in order to obtain informed consent to proceed with the dental hygiene interventions you have planned.

5. Role-play to present the care plan to the patient.

6. Write a progress note documenting that you have presented the care plan and obtained informed consent.

DISCOVERY EXERCISES

1. Remember Jonathon Meyers, the graduate student from the exercises in Chapters 24 and 25? Imagine that you have now completed his initial therapy plan and are evaluating the results. He has reached most of the goals you set together in the plan, and his oral health status has much improved.

   You recommend a 3-month periodontal maintenance interval, but he wants to wait at least 6 months before coming to see you again. He cites recent toothpaste television commercials that recommend seeing a dentist every 6 months. You know that patients with a history of periodontal infection need to be seen more often.

   Conduct a brief review of recent literature to determine what scientific evidence supports a shorter periodontal maintenance interval. Write an outline of points you will cover when you explain to Jonathon why those research findings influence your recommendations for his continuing care plan.

2. Develop a PICO question related to determining the best fluoride regimen to recommend for a preschool-age child with extreme caries risk.

3. Select two or three current articles from your literature search that seem as if they would be useful for helping you decide which fluoride therapies you will recommend for this preschool-age patient. Either go to the library to find the paper journal or use online full-text sources to read the articles you have selected. Read the articles and evaluate the strength and usefulness of the information that is in them.

FOR YOUR PORTFOLIO

1. Using the patient-specific dental hygiene care plan template in Appendix B or the care-plan format used in your dental hygiene program, complete comprehensive dental hygiene care plans for a variety of patients you have assessed in your school clinic. Demonstrate your ability to plan for a diverse selection of patients by selecting care plans prepared for patients with a variety of systemic conditions, risk factors, and levels of dental disease.

2. In your portfolio, include a care plan prepared at the beginning of your education and one for a similar patient prepared near the end of your education. Provide a written statement that reflects on and analyzes the ways in which a comparison of the two care plans demonstrates what you have learned about planning patient care.

Questions Patients Ask

What sources of information can you identify that will help ssyou answer your patient's questions in this scenario?

"I saw something on the Internet recently about new research that proves that a certain new kind of treatment is more effective than the recommendations you have made in my dental hygiene care plan. Can we change my dental hygiene care plan?"

Word Search Puzzle

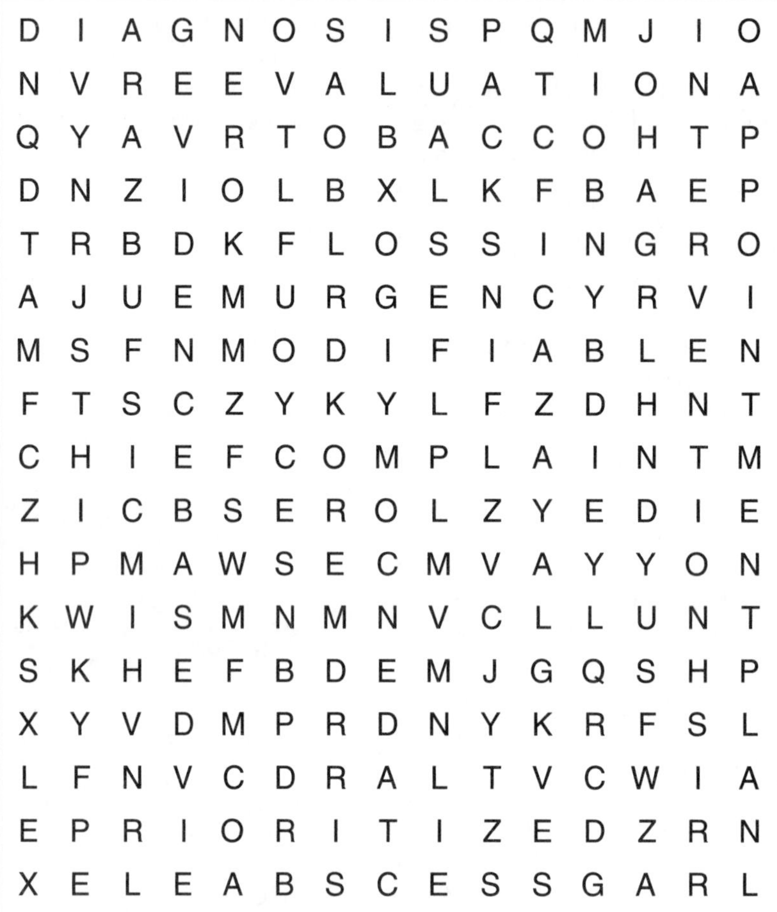

Word Search Clues

- One type of acute gingival or periodontal condition.
- A critical analysis and evaluation or judgment related to patient's medical, dental, and personal health–related data.
- Patient care interventions supported by relevant, scientifically sound research.
- A significant risk factor for poor periodontal outcomes, certain systemic conditions, and oral cancer.
- A dental related example of "activities of daily living."
- The patient's statement regarding the reason for seeking dental care (two words).
- Risk factors influenced by dental hygiene interventions that change health behavior.
- A statement that identifies a patient problem.
- To arrange in order of importance.
- Refers to a dental hygiene treatment or recommendation that is intended to improve a patient's oral health.
- Acronym that refers to a protocol used to determine caries risk level and select interventions based on risk level.
- Discomfort or pain that requires first attention when planning dental hygiene care.
- Assessment to determine whether expected outcomes of treatment have been met.
- The section of the dental hygiene care plan that outlines the sequence of interventions planned in a series of appointments (two words).

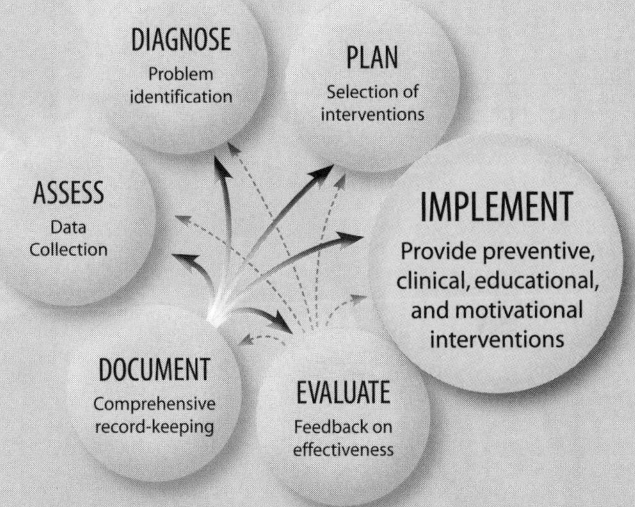

SECTION

VI

Implementation: Prevention

Chapters 26-37

SECTION VI LEARNING OBJECTIVES

Completing the exercises in this section of the workbook will prepare you to:

1. Educate patients regarding the prevention of oral disease.
2. Promote patient behaviors and practices that enhance oral health.
3. Select patient-specific dental hygiene interventions that will prevent oral disease and promote oral health.
4. Document prevention interventions and recommendations.

COMPETENCIES FOR THE DENTAL HYGIENIST (Appendix A)

Competencies supported by the learning in Section V

Core Competencies: C3, C4, C5, C7, C9, C10, C11, C12, C13

Health Promotion and Disease Prevention: HP1, HP2, HP4, HP5

Patient/Client Care: PC10, PC11, PC12, PC13

26

Preventive Counseling and Behavior Change

LEARNING OBJECTIVES

Upon successful completion of these exercises, you will be able to:

1. Explain the steps in a preventive program to motivate patient behavior change, identify the need to conduct preventive counseling, and describe the proper setting.
2. Explain the elements, principles, and processes of motivational interviewing (MI).
3. Describe key factors, core skills, and strategies for implementing a MI approach to patient counseling.
4. Document the outcomes of a patient counseling session.

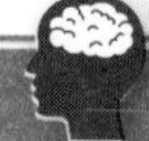

KNOWLEDGE EXERCISES

Write your answers for each question in the space provided. Note: Workbook Appendix D provides an overview of Motivational Interviewing (MI) that may be helpful as you study the questions below.

1. Order the steps in a preventive program.

Order	Description
_______	Evaluate progressive changes
_______	Plan for intervention
_______	Plan short- and long-term continuing care
_______	Perform clinical preventive services
_______	Assess the patient's needs
_______	Implement the plan

2. List the factors that need to be considered during the assessment phase of a preventive program.

3. When is preventive counseling conducted?

4. Describe the role of active listening in the MI approach to patient counseling and behavior change.

5. List the things a good listener *does not* do during patient counseling.

6. Why is it necessary to review the patient's behavior change goals during *each* patient appointment?

7. What body language factors lead to a more successful preventive counseling session?

8. Which two behavior change theories form the basis of MI?

9. What are the two essential characteristics of MI?

10. When is brief motivational interviewing (BMI) effective?

11. List the four interrelated elements of the spirit of MI.

P	
A	
C	
E	

12. List the four patient-centered conditions that demonstrate the clinician's attitude of acceptance.

13. What are the four guiding principles of MI?

R	
U	
L	
E	

14. Explain why it is necessary for the dental hygienist to resist the "righting reflex" during patient counseling.

15. What is the significance of understanding the patient's motivation?

16. In your own words, describe what is meant by "empower the patient."

17. Identify the four processes of MI based on the brief definitions provided in the table below.

________	Establish a helpful connection and working relationship.
________	Develop and maintain a specific direction in the conversation about change.
________	Elicit the patient's own motivations for change.
________	Develop the commitment to change and formulating a concrete plan of action.

18. List three elements of MI implementation.

19. List two elements of information exchange.

20. List two techniques of asking permission.

21. List two reasons why an exploration of the patient's prior knowledge is necessary.

22. Why is it important to let the patient set the agenda for the information and recommendations to be discussed?

23. List the core skills of MI, which are represented by the acronym OARS.

O	________________
A	________________
R	________________
S	________________

24. What is the purpose of asking open-ended questions during a MI session?

25. In your own words, describe affirmation.

26. How does affirmation by the clinician contribute to a patient's health behavior change?

27. Fill in the blank: Good affirmations contain the word ____________. Using statements that begin with the word __________ will focus the conversation more on the clinician than the patient.

28. In your own words, define the term "reflective listening."

29. Describe the difference between the two types of reflection responses used in MI.

30. In your own words, describe the difference between sustain talk and change talk.

____

____

31. ____________________ is the point at which the patient is determining whether the benefits of change outweigh the risks of the current behavior.

32. When the clinician takes a neutral position it allows the patient to:

____

____

33. What is the purpose of the Pro/Con Matrix?

____

____

____

____

34. What is the purpose of the readiness ruler?

____

____

____

____

35. Fill in the blank boxes in Infomap 26-1 to organize concepts related to the four components of preparatory change talk.

36. List the signs that indicate the patient is ready to make changes in a current oral health behavior.

____

____

____

____

INFOMAP 26-1 COMPONENTS OF PREPARATORY CHANGE TALK

COMPONENT		EXAMPLES OF PATIENT STATEMENTS	EXAMPLES OF PHRASES TO STIMULATE CHANGE TALK
D		I wish to, I want to, I would like to...	
A		I could, I might be able to	
R		Statements identifying a rationale for making a change	
N		I must, I need to, I should do...	

37. Match the type of planning scenario to the description.

Plan Type	Description
A. Clear plan	______ The patient is developing the plan from scratch.
B. Several clear options	______ The patient knows what they want or need to do.
C. Brainstorming	______ The patient has determined there is more than one way to move toward the goal.

38. What two factors most influence whether patient counseling is directed to the caregiver, to the child, or to both?

____

____

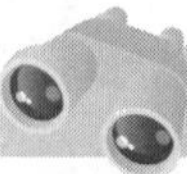

BOX 26-1 MeSH TERMS

Use a combination of MeSH terms and other key words to develop an effective and efficient PubMed literature search strategy.

Health communication	Health behavior
Health education	Motivational Interviewing
Health education, dental	Health knowledge, attitudes, practice

COMPETENCY EXERCISES

Apply information from the chapter and use critical thinking skills to complete the competency exercises. Note: Workbook Appendix D provides an overview of MI that may be helpful.

Each of the following patient conversations contains clinician responses that illustrate MI principles and tools. Complete the exercises below by indicating the appropriate MI skill or tool on the lines provided for each of the clinician's statements.

BMI SESSION #1 | ENGAGING THE PATIENT

PERSON SPEAKING	CONVERSATION STATEMENTS	CORE SKILLS AND TOOLS OF MI
Clinician:	Now that we have updated your medical history and current medications, may I take some time to discuss your systemic health in more detail?	______________
patient:	Sure... that's fine.	
Clinician response:	You are insulin diabetic and on a few medications including a calcium channel blocker and statin cholesterol medication. What do you know about your diabetes and your medications and how they affect your oral health?	______________ ______________
Patient:	Well... I read somewhere that diabetics can have problems with their gums and medications can cause dry mouth. I think my gums are good; I brush and floss two times a day. I do drink a lot of water throughout the day because my mouth is dry.	
Clinician response:	So, you are aware of the link between diabetes and gum health. It is great you are taking the necessary daily home care steps to maintain your gum and bone health. Drinking water throughout the day is also good for your oral and systemic health. May I discuss the connection of your systemic conditions and medications that are relevant to your oral health?	______________ ______________ ______________ ______________
Patient:	Yes please... I do my best to stay healthy. My diabetes is well controlled by the insulin pump I have and I never miss a dose of my blood pressure or cholesterol medications.	
Clinician response:	Your health is very important to you. You are really diligent about taking your medications. Would you like to know more about diabetes and periodontal disease or your medications first?	______________ ______________

BMI SESSION #2	FOCUSING THE DISCUSSION/EVOKING REASONS	
PERSON SPEAKING	CONVERSATION STATEMENTS	CORE SKILLS AND TOOLS OF MI
Patient:	I really hate having my teeth cleaned, they always make me bleed, and my gums hurt for days afterward.	
Clinician response:	Having your teeth cleaned is painful and you don't like the bleeding.	______________
Patient:	I know I need to come, but I just don't like it.	
Clinician response:	You know it's important for your health and to keep your teeth, but it's really uncomfortable for you and you wonder if it's worth it. What can we do to help make it more comfortable for you so you can come more regularly for your preventive care?	______________ ______________

BMI SESSION #3	EVOKING/ELICITING CHANGE TALK	
PERSON SPEAKING	CONVERSATION STATEMENTS	CORE SKILLS AND TOOLS OF MI
Patient:	I'm really upset I have all these new cavities this time.	
Clinician response:	You're not happy with what's going on in your mouth.	______________
Patient:	I never had cavities until I stopped smoking. It must all the candy and gum.	
Clinician response:	It is fabulous you have quit smoking! Your health is really important to you. What do you already know about how snacking habits cause cavities?	______________ ______________
Patient:	Well, I know candy causes cavities, but I have to eat candy or chew gum so I don't smoke.	
Clinician response:	Can I share with you some alternatives that won't cause cavities?	______________ ______________
Patient:	Sure.	
Clinician response:	Gums and mints that are sugarless won't cause cavities. There are many on the market. What do you think about that?	______________ ______________

BMI SESSION #4	EXPLORING AMBIVALENCE/DECISIONAL BALANCE	
PERSON SPEAKING	CONVERSATION STATEMENTS	CORE SKILLS AND TOOLS OF MI
Patient:	I know I shouldn't drink those energy drinks, but I need them to get me through the day.	
Clinician response:	On one hand, you really like the energy you get from them, but, on the other hand, you also realize they're causing your cavities.	________________
Patient:	Yeah, I can't imagine trying to get through the day without them.	
Clinician response:	So, can you tell me some of the good things and bad things about drinking energy drinks?	________________ Exploring decisional balance using the: ________________
Patient:	Well, I drink them all day long and they give me energy and keep me going. Sometimes I don't have time for meals, and they help me get through the day. The problem is that now I have a bunch of cavities that's probably from all the sugar.	
Clinician response:	So, on one hand, you feel powerless over this energy drink, but yet you know it's ruining your teeth.	________________
Patient:	Yeah, I don't know what I'm going to do now.	
Clinician response:	What are some advantages and disadvantages of changing your energy drink habit?	________________
Patient:	Well, I sure will save a lot of money and time coming to the dentist!	
Clinician response:	(laughing) Well, that would make anybody happy, right? What else?	________________ ________________

Now that you have had a bit of practice identifying the MI skills and tools in some clinician's responses, this next exercise will let you practice responding to a patient statement. As you think about what you will say, remember how important it is to "Resist Righting Reflex" in your response.

As you write your response in the space at the end of BMI Session #5 on the next page, make sure to include statements that:

- Indicate you are listening with compassion.
- Reflect empathetically on the patient's beliefs and values.
- Provide affirmation for the patient's current oral health behaviors.
- Help move the conversation forward toward a solution in a way that empowers the patient.
- Compare your response with those developed by your student colleagues.

BMI SESSION #5	RESIST RIGHTING REFLEX	
PERSON SPEAKING	**CONVERSATION STATEMENTS**	**CORE SKILLS AND TOOLS OF MI**
Patient:	I hate getting my teeth cleaned... those metal instruments hurt! My teeth are so sensitive... to ice cream and coffee too, but those instruments are the worst!	
Clinician response:	Your teeth are supersensitive and you would prefer if we didn't use the metal instruments that hurt so much. What do you know about sensitive teeth?	Simple reflection Empathy Open-ended question (elicit)
Patient:	Nothing... and I don't care "why" my teeth hurt all the time. I just want the sensitivity gone!	
Clinician response:	Okay, you don't want to know what causes sensitive teeth, but you would like a solution. May I suggest some products to reduce your sensitivity?	Simple reflection Asking permission
Patient:	Yes... but I don't want to hear anything about fluoride! My last hygienist tried to get me to use fluoride toothpaste and rinses. I use all natural toothpaste because fluoride is *poison!*	
Your response:	____________________ ____________________ ____________________	Reflection Affirmation Asking permission

EVERYDAY ETHICS

Before completing the learning exercises below, reread and reflect on the Everyday Ethics Scenario and Questions for Consideration in this chapter of the textbook. It may also be useful to review the Dental Hygiene Ethics discussion in Chapter 1, the Ethical Applications in the introduction pages for each section in the textbook, as well as the Codes of Ethics in textbook Appendices I–IV.

Individual Learning Activity

Identify a situation you have experienced that presents a similar ethical dilemma. Write about you would do differently now than you did at the time the incident happened—support your discussion with concepts from the dental hygiene codes of ethics.

Collaborative Learning Activity

Answer each of the questions for consideration at the end of the scenario in the textbook. Compare what you wrote with answers developed by another classmate and discuss differences/similarities

Factors To Teach The Patient

This scenario is related to the following factors listed in this chapter of the textbook:

- Elicit from the patient's short- and long-term goals pertaining to what the patient would like to achieve regarding disease status and overall self-care.
- Your patient Melina expresses her desire to implement a daily flossing routine. She understands that her bleeding gums are directly related to the fact that she does not floss and has demonstrated her ability to use the floss. During your discussion today, Melina is able to articulate reasons she *should* floss every day. She tells you she tries hard to remember to floss when she brushes, but states how difficult it is for her to fit the extra time for flossing into her daily routine.

Use a motivational interviewing approach (See Appendix D) and role-play with a student colleague to develop a conversation that can help this patient set both short- and long-term goals for daily oral care.

27

Protocols for Prevention and Control of Dental Caries

LEARNING OBJECTIVES

Upon successful completion of these exercises, you will be able to:

1. Identify and define key terms and concepts related to dental caries.
2. Identify the stages of dental caries and describe the caries process.
3. Plan protocols for prevention, remineralization, and maintenance based on individualized assessment of risk factors for dental caries.

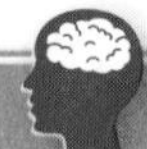

KNOWLEDGE EXERCISES

Write your answers for each question in the space provided.

1. In your own words, describe how the metabolic action of *Streptococcus mutans* and *Lactobacillus* bacteria contributes to the destruction of tooth structure and causes dental caries.

2. A child can be at risk for dental caries as soon as tooth eruption begins. Why?

3. List the types of fermentable carbohydrates.

4. Identify the acids produced during the metabolic process of the bacteria in dental biofilm.

5. The ________________ of carbohydrate ingestion in your patient's diet has a strong influence on the amount of acid produced and the extent of tooth destruction.

6. In what ways does the presence of adequate saliva protect your patient against dental decay?

7. In your own words, describe how fluoride protects your patient against dental decay.

8. Although the incidence of dental caries in the general population has declined in recent years, dental caries is still a major problem that affects the health and welfare of adults and children alike. The dental hygienist's focus in caries detection has changed from identifying only end-stage dental caries that require restoration to identifying patient risk factors and the earliest stages of dental caries. At this point, dental hygiene interventions can help remineralize the natural tooth structure. What tools will you use to identify dental caries at very early stages during an oral examination of your patient?

9. In your own words, describe what you will observe during a visual examination at each of the stages of dental caries on a tooth surface.
   - *Initial infection*
   - *Early subsurface infection*
   - *Early white spot lesion*
   - *Later white spot lesion*
   - *Cavitation*
   - *Radiographic (proximal surface) early dental caries*
   - *Large proximal surface dental caries*

10. In your own words, outline the dental hygienist's role (objectives and interventions) in planning patient care for caries management.

11. What is the purpose of discussing individualized caries risk assessment with each patient?

12. List the five risk factor categories associated with the CAMBRA guidelines for caries management.

13. List the four CAMBRA risk levels.

14. List the four intervention categories identified in the CAMBRA management protocol.

15. How can you best gather data to assess your patient's individual caries risk factors?

16. Outline a protocol for remineralization you can initiate when your patient has evidence of early carious lesions that do not yet require restorative treatment.

COMPETENCY EXERCISES

Apply information from the chapter and use critical thinking skills to complete the competency exercises. Write responses on paper or create electronic documents to submit your answers.

1. Seventeen-year-old Tren Nguyen immigrated to the United States with his family about 6 years ago. Since he arrived, Tren has embraced all things American and spends his free time playing computer games,

snacking on fast food, and hanging out with friends. Tren's history of dental visits has been infrequent. He has been seen in your office only twice before—right after he arrived in the United States and then again about 3 years ago for a prophylaxis. No significant dental findings were charted at either of those visits. He has no history of previous dental restorations. He came to the clinic today because a dental checkup is required as part of his physical examination to play sports when he goes off to college next fall.

When you examine Tren's mouth today, you find significant early and late white spot lesions on the facial surfaces of almost all of his teeth. It is interesting that there are no observable caries in the pits and fissures on the occlusal surfaces of any of his teeth and the surfaces are not deeply grooved. Make a list of the questions you will ask Tren as you gather caries risk assessment data before you write his dental hygiene care plan.

2. Now comes the fun part. You don't usually get to make up answers for all the questions that you ask your patients, but this time we can't go any further with these exercises unless we have some data. In the interest of your own learning, make up reasonable-sounding answers for each of the questions you asked Tren during your discussion of caries risk factors. Using the data you have collected from Tren's caries risk assessment, determine his CAMBRA level.

3. Write two dental hygiene diagnosis statements for Tren's care plan.

4. List the dental hygiene interventions you will plan to help Tren *arrest or control* disease and *regenerate, restore, or maintain* his oral health.

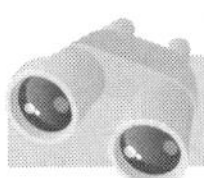

BOX 27-1 MeSH TERMS

Use a combination of MeSH terms and other key words to develop an effective and efficient PubMed literature search strategy.

Dental caries	Risk assessment
Dental caries susceptibility	Risk factors
Diet, cariogenic	Tooth demineralization
Cariogenic agents	Tooth remineralization

EVERYDAY ETHICS

Before completing the learning exercises below, reread and reflect on the Everyday Ethics Scenario and Questions for Consideration in this chapter of the textbook. It may also be useful to review the Dental Hygiene Ethics discussion in Chapter 1, the Ethical Applications in the introduction pages for each section in the textbook, as well as the Codes of Ethics in textbook Appendices I–IV.

Individual Learning Activity

Imagine that you have observed what happened in the scenario, but are not one of the main characters involved in the situation. Write a reflective journal entry that:

describes how you might have reacted (as an observer—not as a participant),

expresses your personal feelings about what happened,

or

identifies personal values that affect your reaction to the situation.

Collaborative Learning Activity

Work with a small group to develop a 2- to 5-minute role-play that introduces the everyday ethics scenario described in the chapter (a great idea is to video record your role-play activity). Then develop separate 2-minute role-play scenarios that provide at least two alternative approaches/solutions to resolving the situation. Ask classmates to view the solutions, ask questions, and discuss the ethical approach used in each. Ask for a vote on which solution classmates determine to be the "best."

Factors To Teach The Patient

This scenario is related to the following factors listed in this chapter of the textbook:

- What causes cavities and how they develop.
- That early dental caries is not a cavity; what demineralization means.
- How remineralization can be accomplished using fluoride toothpaste and drinking fluoridated water daily.
- That the use of fluorides is necessary throughout life.

Use the Motiviational Interviewing approach (see Appendix D) as a guide to write a conversation explaining the components of Tren's care plan to him in such a way that you will motivate him to comply with your recommendations. (This patient was introduced in the Competency Exercises for this chapter.)

Crossword Puzzle

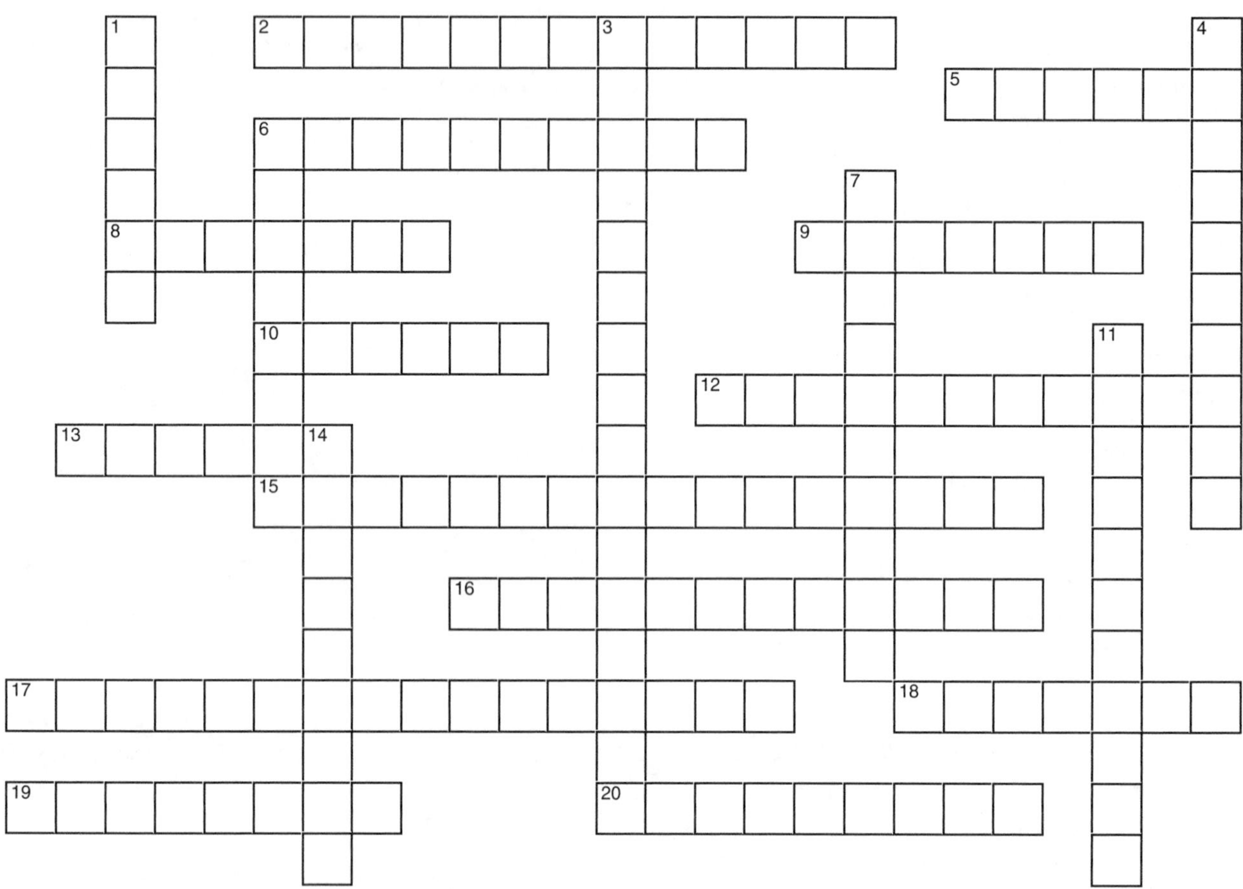

Puzzle Clues

Across

2. A species of bacteria that is more active in the later stages (progression) of decay.
5. A protocol for caries management.
6. Process that determines a patient's risk factors for disease.
8. Designates the highest level of risk for determining dental caries management protocols.
9. Describes rapidly progressing caries in many teeth; an acute condition as opposed to a chronic condition.
10. Buffers acids in the mouth and supplies minerals to replace the calcium and phosphate ions dissolved during demineralization.
12. This lesion gives evidence of subsurface demineralization (two words).
13. Capable of neutralizing acid in a solution; one function of saliva.
15. Process in which minerals are removed from the tooth structure by acids.
16. A specific species of bacteria that predominates in the initial stages of the caries process.
17. Aided by sufficient saliva and by the action of topical fluorides.
18. Ingredient in chewing gum that reduces levels of *Streptococcus mutans* and promotes remineralization.
19. Type of radiograph that can reveal caries on proximal surfaces of teeth.
20. The science and study of dental decay.

Down

1. Professional term for dental decay.
3. Management of dental caries through use of fluoride, calcium phosphate, or other agents.
4. Refers to bacteria that are capable of turning fermentable carbohydrates into acid.
6. Describes the caries process that has been halted.
7. The final stage in the process of caries formation.
11. Habits, behaviors, lifestyles, or conditions that increase the probability of a disease occurring (two words).
14. Another term for secondary caries.

28

Oral Infection Control: Toothbrushes and Toothbrushing

LEARNING OBJECTIVES

Upon successful completion of these exercises, you will be able to:

1. Identify and define key terms and concepts related to toothbrushes and toothbrushing.
2. Describe the characteristics, factors influencing selection, and proper care of manual toothbrushes.
3. Describe indications, procedures, and limitations for a variety of toothbrushing methods and select appropriate toothbrushing methods for individual patients.
4. Discuss indications for use of power toothbrushes and identify important design, technique, and patient instruction factors.
5. Identify indications and methods for supplemental brushing.
6. Select toothbrushing techniques for special conditions.

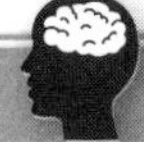

KNOWLEDGE EXERCISES

Write your answers for each question in the space provided.

1. Define *toothbrush abrasion*.

2. In your own words, describe an effective toothbrush handle.

3. Describe a tuft in the head of a toothbrush.

4. List four factors that affect the stiffness or firmness of toothbrush filaments.

5. List four factors that influence the type of toothbrush selected for an individual patient.

6. In your own words, describe the procedure for holding a toothbrush and positioning it in the mouth for effective removal of dental biofilm.

7. Identify methods you can suggest to your patient for timing brushing in order to enhance effectiveness.

8. The Bass method of brushing is widely taught by dental hygienists to enhance effectiveness of their patients' oral cleaning. What problems are sometimes encountered as patients try to learn this technique?

9. Which two methods of toothbrushing are sometimes taught to young children when they have difficulty mastering a sulcular brushing technique?

10. Describe the procedure for the modified Stillman method of toothbrushing.

11. Which toothbrushing methods instruct the patient to direct the brush filaments at a 45° angle toward the gingival margin?

12. Which toothbrushing method instructs the patient to direct the brush filaments at a 45° angle toward the occlusal plane?

13. What are the problems with biofilm removal when the patient uses the method described in question 12?

14. What three factors in toothbrushing are most likely to contribute to gingival recession or tooth abrasion?

15. List two methods for brushing occlusal surfaces.

16. What two anatomic features contribute to retention of dental biofilm on a patient's tongue?

17. Identify two methods for cleaning the tongue.

18. List alterations in the appearance of gingival tissues that require you to recommend a different toothbrushing technique in order to correct or reduce gingival damage.

19. Identify at least three special circumstances in which the use of a powered toothbrush can enhance the removal of bacterial biofilm.

20. In your own words, describe the motion of an oscillating power toothbrush head. (*Hint:* use your hand to demonstrate the motion described in Table 28-3 in the textbook.)

COMPETENCY EXERCISES

Apply information from the chapter and use critical thinking skills to complete the competency exercises. Write responses on paper or create electronic documents to submit your answers.

1. Nicholas Bean, a 12 year old who is your first patient of the day, is going right from his prophylaxis appointment to the orthodontist's office, where they will be placing full-mouth bands and brackets on his teeth. You know that the best toothbrush to recommend for him to use is a bilevel orthodontic toothbrush, but you do not happen to have a sample to give him. You decide to tell his mother what it looks like so she can get one. Using terminology that describes the parts of a toothbrush from Figure 28-1 in the textbook and the pictures from Figure 28-2 in the textbook, develop a brief description of this type of toothbrush trim profile.

2. Mr. Gabriel Chin is one of your favorite patients, and he loves to share stories of his travels around the world. Today when he presents for his recall appointment, he shows you some toothbrushes that he recently brought back from a trip to visit relatives in his native country. The toothbrush, he states proudly, is the type his family has been using for many years and is made from the hairs of wild boars. You want to educate him without belittling his enthusiasm for his family's history. To help him understand about a better alternative, list three reasons why nylon or synthetic filaments are used today for toothbrushes instead of natural bristles.

3. Mrs. Janette Evans has been diagnosed with active periodontal disease. You will be working closely with her once a week for the next 2 months to control oral disease and obtain periodontal health because she will soon be going into the hospital for open-heart surgery. What important information should you give her about how to care for her toothbrush?

4. As you are providing oral hygiene instructions using the Bass method for Mrs. Evans, she asks you how much time she should spend brushing her teeth in order to thoroughly remove all of the biofilm, as you are recommending. Explain one of the methods she can use to monitor her toothbrushing.

5. When you are showing Mrs. Evans how to brush, you note that she needs some extra help with the distal surfaces of tooth 19, the most posterior tooth in that arch. Explain how she should position her toothbrush.

6. Explain how Mrs. Evans can effectively use her toothbrush to clean the mesial surface of tooth 7, which is extremely rotated and tilted in a labial direction.

7. Using your institution's guidelines for writing in patient records, document the oral hygiene instructions you provided for Mrs. Evans. Be sure to include enough detail so that you can use the comments at a subsequent visit to reinforce the information you provided.

8. When you see Mrs. Evans a week later, her biofilm scores are a bit lower but still not up to the levels you would like to see after your extensive oral hygiene instructions. When you do your intraoral examination, you notice a scuffed epithelial surface, several red pinpoint spots, and some generalized redness along the lingual gingival margin of teeth 13–15 and the facial margins of teeth 29–31. You determine that these acute lesions may be the result of toothbrushing activity during the previous week. Identify three possible precipitating factors and explain measures you or Mrs. Evans should take to eliminate the problems.

9. What are some reasons you might recommend a power toothbrush for Mrs. Evans instead of the manual toothbrushing technique you originally taught her?

DISCOVERY EXERCISES

Collaborate with your classmates to gather samples of a variety of different power toothbrushes. (*Hint*: Contacting dental product companies is one way to do this, or you can use models that you, your classmates, or your faculty already own.)

1. For each brand or model of power toothbrush, determine the following information:
   - Motion
   - Brush head shape
   - Filaments
   - Handle size and shape
   - Overall weight
   - Power source
   - Speed

2. Discuss which model would be best for a variety of situations—for example, which one would you

recommend for a child? For a caregiver to use when brushing someone else's teeth? Think of other situations and types of patients.

3. Conduct a PubMed search and review professional literature to evidence to support the recommendation of the type of power toothbrush you like best.

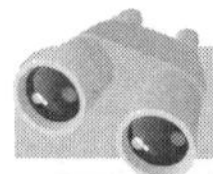

BOX 28-1 MeSH TERMS

Use a combination of MeSH terms and other key words to develop an effective and efficient PubMed literature search strategy.

Dental devices, home care	Toothbrushing
Health education, dental	Gingival recession
Oral hygiene	Tooth abrasion

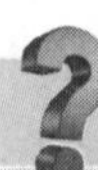

Questions Patients Ask

What sources of information can you identify that will help you answer your patient's questions in this scenario?

"What toothbrush is right for me?" "Is a power toothbrush really worth buying? Will it help keep my teeth cleaner and my gums healthier?" "How do you know that the toothbrushing method you are teaching me is right for me?" You will hear these types of questions from your patients many, many times.

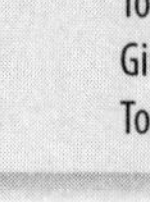

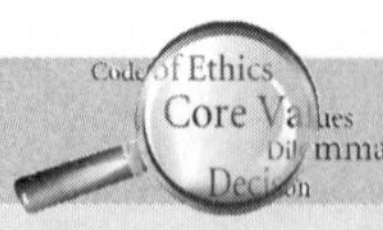

EVERYDAY ETHICS

Before completing the learning exercises below, reread and reflect on the Everyday Ethics Scenario and Questions for Consideration in this chapter of the textbook. It may also be useful to review the Dental Hygiene Ethics discussion in Chapter 1, the Ethical Applications in the introduction pages for each section in the textbook, as well as the Codes of Ethics in textbook Appendices I–IV.

Collaborative Learning Activity

Work with a small group to develop a 2- to 5-minute role-play that introduces the everyday ethics scenario described in the chapter (a great idea is to video record your role-play activity). Then develop separate 2-minute role-play scenarios that provide at least two alternative approaches/solutions to resolving the situation. Ask classmates to view the solutions, ask questions, and discuss the ethical approach used in each. Ask for a vote on which solution classmates determine to be the "best."

Discovery Activity

Ask a friend or relative who is not involved in health care to read the scenario and discuss it with you from the perspective of a "patient" who receives services within the healthcare system. Discuss what you learned from the concerns, insights, or difference in perspective that person expressed.

Factors To Teach The Patient

This scenario is related to the following factors listed in this chapter of the textbook:

- ▷ How dental biofilm forms and its effects on the teeth and gingiva.
- ▷ Why it is necessary to remove dental biofilm from the teeth daily, especially before going to sleep.

Thomas Raveli, 18 years old, is home for the holiday from his first term at college, and his mother has insisted that he keep his appointment with you for his regular 6-month cleaning. As you collect assessment data before providing dental hygiene care, you become very aware that his overall oral status is not the same as it has been at previous visits. You note generalized bleeding on probing and overall red and inflamed gingiva. Fortunately, there is no radiographic evidence of bone level changes.

Further questioning reveals that his overall home-care routine has not been adequate and his eating patterns include frequent snacking because he doesn't particularly like the regular meals served in his dorm. He tells you about how hard it is to keep a regular schedule when he is so stressed by his college workload. He comments that it has been especially tough during the last several weeks when he was writing final exams. That's when he started noticing that his gums were bleeding every time he brushed his teeth! It hurt to brush, so he admits that he has been neglectful of his daily oral care.

Use the motivational interviewing approach (see Appendix D) to write a statement explaining how using the proper brushing techniques can help prevent future problems for Thomas.

Use the conversation you create to role-play this situation with a fellow student. If you are the patient in the role-play, be sure to ask questions. If you are the dental hygienist, try to anticipate questions and provide evidence-based answers for them in your explanation.

Word Search Puzzle

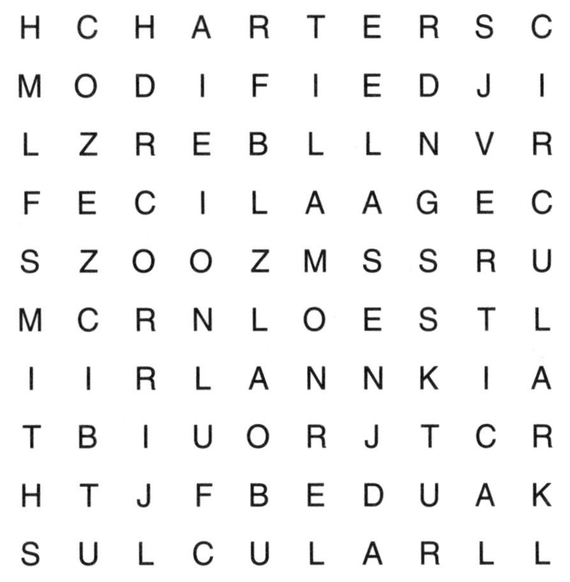

H	C	H	A	R	T	E	R	S	C
M	O	D	I	F	I	E	D	J	I
L	Z	R	E	B	L	L	N	V	R
F	E	C	I	L	A	A	G	E	C
S	Z	O	O	Z	M	S	S	R	U
M	C	R	N	L	O	E	S	T	L
I	I	R	L	A	N	N	K	I	A
T	B	I	U	O	R	J	T	C	R
H	T	J	F	B	E	D	U	A	K
S	U	L	C	U	L	A	R	L	L

Word Search Clues

There are a variety of different toothbrushing methods you can teach your patients. Some are better than others for maximizing biofilm removal and minimizing damage to oral tissues. But all of them are included in this word search puzzle.

- Bass
- Charters
- Circular
- Fones
- Horizontal
- Leonard
- Modified
- Roll
- Scrub
- Smith's
- Stillman
- Sulcular
- Vertical

29

Oral Infection Control: Interdental Care

LEARNING OBJECTIVES

Upon successful completion of these exercises, you will be able to:

1. Identify and define key terms and concepts related to interdental care.
2. Describe the interdental embrasures.
3. Describe the characteristics, indications, and procedures for use of a variety of interdental cleaning devices.
4. Include individualized recommendations for interdental care in dental hygiene care plans.

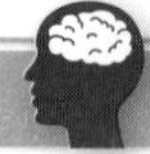

KNOWLEDGE EXERCISES

Write your answers for each question in the space provided.

1. Posterior teeth have __________ papillae with a col, and anterior teeth have __________ papilla that forms a small col under the contact area.

2. Identify tissue and anatomic characteristics of the col, the adjacent teeth, and the surrounding papillae that contribute to the increased risk of gingivitis in the interdental area.

3. Identify the different types of floss that you and your patient can select, based on individual preference and needs.

4. Complete Infomap 29-1 to compare the benefits and limitations of waxed (or PTFE) and unwaxed floss, as noted in the textbook.

INFOMAP 29-1

FLOSS TYPE	BENEFITS	LIMITATIONS
Waxed or expanded PTFE		
Unwaxed floss		

5. Identify the location, cause of, and methods for preventing floss cuts and clefts.

6. List additional flossing aides you can recommend for a patient and identify indications for recommending each one.

7. What kind of flossing motion can be applied with tufted floss, knitting yarn, or gauze strips that is not typically applied with regular floss?

8. Describe the shapes of interdental brushes.

9. Describe a situation in which the interdental brush is a better choice than dental floss for complete biofilm removal or for application of chemotherapeutic agents on proximal surfaces of teeth.

10. End-tuft brushes are usually recommended for a single area that is difficult to reach with a regular toothbrush. In what specific situations might you recommend the use of an end-tuft brush?

11. In your own words, describe a wooden interdental cleaner, state how it is used, and identify factors you must consider when recommending it for a patient.

12. Describe an interdental tip and a toothpick in holder and explain how they are used.

Interdental tip

Toothpick in holder

13. Describe oral irrigation.

14. List the three delivery method categories for oral irrigation.

15. List the advantages of patient-applied daily irrigation measures.

16. List the patient assessment factors that provide information to help you assess your patient's individual needs before recommending a specific device for his or her interdental care.

COMPETENCY EXERCISES

Apply information from the chapter and use critical thinking skills to complete the competency exercises. Write responses on paper or create electronic documents to submit your answers.

1. The best way to learn how to teach a patient about flossing is to practice doing it. Use all of the information you learned in the textbook chapter to teach a family member or friend (but not one of your student colleagues, because he or she has already read this chapter) about how and when to floss.

2. After careful assessment of his current oral hygiene measures, you find that your patient, Mr. Adamson, has very large hands and has a great deal of difficulty maneuvering dental floss in his posterior teeth. He also has an orthodontic band on tooth 3, which positions a temporary appliance being used to maintain an open space for the later placement of a permanent bridge. He has high levels of biofilm on all proximal areas and along the gingival margin of the orthodontic band. Write two dental hygiene diagnosis statements related to these issues.

3. Write a goal for the problems you identified in the dental hygiene diagnoses in question 2. Include a time frame for meeting the goal. How will you measure whether or not your patient met the goal?

4. You decide to recommend a floss holder for regular floss as well as the use of a "Perio-Aid" for

Mr. Adamson. Obtain samples of these interdental devices, if you can, to help you with this exercise (they will also help with the Factors to Teach the Patient section). Write a progress note documenting your recommendations and the oral hygiene instructions that you provided for Mr. Adamson.

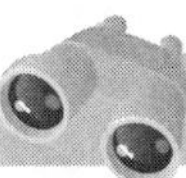

BOX 29-1 MeSH TERMS

Use a combination of MeSH terms and other key words to develop an effective and efficient PubMed literature search strategy.

Oral hygiene
Dental devices, home care
Gingiva

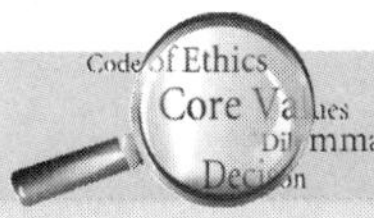

EVERYDAY ETHICS

Before completing the learning exercises below, reread and reflect on the Everyday Ethics Scenario and Questions for Consideration in this chapter of the textbook. It may also be useful to review the Dental Hygiene Ethics discussion in Chapter 1, the Ethical Applications in the introduction pages for each section in the textbook, as well as the Codes of Ethics in textbook Appendices I–IV.

Individual Learning Activity

Imagine that you are the dental hygienist in this scenario. Answer each of the questions for consideration at the end of the scenario.

Discovery Activity

Ask a friend or relative who is not involved in health care to read the scenario and discuss it with you from the perspective of a "patient" who receives services within the healthcare system. Discuss what you learned from the concerns, insights, or difference in perspective that person expressed.

Factors To Teach The Patient

This scenario is related to the following factors listed in this chapter of the textbook:

- By demonstration with disclosing agent, how the toothbrush doesn't clean the interdental area thoroughly.
- About dental biofilm and how it collects on the proximal tooth surfaces when left undisturbed.
- How vulnerable the interdental area is to gingival infection.
- How to use each recommended interdental aid to clean the proximal tooth surfaces.

Use motivational interviewing principles (see Appendix D) to develop a conversation explaining to Mr. Adamson (introduced in question 2 of the Competency Exercises) how to assemble and use the interdental devises you are recommending.

30

Dentifrices and Mouthrinses

LEARNING OBJECTIVES

Upon successful completion of these exercises, you will be able to:

1. Identify and define key terms and concepts related to dentifrices and mouthrinses.
2. Describe the components, action, and therapeutic or cosmetic benefits of a dentifrice.
3. Describe the purpose of, procedure for, and ingredients used in oral rinses.
4. Identify the considerations in selecting patient-specific dentifrices and oral rinses.
5. Define the purpose, requirements, and use of the revised ADA Seal Program.

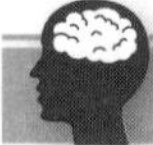

KNOWLEDGE EXERCISES

Write your answers for each question in the space provided.

1. What are the beneficial effects of the active ingredients in dentifrices?

2. Identify the three purposes of a dentifrice.

3. What is the purpose of the humectants in a dentifrice?

4. List at least three types of abrasives used as polishing agents in a dentifrice.

5. What are the purposes of sorbitol or glycerol as an ingredient in a dentifrice?

6. What is the purpose of essential oils (e.g., peppermint) used in dentifrices?

____

____

7. The amount of therapeutic agent in a dentifrice is about ___________.

8. Which therapeutic ingredient in a dentifrice is related to prevention of dental caries?

____

9. Identify four therapeutic ingredients in a dentifrice that are related to reduction of supragingival calculus formation?

____

____

____

____

10. What is the most common ingredient used in dentifrices to aid in reducing sensitivity?

____

11. List the six basic ingredients in commercial mouthrinses.

____

____

____

____

____

____

12. List at least three general types of chemotherapeutic agents found in mouthrinses and identify the purpose of each.

____

____

____

____

____

____

____

____

____

____

13. List at least three characteristics of an effective mouthrinse.

____

____

____

14. Which therapeutic agent available in mouthrinses has the greatest substantivity?

____

15. Which therapeutic agent available in mouthrinses acts by causing bacteriolysis?

____

16. Which therapeutic agent available in mouthrinses acts by inhibiting bacterial enzymes?

____

17. Which therapeutic agent available in mouthrinses is inactivated by a foaming agent frequently contained in commercial dentifrices?

____

18. Which two therapeutic agents available in mouthrinses are associated with the adverse effect of staining?

____

____

19. Describe the action and use of a mouthrinse containing peroxide.

____

____

____

20. Explain why rinsing with a mouthwash that contains an effective therapeutic agent may not be effective for a patient with deep periodontal pockets.

____

____

21. List factors to consider when providing patient-specific recommendations for dentifrices.

____

____

____

____

22. Which mouthrinse agents have no clinical evidence to support their use for reducing gingivitis or biofilm?

23. What is the website for the ADA Seal Program?

24. List the items that should be documented in the patient's chart concerning dentifrices and mouthrinses.

COMPETENCY EXERCISES

Apply information from the chapter and use critical thinking skills to complete the competency exercises. Write responses on paper or create electronic documents to submit your answers.

1. Using the information in the textbook, compare effectiveness, adverse effects, availability to the patient, and any other factors about therapeutic agents that might affect patient acceptance. (*Hint:* Use a separate piece of paper to make a one-page infomap, or table, to aid in your comparison.) What additional information would you like to have about each of these agents that might help you inform your patients about using them?
2. Evan, a 7 year old, has been prescribed a fluoride mouthrinse by Dr. Leiberman. Evan demonstrates a rinsing technique in which he fills his mouth with the liquid and rotates his head in all directions to distribute the rinse to all areas of his mouth.

   You plan to teach him how to rinse using the steps outlined in Box 30-4 of the textbook. Write a dental hygiene diagnosis statement that identifies a problem related to Evan's current rinsing technique.
3. Write a goal for the problem identified in the dental hygiene diagnosis in question 2. How will you measure whether or not Evan met the goal? Include a time frame for meeting the goal.
4. Ms. Greene is a 45-year-old periodontal patient who develops a moderate amount of supragingival calculus. What type of dentifrice might you consider recommending to her?
5. Using your institution's guidelines for writing in patient records, document the recommendation of a toothpaste containing pyrophosphate during patient education.

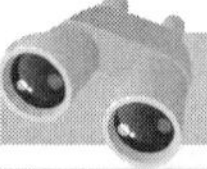

BOX 30-1 MeSH TERMS

Use a combination of MeSH terms and other key words to develop an effective and efficient PubMed literature search strategy.

Dentifrices	Mouthwashes
Denture cleansers	Cariostatic agents
Toothpastes	Fluorides

Questions Patients Ask

What sources of information can you identify that will help you answer your patient's questions in this scenario?

After you answer her questions about the ADA Seal, Ms. Leffler is very impressed with your knowledge, and she clearly believes that *you* are the expert to ask about dental products. Like many of your patients, she has questions about all kinds of oral-care products that she has heard or read about. "Does it really matter which toothpaste I use?" "There are so many different kinds with different ingredients that claim to do different things—which one is really the best?" "Are there any negative side effects that go along with any of those extra ingredients and chemicals?" "Which mouthrinse do you recommend?"

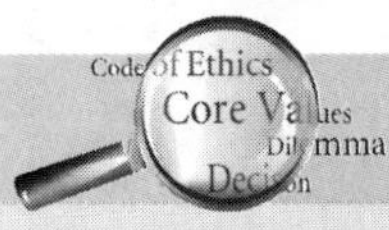

EVERYDAY ETHICS

Before completing the learning exercises below, reread and reflect on the Everyday Ethics Scenario and Questions for Consideration in this chapter of the textbook. It may also be useful to review the Dental Hygiene Ethics discussion in Chapter 1, the Ethical Applications in the introduction pages for each section in the textbook, as well as the Codes of Ethics in textbook Appendices I–IV.

Collaborative Learning Activities

Answer each of the questions for consideration at the end of the scenario in the textbook. Compare what you wrote with answers developed by another classmate and discuss differences/similarities.

Work with a small group to develop a 2- to 5-minute role-play that introduces the everyday ethics scenario described in the chapter (a great idea is to video record your role-play activity). Then develop separate 2-minute role-play scenarios that provide at least two alternative approaches/ solutions to resolving the situation. Ask classmates to view the solutions, ask questions, and discuss the ethical approach used in each. Ask for a vote on which solution classmates determine to be the "best."

Factors To Teach The Patient

This scenario is related to the following factors listed in this chapter of the textbook:

- Significance of ADA product acceptance seal (especially because it is a voluntary program, and no seal on a product does not signify that it is unsafe or not effective).

Ms. Cerene Leffler usually prefers to use all-natural products. She has noticed that the dentifrice she likes does not display the ADA Seal on the package. She asks you during her dental hygiene appointment if that indicates that the toothpaste is not a good choice. Using patient-appropriate language, write a statement explaining to Ms. Leffler what the ADA Seal means.

Word Search Puzzle

R	V	B	C	H	L	O	R	H	E	X	I	D	I	N	E	S
E	D	U	H	H	P	E	A	S	I	Z	E	A	D	S	W	U
M	E	F	E	Y	X	E	X	X	A	R	M	O	Z	Y	A	B
I	N	F	M	G	W	O	M	Y	S	I	M	H	E	N	N	S
N	T	E	O	F	H	F	I	L	T	C	H	O	W	E	T	T
I	I	R	T	D	H	L	N	I	R	X	H	G	L	R	I	A
E	F	B	H	C	Y	U	C	T	I	T	D	A	A	G	M	N
R	R	S	E	A	D	O	O	O	N	Z	N	C	T	I	I	T
A	I	T	R	D	R	R	P	L	G	G	H	I	W	S	C	I
L	C	R	A	A	O	I	O	P	E	S	U	D	K	M	R	V
I	E	I	P	S	K	D	L	O	N	T	M	O	L	I	O	I
Z	N	C	Y	E	I	E	Y	B	T	A	E	G	L	A	B	T
A	G	L	R	A	N	S	M	I	I	N	C	E	C	C	I	Y
T	H	O	X	L	E	S	E	N	U	N	T	N	M	T	A	L
I	N	S	N	F	T	E	R	D	K	O	A	I	X	I	L	C
O	O	A	M	L	I	Z	W	E	K	U	N	C	M	V	V	X
N	C	N	D	E	C	C	L	R	H	S	T	W	W	E	Q	B

Puzzle Clues

- Motions of fluids or the forces that produce or affect such motion.
- The term that means acid forming.
- Substance that retains moisture and prevents hardening upon exposure to air.
- Abbreviation for chlorhexidine.
- A substance with a high molecular weight that results from chemically combining two or more monomers.
- Restoration of mineral elements.
- Treatment of disease by means of chemical substances or pharmaceutical agents.
- A caries prevention agent found in dentifrices and mouthrinses.
- A substance that causes contraction or shrinkage and arrests discharges.
- Indicates that efficacy claims of a product have been tested by research studies and are valid (two words).
- Ability of an agent to bind to surfaces and be released and retain potency over an extended period of time.
- A chemotherapeutic substance usually used with a toothbrush.
- Reduces oral acidity.
- An action in which one agent or drug enhances the effect of another.
- A broad-spectrum antibacterial agent that has the ability to bind and remain in the oral cavity over a period of time.
- A chemical with a bacteriostatic or bactericidal effect.
- Refers to a type of ingredient added to a dentifrice to produce a specific preventive or treatment outcome.
- A substance added to a dentifrice to prevent separation of the solid and liquid ingredients during storage.
- This flavoring agent in dentifrices has been shown to provide anticaries benefits.
- Type of fluoride that has been shown to help reduce oral biofilm.
- This agent has been shown to have a beneficial effect on reducing the bacteria associated with VSC production.
- Description of the amount of toothpaste dispensed on the toothbrush of a 2- to 5-year-old child (two words).

31

The Patient with Orthodontic Appliances

LEARNING OBJECTIVES

Upon successful completion of these exercises, you will be able to:

1. Identify and define key terms and concepts related to care of patients with orthodontic appliances.
2. Identify appliances and instruments used in orthodontic treatment.
3. Describe procedures for placing and removing orthodontic appliances.
4. Provide oral hygiene instructions for a patient before, during, and following orthodontic treatment.

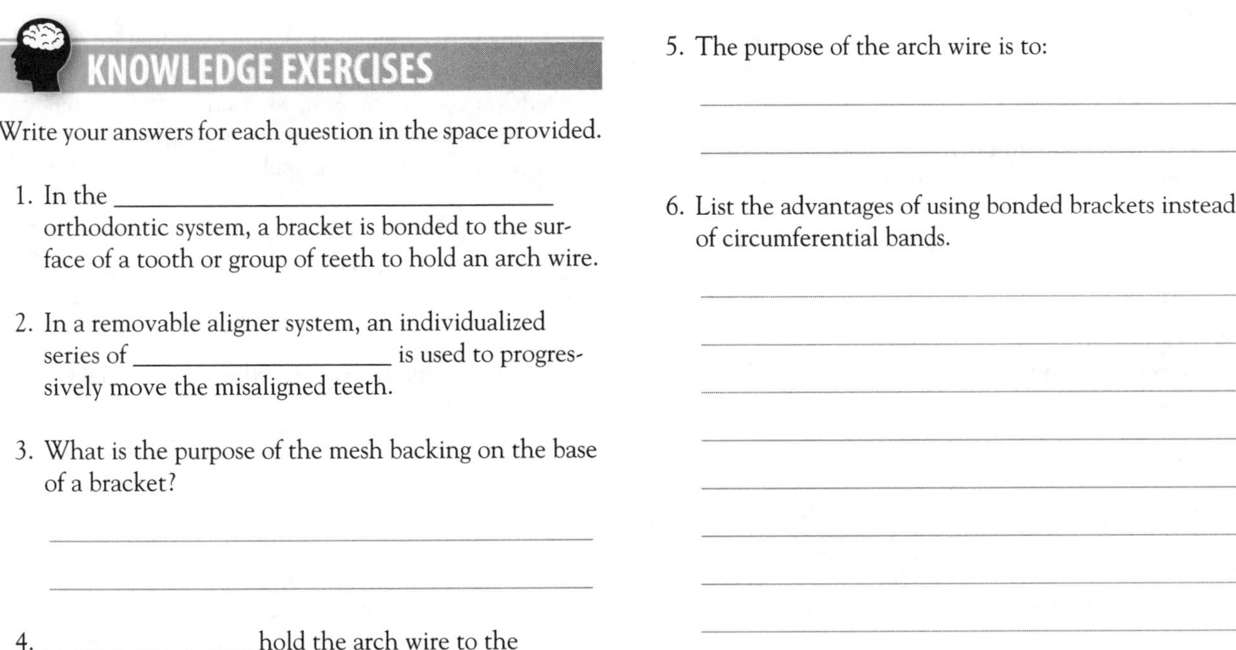

KNOWLEDGE EXERCISES

Write your answers for each question in the space provided.

1. In the ________________________ orthodontic system, a bracket is bonded to the surface of a tooth or group of teeth to hold an arch wire.

2. In a removable aligner system, an individualized series of ________________ is used to progressively move the misaligned teeth.

3. What is the purpose of the mesh backing on the base of a bracket?

4. ________________ hold the arch wire to the bracket.

5. The purpose of the arch wire is to:

6. List the advantages of using bonded brackets instead of circumferential bands.

7. List the disadvantages of bonded brackets.

____

____

____

8. What materials are bonded brackets commonly made from?

____

____

____

9. What is documented for each patient prior to placing bonded orthodontic brackets?

____

____

10. The procedure for applying the bonding agent is similar to the procedure for placing a dental ____________________.

11. The use of filler particles in bonding resin increases ______________________________ ____________(multiple words); therefore, heavily filled resins are used for brackets placed on ____________________ teeth, which are subject to high forces of mastication.

12. Explain the significance of using a fluoride-releasing bonding system.

____

____

____

13. A patient with orthodontic appliances is at risk for a higher incidence of which two oral diseases?

____

____

14. Describe how a regular toothbrush can be adapted on the facial surface of teeth with an orthodontic appliance?

____

____

____

____

____

____

15. Explain how an orthodontic toothbrush, such as that pictured in Figure 31-4 in the textbook, is used.

____

____

____

16. Explain the effect of the debonding process on tooth enamel.

____

____

____

17. Use of a ______________________________________can help reduce the effects of the debonding process on tooth enamel.

18. What is the purpose of frequent rinsing and drying during removal of the bonding resin?

____

____

19. List the final-finish steps so that will leave help restore the pretreatment enamel surface finish following removal of the bonding resin.

____

____

____

____

20. Along with careful periodontal examination, examination for demineralized areas, and removal of leftover composite resin, what other professional assessments and interventions are required after debonding orthodontic appliances?

____

____

____

21. What is the purpose of an orthodontic retainer?

____

____

COMPETENCY EXERCISES

Apply information from the chapter and use critical thinking skills to complete the competency exercises. Write responses on paper or create electronic documents to submit your answers.

1. Ms. Anna Moyer, a real-estate agent who really relies on her smile as she interacts with the public in her job, is very excited and yet extremely nervous on the day the brackets that have hidden her smile for so long are being removed. After the brackets and arch wires are removed from Ms. Moyer's teeth, it is necessary to remove all residual adhesive. Discuss the steps you will take to ensure that all areas of each tooth are thoroughly free from adhesive.

2. Discuss the purpose of post-debonding preventive care that you, the dental hygienist, will provide for Ms. Moyer.

3. Two weeks after her fixed orthodontic appliances are removed, the orthodontist delivers a Hawley appliance to Ms. Moyer. You are responsible for educating and instructing her about the purpose and care of her retainer. What important points will you cover in your discussion?

4. Your next patient is Missy Breckenridge. She has had her orthodontic appliances for about 2 years now, and you notice that her gingiva is not as healthy as it was when you saw her 6 months ago. When you disclose her mouth, there is a large accumulation of dental biofilm between the brackets and her gingival margins. What topics will you be sure to include in your discussion with Missy as you provide oral hygiene instructions that address her need to ensure cleanliness on all surfaces.

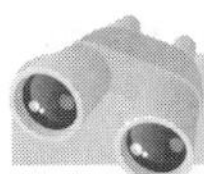

BOX 31-1 MeSH TERMS

Use a combination of MeSH terms and other key words to develop an effective and efficient PubMed literature search strategy.

Orthodontic appliances
Orthodontic appliance design
Orthodontic brackets
Orthodontic extrusion
Orthodontic retainers
Orthodontic space closure
Orthodontic wires
Orthodontics, corrective
Orthodontics, interceptive
Orthodontics, preventive
Orthodontics, corrective
Orthodontics, interceptive
Orthodontics, preventive
Tooth movement
Tooth demineralization
Dental bonding
Dental debonding

EVERYDAY ETHICS

Before completing the learning exercises below, reread and reflect on the Everyday Ethics Scenario and Questions for Consideration in this chapter of the textbook. It may also be useful to review the Dental Hygiene Ethics discussion in Chapter 1, the Ethical Applications in the introduction pages for each section in the textbook, as well as the Codes of Ethics in textbook Appendices I–IV.

Individual Learning Activity

Identify a situation you have experienced that presents a similar ethical dilemma. Write about you would do differently now than you did at the time the incident happened—support your discussion with concepts from the dental hygiene codes of ethics.

Discovery Activity

Ask a dental hygienist who has been practicing for a year or more to read the scenario. Provide them with a copy of the Code of Ethics as well. Share the responses you have made to answer each question and ask that person to discuss the situation with you. What insights did you have or what did you learn during this discussion?

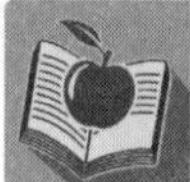

Factors to Teach the Patient

This scenario is related to the following factors listed in this chapter of the textbook:

- ▷ The significance of biofilm around orthodontic appliances and teeth.
- ▷ How, when, and why to use fluoride rinses, toothpastes, and brush-on gels.
- ▷ The frequency for professional follow-up during and after orthodontic therapy.

Nicholas Bean is a 12-year-old patient. He is going directly from his prophylaxis appointment with you to the orthodontist's office, where they will be placing full-mouth bands/brackets and arch wires on his teeth. As they arrive for the appointment, Nicholas's mother comments that they won't be seeing you again until the braces come off. You want to begin to educate Nicholas and his mother right away about the importance of the use of fluorides, thorough daily oral hygiene measures, and especially why regular maintenance appointments are necessary during orthodontic treatment.

Using the information you learned from reading this chapter and the principles of motivational interviewing (Appendix D) as a guide, prepare an outline for a conversation with Nicholas' mother that provides anticipatory guidance about ways to maintain good oral health status while her son is undergoing orthodontic care.

32

Care of Dental Prostheses

LEARNING OBJECTIVES

Upon successful completion of these exercises, you will be able to:

1. Identify and define key terms and concepts related to care of dental prostheses.
2. Identify the components and characteristics of a variety of dental prostheses.
3. Describe the cleaning and care of dental prostheses.
4. Identify procedures to care for the remaining natural teeth, implants, and underlying oral tissues.

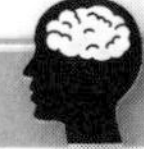

KNOWLEDGE EXERCISES

Write your answers for each question in the space provided.

1. List the components of a fixed partial denture prosthesis.

2. List the criteria for an acceptable fixed partial denture prosthesis.

3. In your own words, describe the procedures for oral cleansing of a fixed dental prosthesis.

4. What characteristic of a removable partial denture prosthesis can negatively affect your patient's gingival health?

5. If your patient is unable to remove his or her own partial denture prosthesis, how do you help the patient remove it?

6. In your own words, describe an obturator.

7. Label Figure 32-1 with the following components.
   - *Denture border*
   - *Impression surface*
   - *Occlusal surface*
   - *Polished surface*

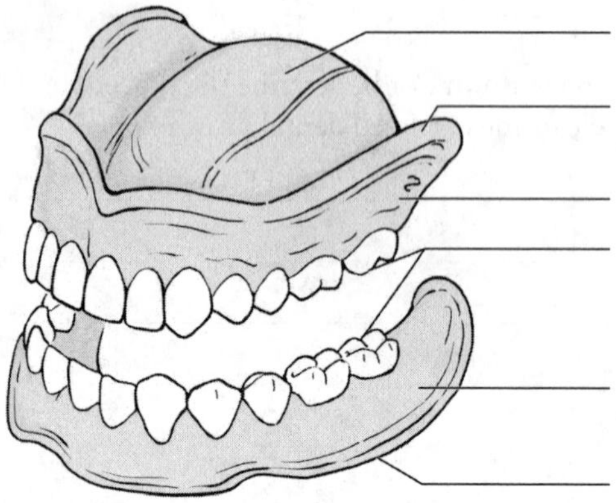

8. Identify two kinds of liners that may be present on the impression surface of a complete denture prosthesis.

9. Identify two kinds of complete overdenture prostheses.

10. What are the advantages of a complete overdenture prosthesis?

11. List factors that contribute to the success of an overdenture prosthesis.

12. What are the advantages of natural tooth and implant-retained overdentures?

13. What dental hygiene interventions provide an added measure of protection for the oral health of a patient with a partial denture, single arch complete denture with natural teeth remaining in the opposite arch, or overdenture supported by natural teeth?

14. What two procedures can be used to clean an oral prosthesis?

15. Describe the process you will use to remove your patient's complete denture if, for some reason, your patient is not able to remove it himself or herself.

- *Maxillary complete denture*

- *Mandibular complete denture*

16. Identify two oral conditions that can be prevented with proper cleansing and care of dental prostheses and underlying tissues.

17. What is the purpose of instructing your patients to remove and properly store their dental prosthesis in liquid while sleeping at night?

18. What are the requirements for a denture cleanser you will recommend to your patient?

19. Complete Infomap 32-1 to compare the various types of cleansers you can recommend for the care of full and partial dentures.

INFOMAP 32-1

TYPE	ACTIVE INGREDIENT	CLEANSER ACTION	DISADVANTAGES
Immersion type			
Alkaline hypochlorite (household bleach)			
Alkaline peroxide (commercial powder or tablet)			
Dilute acids (commercial ultrasonic solutions)			
Enzymes (in various cleansers)			
Abrasive type			
Pastes and powders (various commercial products)			
Household agents (salt, bicarbonate of soda, hand soap, scouring powders)			

COMPETENCY EXERCISES

Apply information from the chapter and use critical thinking skills to complete the competency exercises. Write responses on paper or create electronic documents to submit your answers.

1. Imagine that you have just joined the on-site dental team at a long-term care facility or nursing home. A short time after you begin your position, you discover that many of the residents wear full or partial dentures and those dentures are not being cleaned regularly by the nurses' aides who are responsible for providing daily personal care for the residents. Most of the dentures worn by the residents are complete arch dentures made of acrylic resins. Many are old and stained, and some have calculus buildup on the surfaces of the denture. The dentures are seldom removed from the patients' mouths. When they are, they are often just placed on the bedside table or in the drawer until family members come for a visit and decide that the patient looks better with the denture back in place.

   You plan to provide an in-service presentation for the caregivers about the importance of denture care, and you also plan to provide hands-on training in denture-cleaning techniques for the caregiver staff.
   - *List the information that you will include in your in-service presentation about denture care.*
   - *Create a step-by-step checklist that the aides can use at the bedside to document daily cleaning of each resident's removable prosthesis as well as the resident's oral tissues.*

2. During a dental hygiene appointment, you carefully and completely clean and disinfect your patient's removable maxillary complete denture and mandibular partial denture before returning it to the patient's mouth at the end of the visit. Using your school's guidelines for documenting in patient progress notes, describe the service you provided for this patient.

DISCOVERY EXERCISE

Investigate commercially available denture cleaners so you can make a recommendation to the long-term care center or nursing home staff. What is the active ingredient in each one? What is the relative cost of each type? Which type might be easiest for the caregivers to use in the nursing home setting? Which one (or ones) will you recommend in your in-service presentation? Provide a rationale for your choice(s).

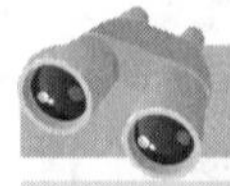

BOX 32-1 MeSH TERMS

Use a combination of MeSH terms and other key words to develop an effective and efficient PubMed literature search strategy.

Dental prosthesis
Denture design
Denture, complete
Denture, complete, immediate
Denture, partial, fixed
Denture, partial, removable
Denture precision attachment
Denture overlay
Denture cleansers

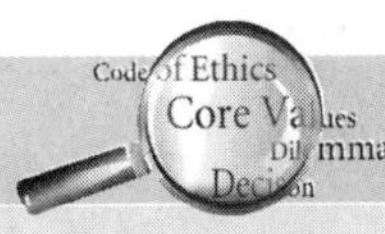

EVERYDAY ETHICS

Before completing the learning exercises below, reread and reflect on the Everyday Ethics Scenario and Questions for Consideration in this chapter of the textbook. It may also be useful to review the Dental Hygiene Ethics discussion in Chapter 1, the Ethical Applications in the introduction pages for each section in the textbook, as well as the Codes of Ethics in textbook Appendices I-IV.

Individual Learning Activity

Imagine that you are the dental hygienist in this scenario. Answer each of the questions for consideration at the end of the scenario.

Discovery Activity

Ask a dental hygienist who has been practicing for a year or more to read the scenario. Provide them with a copy of the Code of Ethics as well. Share the responses you have made to answer each question and ask that person to discuss the situation with you. What insights did you have or what did you learn during this discussion?

Factors To Teach The Patient

This scenario is related to the following factors listed in this chapter of the textbook:

- ▷ How to make a self-examination of the oral tissues.
- ▷ Why all prostheses need cleaning more than once a day.
- ▷ The need to adapt toothbrushing, flossing, and use of other aids to the care of the abutment teeth.
- ▷ How tongue cleaning contributes to complete oral health.
- ▷ The significance of regular maintenance appointments to have the oral tissues checked and the prostheses professionally cleaned.

Evangeline Dada has just received a brand new six-unit anterior bridge, which spans her entire smile from abutment tooth #6 to abutment tooth #11. Before placement of the fixed prosthesis, she had a removable temporary appliance made of plastic. She had no trouble cleaning her teeth when she could remove the old appliance, and she has done a good job of keeping all her oral tissues healthy. She states she is completely at a loss as to how she must take care of this beautiful new smile of hers and asks you to spend some extra time providing oral-hygiene instructions for her today.

Use the principles of motivational interviewing described in Appendix D as a guide to develop a conversation to educate Evangeline about her new bridge, the abutment teeth that support it, and maintaining the health of the oral tissues around and underneath this new fixed prosthesis.

Use the conversation you create to role-play this situation with a fellow student. If you are the patient in the role-play, be sure to ask questions. If you are the dental hygienist, try to anticipate questions and answer them in your explanation.

Word Search Puzzle

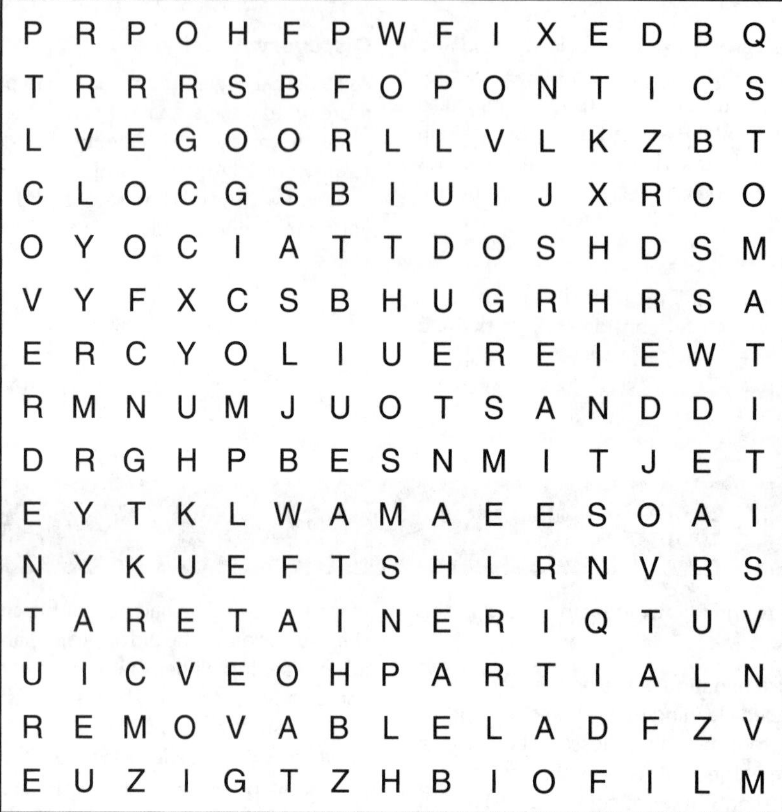

Puzzle Clues

1. A caries preventative agent often placed on teeth that support an overdenture prosthesis.
2. The surface of the dental prosthesis that makes contact with teeth in the opposing arch.
3. A substance that adheres to surfaces of a denture in the same way it can adhere to the surfaces of a natural dentition.
4. An artificial replacement for a body part.
5. A type of oral prosthesis that is cleaned and cared for outside of the oral cavity.
6. Component of a fixed partial denture that replaces a missing natural tooth.
7. A type of partial denture prosthesis that is secured to natural teeth or dental implants and must be cleaned and cared for inside the oral cavity.
8. The type of dental prosthesis that replaces one or more teeth, but not all of the teeth in an arch.
9. The clasp that holds a partial denture around abutment teeth.
10. A type of removable dental prosthesis supported by retained natural teeth or implants and the soft tissue of the alveolar ridge.
11. A type of dental prosthesis that replaces the dentition and associated structures in an entire oral arch.
12. The part of a dental prosthesis that rests on the oral mucosa and to which teeth are attached.
13. A dental prosthesis that closes a congenital or acquired opening in oral tissues.
14. A type of connector that attaches a removal prosthesis to a metal receptacle included within a restoration of an abutment tooth.
15. A tooth or an implant used to support a fixed or removable dental prosthesis.
16. A term commonly used to refer to a fixed partial denture prosthesis.
17. The external or outer surface of a dental prosthesis is a highly ____________ surface, whereas the occlusal and impression surfaces are not.
18. An infection of the oral mucosa that can occur under a removable dental prosthesis.

33

The Patient with Dental Implants

LEARNING OBJECTIVES

Upon successful completion of these exercises, you will be able to:

1. Identify and define key terms and concepts related to care of the patient with implants.
2. Discuss types, preparation and placement, and maintenance care for dental implants.
3. Discuss the components of a postrestorative evaluation of a dental implant.
4. Identify the factors that contribute to implant complication and failure.
5. Plan dental hygiene care for a patient with a dental implant.

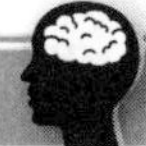

KNOWLEDGE EXERCISES

Write your answers for each question in the space provided.

1. Match the type of bone cell with its appropriate function.

Bone Cell	Function
___ Osteocyte	A. Repair and regeneration
___ Osteoblast	B. Remodeling and homeostasis
___ Osteoclast	C. Mediate activity

2. Explain how Wolff's law is related to dental implants.

____

____

____

3. Identify the bone density classification for each of the following descriptions.

Bone Density Classification	Description
_______________	Immature, nonmineralized bone
_______________	Dense cortical bone
_______________	Thin cortical bone crest/fine trabecular bone
_______________	Thick to porous cortical bone crest/ coarse trabecular bone
_______________	Fine trabecular bone

4. In your own words, define the following types of bone graft options.

Bone Graft Option	Definition
Zenograft	_______________
Autograft	_______________
Allograft	_______________
Alloplast	_______________

5. How long does it take for a newly placed dental implant to reach a steady state of osseointegration?

____

6. What is the significance of fibrous encapsulation?

____

____

7. In your own words, describe the connection between the implant and the patient's oral soft tissue.

____

____

____

____

____

____

____

____

8. In your own words, briefly describe each of the three types of dental implants.

Subperiosteal:

____

____

Transosseous (Transosteal):

____

____

____

____

Endosseous (Endosteal):

____

____

____

____

9. The most common current form of dental implant is the ______________ type that has a ______________ shape.

10. Identify factors that can increase a patient's risk for poor outcomes if dental implants are placed.

____

____

____

____

____

____

____

____

____

____

____

____

____

____

____

____

11. What are the components of a postrestorative evaluation?

____

____

____

____

____

____

____

____

12. Each time the patient with dental implants is scheduled for routine continuing care, you will examine the implant area carefully. List the basic criteria that indicate a healthy implant.

____

____

____

____

____

13. Briefly describe the basic technique for routine probing to check for tissue integrity and bleeding around the dental implant during a continuing care appointment.

14. Briefly described methods of removing calculus from the surface of a dental implant.

15. Explain why it is important to instruct a patient with dental implants to select self-cleaning implements and agents carefully.

16. Identify two prominent contributing factors in the breakdown of the peri-implant environment.

17. What are some systemic factors that can contribute to implant failure?

18. What maintenance phase issues can contribute to implant failure?

19. In your own words, briefly describe each of the three classifications of peri-implant disease.

Peri-implant mucositis:

Peri-implantitis without mobility:

Peri-implantitis with mobility:

20. When signs of peri-implant disease are noted during an oral examination, at what point is the patient referred back to the oral surgeon for intervention?

COMPETENCY EXERCISES

Apply information from the chapter and use critical thinking skills to complete the competency exercises. Write responses on paper or create electronic documents to submit your answers.

1. Describe the dental hygienist's role in collaborative treatment planning and preparing the patient for dental implant procedures.
2. Matthew Glenn, aged 45 years, is scheduled today for a periodontal maintenance appointment. You are very excited and anxious to check the area of his dental implant–supported bridge. The prosthesis he received 6 months ago is a three-unit replacement for teeth 3, 4, and 5, with each pontic supported by an individual dental implant. You provided oral hygiene instructions for him both before and after his implant procedure, but you haven't seen him since.

During your assessment today, you find out that he is not having any oral problems, and the implants have been comfortable and feel just fine. In fact, he is delighted with the implants. His daily oral care is generally very good, but you notice small areas of biofilm in the hard-to-reach areas of the prosthesis, such as the embrasure between teeth 4 and 5 and the distal surface of tooth 3. To your surprise, there is also significant calculus buildup on the facial and mesial surfaces of tooth number 2.

The gingival tissue around the implant looks generally healthy. Mr. Glenn also exhibits some very slight calculus buildup on the facial surfaces of the left side maxillary molars and on the lingual surfaces of his lower anterior teeth. You find no other significant medical history, dental history, or dental examination findings for Mr. Glenn today.

Use a copy of the Individualized Patient Care Plan template (Appendix B) to develop a care plan for Mr. Glenn that emphasizes daily care techniques to ensure long-term success for his implants and prosthesis.

DISCOVERY EXERCISE

- Research websites for viewing a dental implant procedure.
- Research implant manufacturers and supply companies to discover the cost of the instruments.
- Research the current dental terminology codes from the American Dental Association to identify the correct insurance billing codes for implant maintenance procedures.
- Go to the American Association of Periodontolgy website to find more information about dental implants.

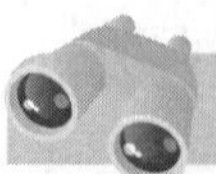

BOX 33-1 MeSH TERMS

Use a combination of MeSH terms and other key words to develop an effective and efficient PubMed literature search strategy.

Dental implantation
Dental implantation, endosseous
Dental implantation, subperiosteal
Dental implants
Dental implants, single-tooth
Osseointegration
Peri-implantitis

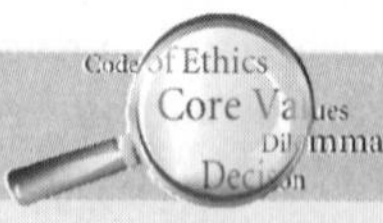

EVERYDAY ETHICS

Before completing the learning exercises below, reread and reflect on the Everyday Ethics Scenario and Questions for Consideration in this chapter of the textbook. It may also be useful to review the Dental Hygiene Ethics discussion in Chapter 1, the Ethical Applications in the introduction pages for each section in the textbook, as well as the Codes of Ethics in textbook Appendices I–IV.

Individual Learning Activity

Identify a situation you have experienced that presents a similar ethical dilemma. What did you learn from how the situation was (or was not) resolved at the time it happened?

Collaborative Learning Activity

Work with a small group to develop a 2- to 5-minute role-play that introduces the Everyday Ethics scenario described in the chapter (a great idea is to video record your role-play activity). Then develop separate 2-minute role-play scenarios that provide at least two alternative approaches/solutions to resolving the situation. Ask classmates to view the solutions, ask questions, and discuss the ethical approach used in each. Ask for a vote on which solution classmates determine to be the "best."

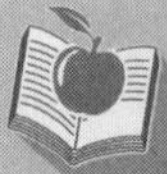

Factors to Teach the Patient

▷ How to care for implants: special needs related to titanium surfaces.
▷ How the health of the periodontal tissues and the duration of the implants and prostheses depend on meticulous daily self-care by the patient and regular professional maintenance.
▷ The role of biofilm in periodontitis and peri-implantitis; vulnerability of the implant to infection from periodontal pathogens that may be present on adjacent natural teeth.
▷ How cleaning a mouth with complex restorations takes longer.

Use the individualized patient care plan you developed for Mr. Glenn (introduced in Competency Exercise question 2) and the principles of motivational interviewing (see Appendix D) as a guide to prepare a conversation to provide oral hygiene instructions for Mr. Glenn during his dental hygiene appointment today.

34

The Patient Who Uses Tobacco

LEARNING OBJECTIVES

Upon successful completion of these exercises, you will be able to:

1. Identify and define key terms and concepts related to the use of tobacco.
2. Explain the systemic and oral effects of tobacco use.
3. Describe the effects of nicotine addiction.
4. Describe strategies for tobacco cessation.
5. Plan dental hygiene care and tobacco cessation interventions for patients who use tobacco.
6. Identify the role of the community-based dental hygienist in community-based tobacco-free initiatives.

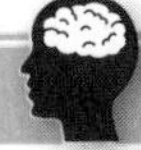

KNOWLEDGE EXERCISES

Write your answers for each question in the space provided.

1. Tobacco contains many components that are __________ to humans. Tobacco use is the single most __________ cause of disease and premature death in the world.

2. The drug in tobacco products that causes addiction is __________.

3. **True or false** (circle one and provide a rationale for your answer.) Tobacco use with a water-cooled hookah device is a safe alternative to traditional smoking.

4. **True or false** (circle one and provide a rationale for your answer.) The electronic nicotine delivery device is *not* an approved method of smoking cessation.

5. List factors that affect the amount of nicotine absorbed into the bloodstream when smoking tobacco.

6. Nicotine from smokeless tobacco can be absorbed through which tissues?

____

____

7. After the onset of smoking a cigarette, peak concentration of nicotine in the blood plasma occurs within approximately __________ and rapidly __________ over the next 20–30 minutes.

8. With the use of moist snuff, plasma concentration of nicotine in blood plasma reaches a peak at about __________ and then slowly declines.

9. How is nicotine eliminated from the body?

____

____

10. Match each of the following descriptive statements with the appropriate component of tobacco. Each term may be used more than once.

Tobacco-Related Terms	Descriptive Statements
A. Cotinine	____ By-product of nicotine is found in body fluids
B. Nicotine	____ The chief psychoactive ingredient in tobacco
C. Nitrosamines	____ The chief addictive agent in tobacco
D. Pyrolysis	____ Refers to a group of cancer-causing chemicals found in tobacco
	____ The process of breaking down chemicals contained in tobacco by heat created at the end of a burning cigarette
	____ Substances measured to determine recent use of nicotine-containing products
	____ Substance found in the various aids used for smoking cessation
	____ Intensifies the release of dopamine by the brain
	____ Although addictive, this chemical is *not* the most physically harmful substance found in tobacco
	____ Released with other substances when the tobacco is ignited

11. In your own words, briefly summarize the systemic effects of tobacco use.

____

____

____

____

____

____

12. List as many negative health effects of tobacco use and/or exposure to second-hand ETS as you can.

____

____

____

____

____

____

____

____

____

____

13. Identify as many potential oral health consequences of tobacco use as you can.

____

____

____

____

____

____

____

____

____

____

14. Match each of the following descriptive statements with the appropriate tobacco-related term.

Tobacco-Related Terms	Descriptive Statements
A. Tolerance B. Dependence C. Abuse D. Addiction E. ETS F. TSNAs	____ The use of any drug in a way that causes harm to the person or other persons who are affected by the user's behavior ____ Refers to the user's need for increased tobacco use over time to create the desired feeling of well-being ____ Loss of control over the amount and frequency of use of tobacco and withdrawal symptoms occur when use of tobacco is discontinued ____ Formed by tobacco smoke reaction with nitrous acid on indoor surfaces. ____ Chronic, progressive, relapsing disease characterized by compulsive use of a substance ____ Refers to passive exposure to second- or third-hand tobacco smoke

15. An individual dependent on nicotine who ceases use of tobacco products will experience significant and unpleasant ______________________ (two words) within 24 hours.

16. Why are children of parents or caregivers who use tobacco also at high risk for disease?

17. In your own words, explain each of the following terms as they relate to your role during dental hygiene care for your patient who uses tobacco products.

Detect:

Explain:

Motivate:

Refer:

Document:

18. Explain two strategies you can use to support a patient who is ready to quit using tobacco.

19. The 5 A's provide the basis for a simple but effective tobacco dependence–intervention approach. Number the 5 A's in the appropriate order (from 1 to 5) and then *briefly* outline the basic premise of each one.

_____ *Advise:*

_____ *Arrange:*

_____ *Ask:*

_____ *Assess:*

_____ *Assist:*

20. List methods available for delivering nicotine-replacement therapy if your patient is considering pharmacotherapy as a treatment for nicotine addiction.

21. Identify nonnicotine pharmacotherapies approved by the FDA for tobacco cessation.

22. In your own words, state the objectives and rationale for using pharmacotherapies to help your patient stop using tobacco.

23. What factors are considered when recommending pharmacotherapies to help your patients stop using tobacco?

24. What are the contraindications for use of pharmacotherapy-assisted tobacco cessation?

25. What are the most common *oral* side effects of the pharmacotherapies used for treatment of nicotine addiction?

COMPETENCY EXERCISES

Apply information from the chapter and use critical thinking skills to complete the competency exercises. Write responses on paper or create electronic documents to submit your answers.

1. Use the Tobacco Use Assessment Form (Figure 34-3 in the textbook) to assess the tobacco-using habits of a friend or relative. Use the methods outlined in the Tobacco Cessation Flowchart (Figure 34-4 in the textbook) and a motivational interviewing approach (see Appendix D) to explore the readiness of this individual to quit.

2. The Section V Summary exercises section of this workbook contains a Patient Assessment Summary for Mrs. Diane White, who is in her first trimester of pregnancy. Although Mrs. White does not smoke, her husband does. Describe the tobacco use and cessation information you would like to be able to provide as you talk to Mrs. White during her dental hygiene

and re-evaluation appointments. Describe how you will use motivational interviewing principles (see Appendix D) as you educate Mrs. White on the detrimental health effects of her husband's tobacco habit.

3. Using your institution's guidelines for writing in patient records, document that you have provided education and counseling related to the health effects of tobacco use during Mrs. White's appointment.

4. As a dental hygienist, your role in addressing the oral and systemic health damage of tobacco use is wider than simply providing assessment, information, motivation, and guidance to individual patients in your clinical practice. Discuss your role in tobacco education and cessation from a personal and community-based or advocacy perspective.

DISCOVERY EXERCISE

Collect a variety of patient education materials—such as brochures, posters, or videotapes—that address the health and/or oral health effects of tobacco use. Encourage each of your student colleagues to collect as many materials as possible from a variety of different sources. Get together in small groups to discuss the materials.

- Determine the scientific accuracy of the information included in the patient-education materials.
- Determine which type of patient each of the materials is best suited for.
- Determine how each of the materials might best be used as part of tobacco-cessation initiatives in your clinic.

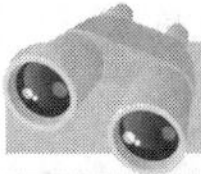

BOX 34-1 MeSH TERMS

Use a combination of MeSH terms and other key words to develop an effective and efficient PubMed literature search strategy.

Smoking	Carcinogens
Tobacco	Head and neck neoplasms
Tobacco products	Mouth neoplasms
Tobacco smoke pollution	Lip neoplasms
Tobacco, smokeless	Tongue neoplasms
Tobacco use	Gingival neoplasms
Tobacco use cessation	Palatal neoplasms
Tobacco use cessation products	Laryngeal neoplasms
Tobacco use disorder	Leukoplakia, oral

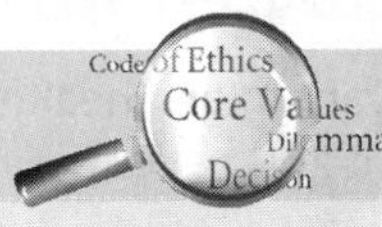

EVERYDAY ETHICS

Before completing the learning exercises below, reread and reflect on the Everyday Ethics Scenario and Questions for Consideration in this chapter of the textbook. It may also be useful to review the Dental Hygiene Ethics discussion in Chapter 1, the Ethical Applications in the introduction pages for each section in the textbook, as well as the Codes of Ethics in textbook Appendices I–IV.

Collaborative Learning Activity

Answer each of the questions for consideration at the end of the scenario in the textbook. Compare what you wrote with answers developed by another classmate and discuss differences/similarities.

Discovery Activity

Summarize this scenario for faculty member at your school and ask them to consider the questions that are included. Is their perspective different than yours or similar? Explain.

Factors to Teach the Patient

This scenario is related to the following factors listed in this chapter of the textbook:

▷ Nonsmokers who breath ETS can incur the same serious health problems as smokers. Children are especially susceptible.

Mrs. White's husband (see Competency Question #2 above) arrives to pick up his wife following her dental hygiene appointment. He wants to discuss their insurance coverage with the office manager, but she is on the telephone, so he must wait for a few minutes to speak with her. He sits down in a chair and immediately takes out a pack of cigarettes and some matches. He asks you for an ashtray.

Use the motivational interviewing principles (see Appendix D) as a guide to prepare an outline for explaining the tobacco-free policy in your office to Mr. White. Mr. White is not your patient—how far can you go in approaching him about the dangers of his tobacco use for his unborn child or providing recommendations for smoking cessation measures?

Use the conversation you create to role-play this situation with a fellow student. If you are the patient in the role-play, be sure to ask questions. If you are the dental hygienist, try to anticipate questions and answer them in your explanation.

35

Diet and Dietary Analysis

LEARNING OBJECTIVES

Upon successful completion of these exercises, you will be able to:

1. Identify and define key terms and concepts related to providing a dietary assessment.
2. Identify vitamins and minerals relevant to oral health.
3. Plan and provide dietary assessment and patient counseling for caries control.

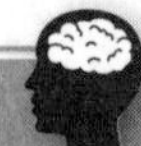

KNOWLEDGE EXERCISES

Write your answers for each question in the space provided.

1. List the major food categories included in the MyPlate icon (Figure 35-1 in the textbook).

____

____

____

____

____

2. Identify two additional food categories listed in Table 35-2, USDA Food Patterns that contribute to an individual's caloric intake.

____

____

3. The food intake patterns sheet contains a table that outlines daily amount of food that is appropriate based on 12 different __________ (two words).

4. Identify three characteristics used to determine the appropriate calorie intake level for an individual person's diet.

____

____

____

5. Look at Table 35-2 in the textbook to find the appropriate calorie level for yourself. Then identify the daily amount of food from the vegetable group that is suggested to meet your nutritional needs.

____

____

6. What amount of food from the dark green vegetable subgroup is suggested for your diet?

7. Table 35-3 in the textbook provides a comprehensive list of nutrients with their functions, associated disease states, and food sources. Your instructor will let you know the level of detail you are expected to recall from the information in that table. It is most important for you to be able to link deficiencies in nutritional intake with oral manifestations you may observe while providing dental hygiene care for your patients. Table 35-4 provides some oral manifestations that are associated with nutritional deficiencies.

   Infomap 35-1 (on the next page) reorganizes information from the textbook to help you associate nutrient deficiencies with specific intraoral findings. Use information throughout Chapter 35 of the textbook to help you complete the infomap with (a) the oral findings you might observe if your patient is deficient in each listed nutrient and (b) food sources for that nutrient you can recommend to your patient.

8. Which vitamins and minerals are associated with healthy skin and mucous membrane?

9. Which nutrients are important for healthy wound healing and tissue repair?

10. Which nutrients are essential for development of healthy tooth structure?

11. Dental caries is the result of intake of _________ foods and is not due to nutrient deficiency.

12. Identify four factors that interact to result in dental caries.

13. Any incident of sucrose intake lowers the pH in the dental biofilm. But what two major factors interact to enhance cariogenic exposure and increase your patient's risk for developing dental caries?

14. In your own words, discuss the purposes of a dietary assessment.

15. Summarize the information you will provide for your patient when you are explaining your dietary assessment intervention prior to asking the patient to complete a food diary.

16. Identify some common dietary omissions that you will want to be sure to review with your patient as you explain the food diary form.

INFOMAP 35-1

NUTRIENT	ORAL MANIFESTATIONS OF DEFICIENCY	FOOD SOURCES
Vitamin A		
Thaimin (vitamin B_1)		
Niacin (vitamin B_3)		
Riboflavin (vitamin B_2)		
Pyridoxine (vitamin B_6)		
Cobalamin (vitamin B_{12})		
Ascorbic acid (vitamin C)		
Vitamin D		
Calcium		
Fluoride		
Folate		
Iron		
Magnesium		
Phosphorus		
Zinc		
Protein		

17. In your own words, explain how to calculate a patient's caries risk using the Sweet Score. (Hint: Use the information in Table 35-7 in the textbook to guide your answer.)

18. If, after calculating the Sweet Score, you determine that your patient is at moderate or high risk for dental caries, what recommendations will you be sure to provide during your oral health education session with that patient?

19. Identify *patient* factors that can affect your success in providing nutritional counseling for your patients.

20. Identify *communication* factors that can affect your success in providing nutritional counseling for your patients.

21. For a patient who is especially caries susceptible, what ingredient in chewing gum will help promote remineralization if chewed immediately after each meal?

22. In your own words, describe the term "nutrition" in terms your patient could understand.

COMPETENCY EXERCISES

Apply information from the chapter and use critical thinking skills to complete the competency exercises. Write responses on paper or create electronic documents to submit your answers.

1. Make a food diary table similar to Table 35-5 in the textbook and create a food diary for everything you ate yesterday. (No cheating, now; no one will ever see this but you.) What nutrients are missing from your diet?

2. Make a copy of the scoring the sweets form (Table 35-7 in the textbook). Use the information in your 24-hour food diary to calculate your personal risk for dental caries. What recommendations will you give yourself to reduce your caries risk?

3. Ask a student colleague, friend, or member of your family to complete a 3- or 5-day food diary. Make a copy of the dietary analysis recording form (Table 35-6 in the textbook) to complete a dietary analysis for that person. Use the SuperTracker web-based analysis program available at http://www.choosemyplate.gov/supertracker-tools/supertracker.html to analyze the diary. This online dietary analysis program is not difficult to learn and the website has a tutorial that will help you get started.

4. Identify topics you would include in a patient education program based on the dietary analysis you completed for question 3.

5. Use the MyPlate nutritional guidelines to create *your* ideal caries-control diet that contains foods you like to eat. Create menus for several days and make sure that your diet provides adequate nutrition for a person who is just like you. Compare your menus with the menus created by your student colleagues.

   Discuss how your colleagues' food preferences, cultural considerations, or personal eating practices compare with yours. What does this exercise help you realize about possible barriers when you are providing diet counseling for your diverse, individual patients?

6. Because individualized dental hygiene care plans are based on individualized patient needs determined by assessment data, not every dental hygiene care plan you write will include dietary assessment or dietary counseling. Discuss patient assessment findings that would indicate the need to include a 24-hour or 3- to 7-day dietary assessment as part of your patient's dental hygiene care plan.

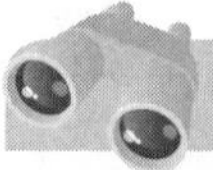

BOX 35-1 MeSH TERMS

Use a combination of MeSH terms and other key words to develop an effective and efficient PubMed literature search strategy.

Diet	Nutritional requirements
Food habits	Dietary carbohydrates
Diet surveys	Dietary sucrose
Nutritional status	Diet, cariogenic
Nutrition assessment	Cariogenic agents
Nutrition disorders	

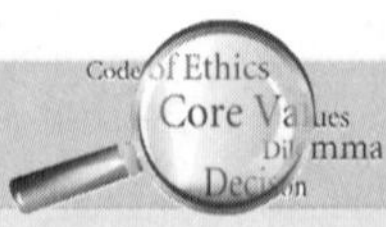

EVERYDAY ETHICS

Before completing the learning exercises below, reread and reflect on the Everyday Ethics Scenario and Questions for Consideration in this chapter of the textbook. It may also be useful to review the Dental Hygiene Ethics discussion in Chapter 1, the Ethical Applications in the introduction pages for each Section in the textbook, as well as the Codes of Ethics in textbook Appendices I–IV.

Individual Learning Activity

Imagine that you are the dental hygienist in this scenario. Answer each of the questions for consideration at the end of the scenario.

Discovery Activity

Ask a dental hygienist who has been practicing for a year or more to read the scenario. Provide them with a copy of the Code of Ethics as well. Share the responses you have made to answer each question and ask that person to discuss the situation with you. What insights did you have or what did you learn during this discussion?

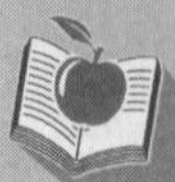

Factors To Teach The Patient

This scenario is related to the following factors listed in this chapter of the textbook:

- ▷ Reasons to avoid frequent daily use of medications with sucrose.
- ▷ Reasons for rinsing with water after a medication contained in a syrupy sucrose mixture.
- ▷ How dental caries on the tooth surface starts and progresses.
- ▷ How the interaction of cariogenic foods, tooth surface, saliva, and microorganisms act together in the dental caries process.
- ▷ How repeated, frequent acid production and the pH in the dental biofilm adversely affect the teeth.

Your next patient, Nathan, is a 7 year old with a lot of serious medical health issues. Because he often has a queasy stomach, his mother fixes him many small meals each day and states that mostly all he will eat are high carbohydrate foods. In addition, Nathan is frequently placed on a (sucrose-enhanced) antibiotic liquid preparation prescribed by his physician. His mother states he absolutely refuses to take any medication in a pill form, so the antibiotic syrup is the only answer.

Use the principles of motivational interviewing (Appendix D) as a guide to prepare an outline for a conversation with Nathan's mother explaining his risk for caries and the importance of changing the boy's daily dietary habits. Make sure to adapt your recommendations for the barriers to behavior change that have been identified in the scenario.

Use the conversation you create to role play this situation with a fellow student. If you are Nathan's mother in the role-play, be sure to ask questions and try to identify additional real-life barriers to behavior change. If you are the dental hygienist, try to anticipate questions and answer them in your explanation.

Crossword Puzzle

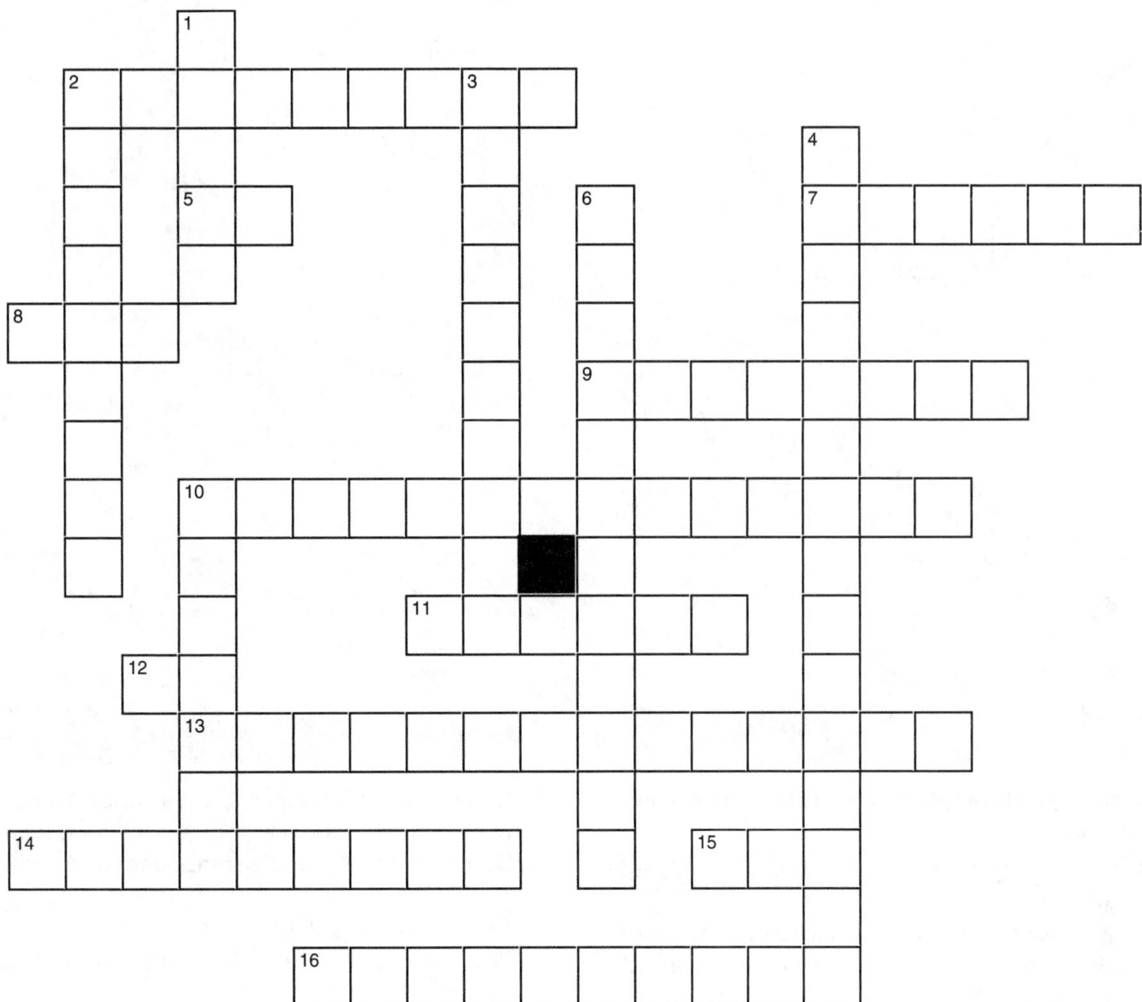

Puzzle Clues

Across

2. A factor in exposure to cariogenic food that is very significant for increasing risk for dental caries.
5. Recommendations for adequate intake of essential nutrients (acronym).
7. United States Department of Health and Human Services (acronym).
8. Average amounts of nutrients that should be consumed daily by healthy individuals (acronym).
9. Chemical substance in foods that is needed by the body for building and repair.
10. Carbohydrate, protein, and fat are examples.
11. Lifestyle that includes an increased amount of physical activity.
12. Maximum intake of a specific nutrient that is unlikely to create adverse health risks for an individual (acronym).
13. Foods that do not lower the pH of biofilm or foods that encourage remineralization.
14. Lifestyle that includes only light physical activity on a day-to-day basis.
15. Comprehensive term that encompasses all categories of dietary reference guidelines (acronym).
16. Term that refers to nutritional inadequacy of specific nutrients in body tissues.

Down

1. Diet consisting only of plant foods.
2. Listing of various foods and measurements of amounts eaten during a specific time period (two words).
3. Foods that lower the pH of oral biofilm and increase risk for dental caries.
4. Refers to comparing the nutrient content of a food with the amount of energy it provides (two words).
6. Poor nourishment resulting from improper food intake.
10. Developed by the USDA to illustrate the food groups important for a balanced diet.

36

Fluorides

LEARNING OBJECTIVES

Upon successful completion of these exercises, you will be able to:

1. Identify and define key terms and concepts related to the use of fluorides.
2. Explain fluoride metabolism, mechanism of action, and effect/benefits of fluoride on pre-eruptive and posteruptive teeth.
3. Describe historical aspects, water supply components, and effects/benefits of water fluoridation.
4. Describe topical fluoride compounds and application methods.
5. Discuss fluoride safety.
6. Plan individualized fluoride prevention interventions.

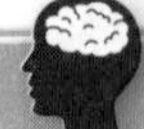

KNOWLEDGE EXERCISES

Write your answers for each question in the space provided.

1. Fluoride is made available to the tooth surface in two ways. Which method has the primary beneficial effect throughout life?

____

____

2. **True or false** (circle one) Fluoride can be lost slowly from the teeth over time due to resorption or remodeling.

3. Describe how dietary fluoride is absorbed by and distributed to body tissues.

____

____

____

4. Dietary fluoride is excreted mostly through the ___________.

5. Approximately 99% of fluoride in the body is located in ___________ tissues, such as ___________ and ___________.

6. During the formation of enamel, fluoride is deposited starting at the ___________.

7. Fluoride concentration is greatest in the area of dentin nearest the ______________. (*Hint*: see Figure 36-1.)

8. Too much fluoride ingested during tooth development can result in ___________.

9. Before the tooth erupts but after the crown is completely mineralized, systemic fluoride is deposited on the ___________.

10. Fluoride, from drinking water or from topical fluoride treatments, continues to be deposited on the surface of the tooth after the tooth has __________.

11. Topical fluoride uptake on the tooth surface is most rapid during __________.

12. Topical fluoride concentration in the enamel is highest at the __________ of the enamel.

13. Fluoride level in cementum is high and increases __________.

14. In your own words, describe demineralization.

15. Where does demineralization occur?

16. In early stages of demineralization, which area of the enamel has the greatest fluoride concentration?

17. In your own words, describe remineralization.

18. What is the role of fluoride in the demineralization–remineralization process?

19. What is the effect of fluoride on bacteria?

20. What is dental fluorosis?

21. Who identified fluorine as the element related to the observed changes in tooth enamel and risk for dental caries?

22. Who was Dr. H. Trendley Dean?

23. What is the optimal level of fluoride concentration in community drinking water currently advised by the US Department of Health and Human services for caries prevention?

24. Adding fluoride to the school water supply in communities that do not have access to a fluoridated community water system is one way to benefit children in rural areas. Why is the concentration of fluoride increased from the optimum level when fluoride is added to only the school water supply?

25. When fluoride is removed from the water in a community, one of two possible effects is noted. What are the two possible effects?

26. What compounds are used to fluoridate community water supplies?

27. List factors to investigate when you are trying to determine whether a child needs dietary fluoride supplements.

28. What level of fluoride is typically found in ready-to-feed and reconstituted infant formulas?

29. In what forms can supplementary fluoride be given?

30. If the fluoride water concentration in the community is 0.45 ppm and there is no additional fluoride in the water supply at school, what is the dose of supplemental fluoride that is recommended for a 5-year-old child and her 12-year-old brother?

31. The ideal fluoride regimen for most patients is high frequency, low concentration. That is why fluoridated water is so effective in preventing dental decay for most people. What factors indicate the need for you to include a professionally applied fluoride treatment in your patient's care plan?

32. What are the objectives for a professionally applied topical fluoride?

33. What is the concentration of fluoride ions in a 1.23% acidulated phosphate gel, which you apply to your patient's teeth using a tray?

Which professional fluoride preparation contains the highest concentration of fluoride ions?

34. What professionally applied solution is recommended for infants and small children who are at high risk for dental caries?

35. Which type of fluoride application is considered effective to reduce dentinal hypersensitivity?

36. If your patient presents with a four-unit porcelain anterior bridge, which fluoride preparation is *not* appropriate for you to recommend and why?

37. How are the patient's teeth prepared before painting on a fluoride solution, applying a fluoride varnish, or placing the trays during a professional fluoride application?

38. Briefly list the steps for applying a fluoride varnish.

____

____

____

____

____

____

____

____

____

____

39. Briefly describe techniques for using self-applied fluorides.

____

____

40. Match each of the following descriptions with the appropriate self-applied fluoride *mouthrinse* preparation. Each type of mouthrinse is described more than once in the description column.

Description	Mouthrinse Type
____ Once per week use	A. Low potency/high frequency
____ Recommended for daily use	B. High potency/low frequency
____ Available only as a sodium fluoride preparation	
____ Available as a sodium fluoride, acidulated phosphate fluoride, or a stannous fluoride preparation	
____ Can be purchased as an over-the-counter preparation	
____ Is available in a 0.5% solution	
____ Is available in a high-potency solution that is commonly diluted with water before use	
____ Is sometimes used in school-based fluoride rinse programs	
____ Has been shown to reduce the incidence of dental caries by 30–40% with reports of a 42.5% reduction in caries in primary teeth	

41. Use Infomap 36-1 to help you compare type of fluoride ion and concentrations available in each type of preparation available for recommendation to patients who are at risk for dental caries.

INFOMAP 36-1

PREPARATION TYPE	APF	NAF (OR SODIUM MONOFLUOROPHOSPHATE)
Professional topical fluoride foam or gel preparations		
Self-applied fluoride gel preparations		
Self-applied fluoride rinse preparations		
Fluoride dentifrice preparations		
Fluoride varnish preparations		
Optimally fluoridated water		

42. In your own words, briefly list important safety measures to discuss with your patient when educating about the use of home fluorides.

43. Briefly describe the signs and symptoms of a toxic dose of fluoride.

44. If your patient feels nauseated and has stomach pain after receiving a professional fluoride treatment in your clinic, what is the first thing you should do?

45. What tooth-related, observable symptom is linked to a larger-than-safe dose of systemic fluoride ingested over a long period of time?

46. Supply the acronym or chemical formula that can be used to document each type of fluoride preparation in a patient progress note—just one more time to help you remember!

- *Acidulated phosphate fluoride*
- *Sodium fluoride*
- *Stannous fluoride*

COMPETENCY EXERCISES

Apply information from the chapter and use critical thinking skills to complete the competency exercises. Write responses on paper or create electronic documents to submit your answers.

1. Refer to the patient assessment summary for Melody Crane (aged 15 months). Use the information in the summary to develop dental hygiene diagnosis statements and a plan for interventions related to her risk for early childhood caries.

2. A dental hygienist experienced an unfortunate incident a few days ago while preparing a fluoride treatment for a 6-year-old child patient who weighs 45 pounds. She filled a set of trays with the maximum allowable amount of 2.0% neutral sodium fluoride gel for children (*Hint*: Consult the legend for Figure 36-5 in the textbook) and left the trays sitting on the counter while she exited the room briefly to get permission for the fluoride treatment from the child's mother. She returned moments later to find that the child had picked up the trays and licked every bit of the fluoride gel out of both the upper and the lower tray.

   Calculate the dose of fluoride that the child received in this incident. Does this amount exceed the safely tolerated dose or the certainly lethal dose? *Hint*: Consult textbook Box 36-5B (STDs and CLDs for children) and Figure 36-6 (how to calculate amounts of fluoride).

3. What type of toxic reaction might the child described in the previous scenario experience after ingesting this dosage of fluoride?

4. Give an example of a situation that could lead to chronic fluoride toxicity and discuss what you would include in an education presentation for your patient (or patient's parent) to prevent this from happening.

CHAPTER 36 – PATIENT ASSESSMENT SUMMARY

Patient Name: *Melody Crane* | Age: *15 Months* | Gender: M [F] | ☑ Initial Therapy

☐ Maintenance

Provider Name: *D.H. Student* | Date: *Today* | ☐ Re-evaluation

Chief Complaint:
Toothache and swollen area in lower left jaw. Ulcerated lesion on upper left lip.

Assessment Findings

Health History
- *Frequent Ear Infections – three since birth*
- *Frequent use of liquid antibiotics – contain sweeteners*
- *ASA Classification - II*
- *ADL level - 3*

At Risk For:
- *Early childhood caries*

Social and Dental History
- *Initial dental visit—first teeth present at 6 months*
- *Family drinks mostly bottled or filtered water.*
- *Fluoride toothpaste used 4X per week—unspecified amount of paste*
- *Bottle used two times daily at naptime and bedtime, at-will use of "sippy-cup" for juice*
- *Five–year-old brother with restorations on all primary molars and some anterior teeth.*

At Risk For:
- *Early childhood caries*

Dental Examination
- *Moderate dental biofilm along cervical margins of maxillary incisors*
- *White-spot lesions at cervical of four maxillary incisors*
- *Red maxillary anterior gingiva*

At Risk For:

Periodontal Diagnosis / Case Type and Status
Gingivitis

Caries Management Risk Assessment (CAMBRA) Level:
☐ Low ☐ Moderate ☐ High ☑ Extreme

Dental Hygiene Diagnosis

Problem	Related to (Risk Factors and Etiology)

Planned Inteventions
(to arrest or control disease and regenerate, restore or maintain health)

Clinical	Education/Counseling	Oral Hygiene Instruction / Home Care

EVERYDAY ETHICS

Before completing the learning exercises below, reread and reflect on the Everyday Ethics Scenario and Questions for Consideration in this chapter of the textbook. It may also be useful to review the Dental Hygiene Ethics discussion in Chapter 1, the Ethical Applications in the introduction pages for each section in the textbook, as well as the Codes of Ethics in textbook Appendices I–IV.

Individual Learning Activity

Imagine the scenario from the patient's perspective. How might the patient's response to the questions following the scenario be different from those of the dental hygienist involved?

Collaborative Learning Activity

Work with another student colleague to role-play the scenario. The goal of this exercise is for you and your colleague to work though the alternative actions in order to come to consensus on a solution or response that is acceptable to both of you.

Factors To Teach The Patient

This scenario is related to the following factors listed in this chapter of the textbook:

- ▷ Personal use of fluorides.
- ▷ Need for parental supervision.
- ▷ Determining need for fluoride supplements.
- ▷ Fluorides being a part of the total preventive program.
- ▷ Fluoridation.
- ▷ Bottled drinking water.

In Competency Exercise question #1, you developed a plan for a patient-specific fluoride intervention for Melody Crane. Use the plan you developed and the example conversations in Appendix D as a guide to prepare a conversation that you might use to educate Melody's mother about the fluoride intervention you have planned and about her role in preventing further caries activity for her children.

Word Search Puzzle

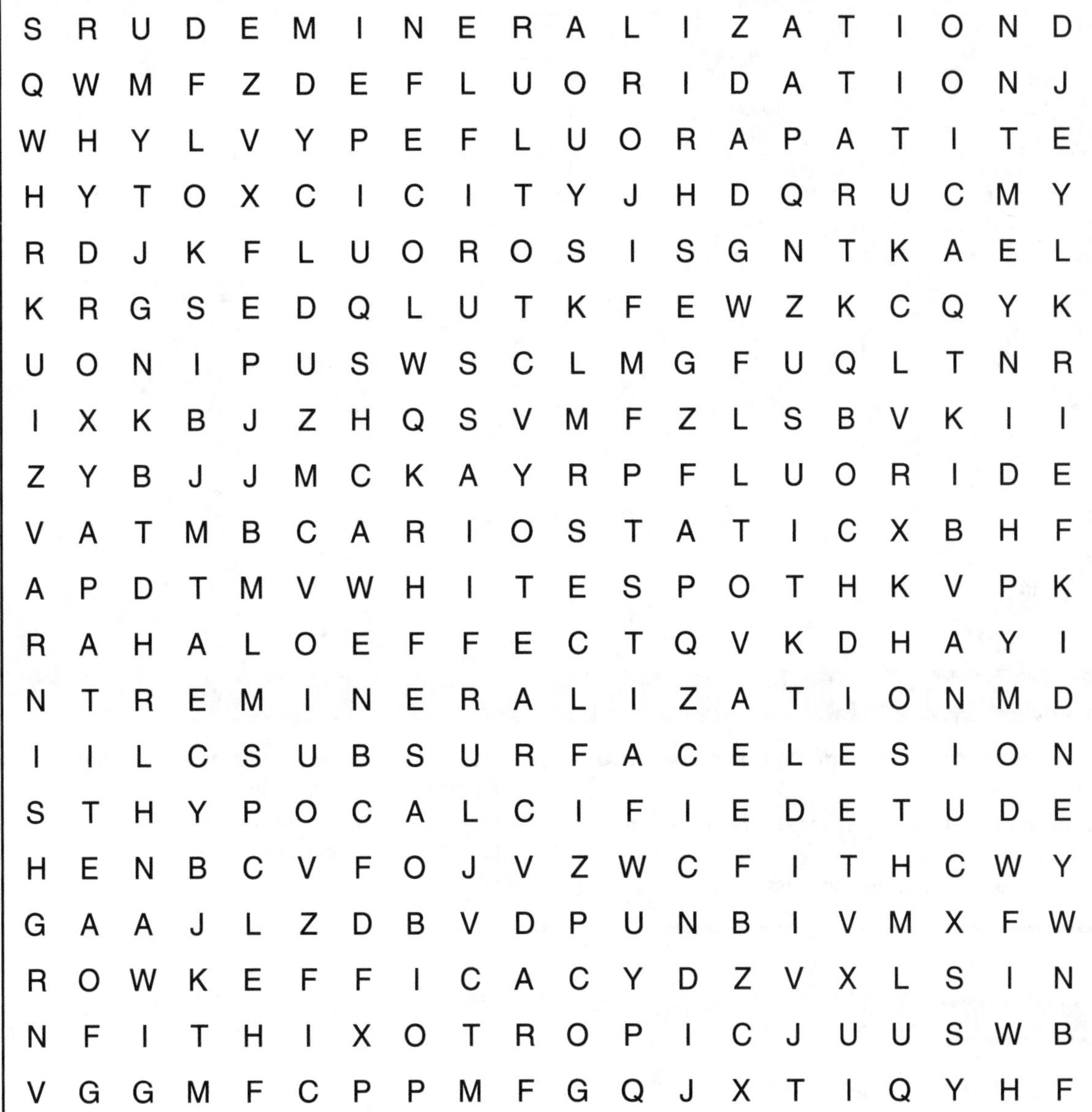

Puzzle Clues

1. Refers to a fluoride preparation with a pH of 3.5 that may etch porcelain (acronym).
2. The researcher who associated Colorado brown stain with drinking water.
3. The result, in an unfluoridated community, of consuming fluoride that has been incorporated into food or beverages during processing (two words).
4. Over the counter (acronym).
5. A small area on the tooth that may be the first clinically detectable caries lesion or an area of demineralization (two words).
6. An area of demineralization below the enamel surface that can become remineralized with fluoride application (two words).
7. $Ca_{10}(PO_4)_6O_2$
8. Inhibiting dental caries
9. The removal of fluoride from a water supply that has a naturally occurring higher-than-optimum fluoride level
10. Breakdown of the tooth structure with a loss of calcium and phosphorus
11. Term referring to the ability of clinically tested products to produce a significant health benefit
12. A less-soluble apatite that is more resistant to acids
13. A systemic nutrient that enhances tooth remineralization
14. Small white spots to severe brown staining and pitting of the enamel caused by pre-eruptive ingestion of excessive amounts of fluoride
15. Most fluoride is excreted from the body through this organ
16. Refers to enamel with deficient calcification
17. Parts per million (abbreviation)
18. Fluoride enhances this process, which returns minerals to the tooth
19. A type of gel that becomes fluid under stress to permit flow
20. This can occur as a result of a rapid intake of high concentration fluoride over a short period of time
21. A form of professional topical fluoride application that is easily applied to root surfaces and sets up in the presence of saliva.

37

Sealants

LEARNING OBJECTIVES

Upon successful completion of these exercises, you will be able to:

1. Identify and define key terms and concepts related to dental sealants.
2. Identify sealant materials and classifications.
3. Describe how dental sealants work to penetrate and fill tooth pits and fissures.
4. Discuss indications for use, clinical procedures for application, and maintenance of dental sealants.

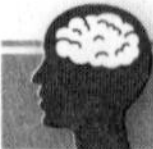

KNOWLEDGE EXERCISES

Write your answers for each question in the space provided.

1. In your own words, describe the purpose of placing a dental sealant.

___

___

___

2. How does the placement of an acid etchant prepare the tooth for a dental sealant?

___

___

___

3. List the criteria for an ideal dental sealant.

___

___

___

___

___

4. The many types of dental sealants have, to some extent, combined or overlapping characteristics. For example, autopolymerized dental sealants can be either clear or opaque in color. Briefly describe the classifications and types of dental sealants.

___

___

___

5. What criteria determine that sealant placement is indicated for a specific patient or tooth?

6. Study Table 37-1 in the textbook and review the section "Clinical Procedures" in Chapter 37 of the textbook to learn the basic procedures for application of dental sealants. List some general rules for sealant application.

7. Number from 1 to 10 to place the action steps for application of dental sealants in the correct order.

Order	Description of Action Step
	___ Check occlusion ___ Isolate tooth (or teeth in a quadrant) ___ Rinse and dry tooth ___ Evaluate (this step occurs twice) ___ Cure or wait for self-polymerization ___ Prepare tooth ___ Place sealant material ___ Dry area and place etchant ___ Prepare patient

8. What is the purpose of debriding and cleaning the tooth surface before etching for sealant placement?

9. What materials can be used to isolate the area receiving a dental sealant?

10. After the tooth surface is etched, rinsed, and completely dried, what should you observe?

11. What anatomic feature may prevent the dental sealant material from penetrating to the bottom of the occlusal fissure?

12. Identify the factors that affect sealant retention.

13. What is documented in the patient record following the placement of a dental sealant?

COMPENTENCY EXERCISES

Apply information from the chapter and use critical thinking skills to complete the competency exercises. Write responses on paper or create electronic documents to submit your answers.

1. You are collecting assessment data during an initial dental hygiene appointment for Dimitri Albergo, who is 12 years old. Dr. Donovan expects you to evaluate the need for dental sealants, record your findings on an assessment form, and then discuss your specific recommendations when he comes in to examine the patient. Together, you will make decisions for including sealants in Dimitri's dental hygiene care plan. What oral findings indicate a potential need for the placement of dental sealants?

2. Discuss why Dimitri's second molars are the most important teeth to evaluate for sealant placement.

3. During your oral examination of Dimitri, you find a pit-and-fissure area on tooth 30 that is questionable for the placement of a dental sealant. What next step will you take to determine whether that specific tooth surface is appropriate for sealant placement?

4. When you evaluate Dimitri's bitewing radiographs, no occlusal or proximal surface dental caries are present on tooth 14. What is the next step in deciding whether or not to select that tooth for placement of a dental sealant?

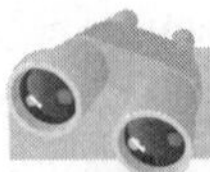

BOX 37-1 MeSH TERMS

Use a combination of MeSH terms and other key words to develop an effective and efficient PubMed literature search strategy.

- Pit-and-fissure sealants
- Acid etching, dental
- Curing lights, dental
- Light curing of dental adhesives
- Resins, synthetic
- Self-curing of dental resins

EVERYDAY ETHICS

Before completing the learning exercises below, reread and reflect on the Everyday Ethics Scenario and Questions for Consideration in this chapter of the textbook. It may also be useful to review the Dental Hygiene Ethics discussion in Chapter 1, the Ethical Applications in the introduction pages for each section in the textbook, as well as the Codes of Ethics in textbook Appendices I–IV.

Individual Learning Activity

Imagine that you are the dental hygienist in this scenario. Answer each of the questions for consideration at the end of the scenario.

Collaborative Learning Activity

Answer each of the questions for consideration at the end of the scenario in the textbook. Compare what you wrote with answers developed by another classmate and discuss differences/similarities.

Factors To Teach The Patient

This scenario is related to the following factors listed in this chapter of the textbook:

- ▷ Sealants as part of a preventive program but not as a substitute for other preventive measures (e.g., limiting dietary sucrose, using fluorides, and controlling dental biofilm).
- ▷ What a sealant is and why such a meticulous application procedure is required.
- ▷ What can be expected from a sealant, including how long it lasts and how it prevents dental caries.

The dental hygiene care plan you develop for Dimitri (introduced in Competency Exercise question 1) recommends dental sealants for all four of his second permanent molars, plus teeth 14 and 3. Dimitri's mother has heard of dental sealants but does not understand why she should spend so much money to "fix" a tooth that has nothing wrong with it. In order to obtain consent from Dimitri's mother to apply the dental sealants, you must educate her.

Use the motivational interviewing principles (see Appendix D) as a guide to develop a conversation to explain dental sealants to Mrs. Albergo.

Crossword Puzzle

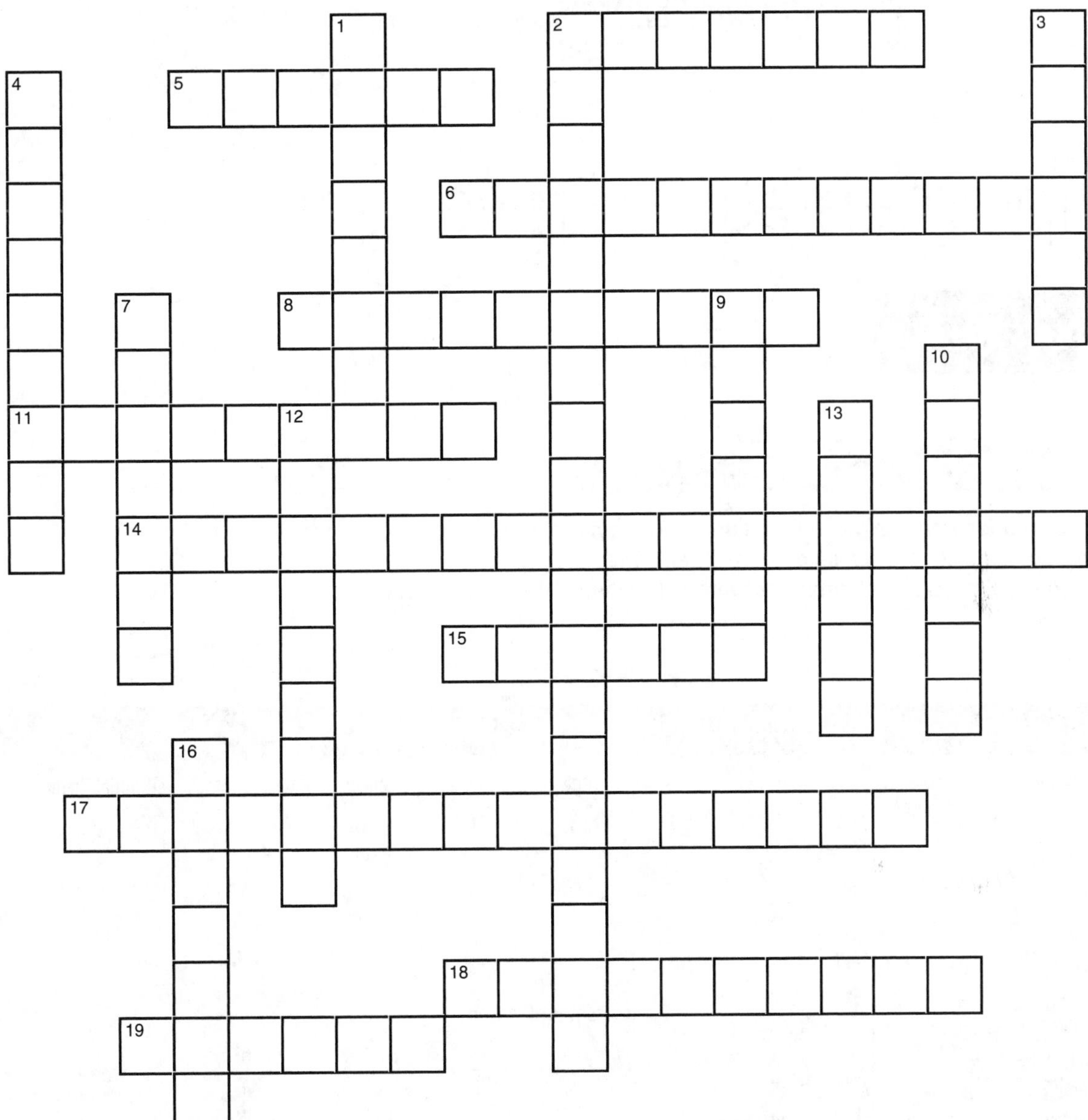

Puzzle Clues

Across

2. A compound of high molecular weight formed by a combination of a chain of simpler molecules.
5. The type of sealant that contains glass, quartz, silica, and other composite materials make the sealant more resistant to abrasion.
6. A type of inked paper ribbon used to determine high spots by marking contacts between maxillary and mandibular teeth.
8. Tiny openings created during the acid etch step of sealant placement.
11. Caries limited to the enamel.
14. The self-curing, hardening process of pit-and-fissure sealants.
15. The process by which the plastic dental sealant becomes rigid.
17. The ability of things to exist together without harm.
18. The type of acid used in a 15%–50% solution to etch the tooth before placement of a dental sealant.
19. Within the living body (two words).

Down

1. Ingredient released by some dental sealants that enhances caries resistance.
2. Polymerization with the use of an external light.
3. Bisphenol A-glycidyl methacrylate (abbreviation, without the hyphen).
4. Resistance to flow as a result of molecular cohesion.
7. Refers to the phosphoric acid solution used to prepare the enamel surface of the tooth prior to placement of dental sealants.
9. Refers to the process of creating irregularities or micropores in the enamel.
10. Under laboratory conditions (two words).
12. Refers to procedures that maintain a dry field during placement of dental sealants to keep saliva from contaminating the area to be etched.
13. The appearance of the surface of a tooth after it is adequately etched and thoroughly dried during sealant application.
16. The physical adherence of a dental sealant to the microspaces between the enamel rods of the tooth structure.

SECTION VI Summary Exercises

Implementation: Prevention

Chapters 26–37

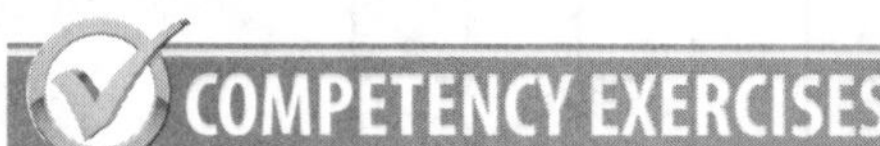

COMPETENCY EXERCISES

Apply information from the chapters and use critical thinking skills to complete the competency exercises. Write responses on paper or create electronic documents to submit your answers.

SECTION VI – PATIENT ASSESSMENT SUMMARY			
Patient Name: *Harold Wilmot*	Age: *44*	Gender: M F	☑ Initial Therapy ☐ Maintenance
Provider Name: *D.H. Student*	Date: *Today*		☐ Re-evaluation
Chief Complaint: *Recently moved into this community—"I need my teeth cleaned."*			
Assessment Findings			
Health History • *Asthma; uses steroid inhaler* • *Hypertension (148/82): controlled with beta-blocker medication* • *Tobacco use: ½ to 1 pack per day for about 25 years* • *ASA classification—II* • *ADL level—0*	**At Risk For:**		
Social and Dental History • *Has had regular dental visits (1 per year); last visit 1 year ago.* • *Has received tobacco cessation education and regular oral hygiene instructions at previous dental visits.* • *Has tried twice to quit smoking, but relapsed because of withdrawal symptoms.*	**At Risk For:**		
Dental Examination • *Complete upper denture; lower partial denture (replaces 23-26, 19, and 30).* • *Generalized recession 1 – 3 mm on remaining teeth; radiographic evidence of generalized slight horizontal bone loss.* • *Probing depths = 5 mm on 31 distal and on mesial and distal surfaces of all premolars; generalized slight bleeding on probing.*	**At Risk For:**		

- *History of coronal and root caries; all current restorations intact; no new cavitated carious lesions.*
- *Moderate calculus on mandibular anterior prostheses; proximal biofilm noted in premolars.*
- *3 mm × 3mm area of leukoplakia on alveolar ridge distal to tooth # 18.*

Periodontal Diagnosis/Case Type and Status	**Caries Management Risk Assessment (CAMBRA) Level:** ☐ Low ☐ Moderate ☐ High ☐ Extreme

DENTAL HYGIENE DIAGNOSIS statements related to PREVENTION interventions	
Problem	**Related to (Risk Factors and Etiology)**

PLANNED INTEVENTIONS related to PREVENTION **(to arrest or control disease and regenerate, restore or maintain health)**	
Education/Counseling	**Oral Hygiene Instruction/Home Care**

Review the Section VI Patient Assessment Summary for Mr. Harold Wilmot to help you answer questions 1–3. The template included with his assessment summary will provide spaces for you to record your answers for these questions.

1. Complete the blank "At Risk For," "Periodontal Diagnosis," and "CAMBRA" sections of the assessment form as best you can with the information in the patient assessment.

2. Write at least three dental hygiene diagnosis statements for Mr. Wilmot's dental hygiene care plan.

3. List the *prevention* interventions you will plan to help Mr. Wilmot *arrest or control disease* and *regenerate, restore, or maintain* oral health.

4. Maria Hernandez is a 19-year-old single mother who has just received health insurance, including dental insurance. This is only her second visit ever to a dentist. The first was when she had a tooth extracted, because of dental caries, at age 14. She presents with swollen gingiva, multiple areas of severe dental caries, and extensive biofilm along the gingival margins of all her teeth. She is 5 months pregnant with her second child and has no other health issues.

   Maria is nearly fluent in English, although Spanish is her first language; she lives with her mother and younger siblings. Maria's first child, who is 4 years old, has been receiving care in the clinic and has, within the last 6 months, had extensive dental work, including crowns and extractions because of dental caries.

   What aspects of prevention will you focus on during a series of perhaps four dental hygiene appointments with Maria?

5. Today you examine Victor Azure, an 11-year-old child who lives on the nearby Navajo reservation with his mother, father, and two older brothers, who attend high school. The results of Victor's dental examination reveal multiple restorations in primary molars and dental sealants on first molars provided by the

dental practice located on the reservation. He has no currently active caries, but you observe a few demineralized areas on the maxillary incisors. You also observe swollen gingiva and extensive biofilm along the gingival margins of all of Victor's teeth.

Victor states that he brushes nearly every day with fluoridated toothpaste but really hates to do it because it is boring. Victor sometimes uses a home fluoride rinse but more often uses a strong-tasting mouthwash that his father likes. Victor states that his father uses the mouthwash because he has bad breath and some of his teeth wiggle. Victor knows some of his remaining primary teeth are getting loose and hopes that the mouthwash will keep him from losing them.

The interview with Victor's mother, Skye, regarding his dental history indicates that Victor was exposed to fluoridated water for only the first 3 years of his life, before the family came back home from Chicago to live on the reservation, which does not have fluoridated water. Victor did not ever visit a dentist until last year, when all the restorative work was done, and his mother states that she plans to try to maintain the regular schedule of visits to the dentist that was recommended when Victor was there 6 months ago.

Skye states that the dentist told her that Victor's high rate of decay is linked to his diet, which is high in frequent carbohydrate intake, including large amounts of carbonated beverages, which he drinks all day long. But she also states that she isn't worried about the high rate of decay in the primary teeth because those are going to fall out soon anyway. She states proudly that she allowed the placement of the sealants to protect his adult teeth from decay.

When you go over Victor's medical history with his mother, you find that except for the fact he is extremely overweight, there are no current health problems. There is, however, a family history of diabetes.

Identify the factors in this case scenario you will address in your plan for preventive dental hygiene care for Victor.

6. Your patient, Mrs. Edmons, makes a frantic telephone call to the clinic this morning. Her normal, healthy, very curious 2-year-old son, Nick, has sucked out and eaten most of a small tube of fruit-flavored toothpaste. She estimates he has consumed about 3 oz. of toothpaste. You ask her to identify the kind and amount of fluoride in the toothpaste. She states the back of the tube indicates 0.15% sodium fluoride. The first step will be to determine the amount of toothpaste Nick has eaten in milliliters. Calculate the amount of fluoride Nick has ingested (see Figure 36-1 in chapter 36). What will you tell Mrs. Edmons?

7. Get together with a group of your student colleagues and gather examples/samples of a variety of adjunctive dental hygiene aids, such as flossing aids or holders, oral irrigators, and different types of interdental cleaners. Each one of you will then be responsible for learning how to use one oral hygiene aid, demonstrating it to all the others in the group and providing feedback to each individual as he or she practices the technique for using the aid.

8. Explore the patient records available in your school clinic to find patients for whom the assessment data indicate a need for preventive interventions. A patient that you have personally collected the assessment data for is probably the best choice, but any patient record will do for this exercise. Use the assessment data to develop a patient-specific dental hygiene care plan for that patient that addresses all the relevant aspects of oral-disease prevention and oral-health promotion discussed in this section of the textbook.

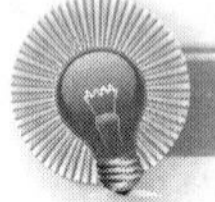

DISCOVERY EXERCISES

1. Identify teaching materials currently available in your school to use for patient education in your clinic. Investigate sources for new or additional materials, and request samples. When you receive them, analyze them for accuracy, readability, and appeal. Decide which ones are most appropriate and valuable for providing information for the patients you will see in your school clinic.

2. Create a product-comparison infomap. This discovery exercise will help you compare chemotherapeutic agents used in dentistry and is best done by working together in small groups of three to six students.

   Step 1: Gather together a variety of mouth rinses, dentifrices, or other dental products that contain chemotherapeutic ingredients recommended by dental hygienists for prevention of dental disease. Have each group member be responsible for finding particular products. You can gather over-the-counter products as well as those that are commonly dispensed only by prescription. You will need to make sure that you have the available packaging information for each product.

   Step 2: Assemble small plastic cups, long cotton swabs, and some paper towels so that you can do a taste test.

   Step 3: Develop an infomap to help you compare these products. There are examples of infomaps throughout this workbook to give you ideas as you develop this one. Your infomap should allow you to compare similar products in such areas as active chemotherapeutic ingredients, alcohol content, ADA Seal of Approval, cost, taste, efficacy of the product based on current research findings, and any other topic areas you think are important for your comparison.

The infomap you create can be used to help you compare products when you are making recommendations to your patients. After your student group develops the basic framework for the infomap, you can continue to add products as you become aware of them in order to keep a currently updated review of products for recommending to your patients.

3. Use the information in the textbook to create an infomap that compares various kinds of manual toothbrushes you can recommend for your patients. How about an infomap comparing the various brands and types of dental floss? What other prevention products could you compare in an Infomap format?

4. Being able to apply evidence-based prevention protocols as we make recommendations for patients requires practice in accessing, analyzing, and applying information from the dental and oral-health literature. Select a prevention topic, and perform a PubMed search to obtain a list of current scientific research articles related to that topic. Obtain the full-text articles either online or at the library.

   Write a short review of the literature to summarize what you learned from reading the articles. Be sure to include recommendations for patient care based on your analysis of the literature.

5. Work with your student colleagues to create an annotated list of websites that provide information on topics related to the prevention of oral disease. Each student should select a topic, and then perform an Internet search using the search engine of his or her choice. Make sure the websites you select provide valid, scientific, and reliable information.

   Write a brief summary of the information you learned from the website, and be sure to include the correct Internet address (URL) at the top of the page. Provide electronic copies of your brief description of the website to your instructor or to a student colleague who is willing to compile the information into one document that can be shared by all students.

6. Investigate prevention in the news. Collect articles from the current popular literature—such as newspapers, magazines, and television or radio announcements—that provide information on prevention of oral diseases. Also look for dental product advertisements that appear in the popular press. This is the information that your patients see and will probably ask you about when you are providing patient education.
   - Is the information that you find presented in the popular media valid and scientifically accurate?
   - How can this information affect the way in which the dental profession is perceived?
   - Does the media information you find agree with the recommendations you make for dental preventive care?

FOR YOUR PORTFOLIO

1. Read the definitions of *behavior change*, *communication style*, *preventive counseling*, and *motivational interviewing* provided in Box 26-1 (in Chapter 26). Combine these definitions to write a personal "Dental Health Educator" philosophy statement.

2. Include a copy of the original product comparison infomap your student group created in the discovery exercise above. As you update the infomap with new product information, also include your most currently updated infomap in your portfolio. Having both the original and the updated infomaps will help demonstrate your commitment to continued learning.

3. Provide written examples to describe dental hygiene education and counseling interventions you have provided for specific patients. Select examples that illustrate your ability to communicate, motivate, and educate particular patients so that positive health outcomes result. Structure your examples so that each includes a discussion of the following:
   - Significant assessment findings
   - Use of the principles of motivational interviewing during patient discussions
   - Prevention topics and methods presented
   - Oral-health techniques demonstrated
   - Method of patient practice used
   - Methods for evaluating success of the patient's compliance, motivation levels, and learning styles (Discuss any factors that affected your ability to communicate with the patient and factors that affected compliance with your recommendations.)

4. Include copies of patient-specific care plans you have developed to illustrate your ability to plan individualized prevention for specific patient cases. Include some early attempts at developing care plans and also some care plans you developed near the end of your student career. Provide a short written analysis of how the early examples compare with the later examples of care planning to demonstrate your growth toward competency in care planning for prevention.

5. Include the literature review you wrote in the discovery exercise above. Later you can update your search to see if there is new information available that might change any recommendations you made in your first review.

6. Collect as many examples of prevention in the news as you can during the time you are a student and jot down notes analyzing each example. Later on you can use your notes to write an analysis of all the examples you collected. Take time to identify trends in how preventive dentistry is presented in the popular media. How does the popular view of dentistry affect the way your patients perceive and are motivated by your prevention interventions and recommendations?

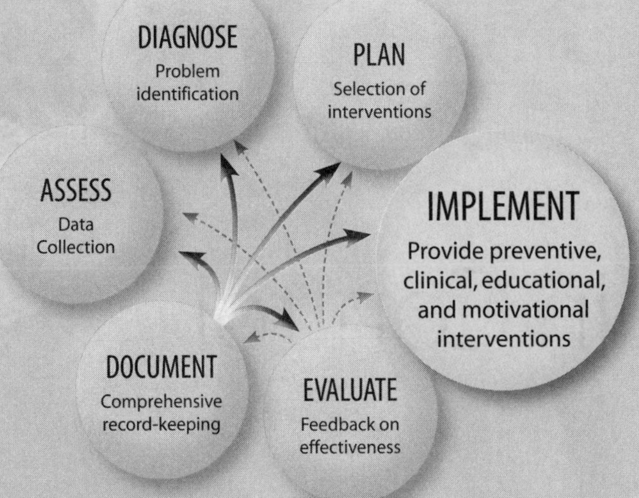

SECTION VII

Implementation: Treatment

Chapters 38-46

SECTION VII LEARNING OBJECTIVES

Completing the exercises in this section of the workbook will prepare you to:

1. Manage patient anxiety and pain during dental hygiene treatment.
2. Provide a variety of dental hygiene treatment interventions.
3. Document clinical dental hygiene treatment.

COMPETENCIES FOR THE DENTAL HYGIENIST

Competencies supported by the learning in Section VII

Core Competencies: C3, C4, C5, C7, C9, C10, C11, C12, C13

Health Promotion and Disease Prevention: HP1, HP2, HP4, HP5, HP6

Patient/Client Care: PC4, PC10, PC11, PC12, PC13

38

Anxiety and Pain Control

LEARNING OBJECTIVES

Upon successful completion of these exercises, you will be able to:

1. Identify and define key terms and concepts related to controlling pain and anxiety.
2. Identify the components of pain and describe a variety of mechanisms for control of dental pain.
3. Describe procedures for nitrous oxide sedation.
4. Describe the pharmacology and method of action of local anesthetics.
5. Describe clinical procedures for administration of anesthesia during dental hygiene treatment.
6. Identify and explain the indications and contraindications for use of anesthesia during dental hygiene treatment.
7. Document pain control measures in patient records.

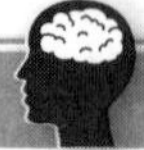

KNOWLEDGE EXERCISES

Write your answers for each question in the space provided.

1. In your own words, describe the interaction between the two components of pain.

2. Describe the difference between an individual with a low pain threshold and a high pain threshold.

3. List the factors that can influence your patient's reaction to dental pain.

4. Which of the five pain-control mechanisms alter pain reaction?

5. Which of the pain-control mechanisms relies for success on your ability to communicate with and educate your patient?

6. Figure 38-1 shows a nitrous oxide delivery system. Label the following components on the figure. It might be useful to use colored pencils (use green for oxygen and blue for nitrous oxide, of course!). Note that some components may not be easy to identify or locate on the figure, but do your best; then investigate or ask your instructor to find out if your idea was correct.
   - *Oxygen tank (add a notation to identify the gas pressure)*
   - *Nitrous oxide tank (add a notation to identify the gas pressure)*
   - *Cylinder valves used to open and close each tank (Hint: There is one on each tank.)*
   - *Hoses that carry only oxygen gas*
   - *Hoses that carry only nitrous oxide gas*
   - *Hoses that can carry both nitrous oxide gas and oxygen*
   - *Regulator or reducing valve (location not discussed in the textbook)*
   - *Flow meter (location not discussed in the textbook) (Hint: The clinician uses this to control the level of each gas administered to the patient.)*
   - *On-demand valve (Hint: Probably located near the flow meter.)*
   - *Reservoir bag*
   - *Nasal hood, nose piece, or mask*
   - *Scavenger system*
   - *Areas where there are connectors (It is important to know where these are because you will regularly need to inspect and test them for potential leaks.)*

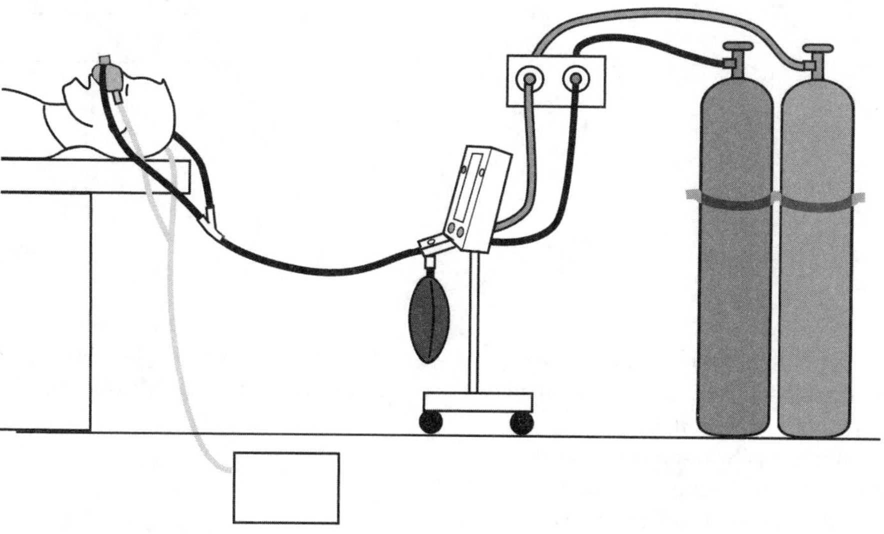

FIGURE 38-1

7. Conscious sedation, produced by administration of a combination of nitrous oxide and oxygen, is frequently used to reduce patient anxiety and perception of pain during short dental procedures that are expected to cause a low level of pain. Identify the two properties of nitrous oxide useful for reducing pain.

8. Why is nitrous oxide sedation especially useful for control of soft tissue discomfort during dental hygiene procedures?

9. What is the appropriate range for percentage of nitrous oxide during dental hygiene procedures?

10. During administration of nitrous oxide analgesia, how much time is usually required for primary saturation of blood to occur?

11. What is the minimum amount of oxygen flow that is maintained by the gas delivery system for patient safety?

12. Describe diffusion hypoxia.

13. How can oxygen hypoxia be prevented?

14. List contraindications for the use of nitrous oxide during dental hygiene care.

15. Attention to the details for providing an effective scavenging system, rigorous equipment maintenance, and the initiation of other methods for preventing overexposure are imperative when nitrous oxide is used during patient care. What are the potential health hazards for clinicians who are exposed to excessive levels of nitrous oxide?

16. Without looking in the textbook, list the steps you will use to administer nitrous oxide–oxygen analgesic during patient care. For each step, when appropriate, indicate the time frame and the amount of oxygen or nitrous flow.

17. In your own words, explain how the nitrous oxide gas is titrated during administration.

18. Identify at least three advantages and three disadvantages of using conscious sedation anesthesia (such as nitrous oxide) to reduce patient pain and anxiety during dental hygiene treatment.

Advantages:

Disadvantages:

19. List three important components to document in your patient's progress notes after you administer nitrous oxide during dental hygiene treatment.

20. Which of the five basic pain-control mechanisms alter pain perception?

21. Describe how a nonopioid analgesic alters pain perception.

22. If pretreatment analgesics are indicated, when should they be administered?

23. List the indications for applying topical anesthetic to reduce your patient's perception of intraoral pain.

24. Identify the active ingredients available as noninjectable or topical anesthetic preparations and the amount of time that each provides anesthesia to the tissues.

25. Match each description below with the correct amide type of local anesthesia. Each type of anesthesia is used more than once; some descriptions apply to more than one type of anesthesia.

Type of Amide Anesthetic	Description
A. Articaine	___ Long-acting amide drug
B. Bupivacaine	___ Short- or medium-acting amide drug
C. Etidocaine	___ Citanest plain and Citanest forte
D. Lidocaine	___ Carbocaine, Polocaine, Isocaine
E. Mepivacaine	___ Duranest
F. Prilocaine	___ Marcaine
	___ Septocaine, Septanest, and Ultracaine
	___ Xylocaine, Octocaine, Lignospan
	___ Available in 1.8 mL of solution in cartridge
	___ Most widely used amide; also available as a topical
	___ Causes less vasodilation, so can be used without a vasoconstrictor
	___ Diffuses best through soft and hard tissues
	___ Provides extended period of analgesia to manage postcare pain
	___ Metabolic by-products can temporarily reduce the oxygen-carrying capacity of blood
	___ Potential drug interaction if patient is taking the drug cimetidine

26. Match each description below with the correct dental cartridge ingredient.

Dental Cartridge Ingredient	Description
A. Amide anesthetic	____ Creates isotonic match with the body
B. Antioxidant	____ Blocks the transfer of ions across the nerve membrane
C. Sodium chloride	____ Constricts blood vessels
D. Sterile water	____ Preservative for the vasoconstrictor
E. Vasoconstrictor	____ Diluting agent

27. Match each description below with the correct group of local anesthesia drugs. Each group is used more than once.

Local Anesthesia Drug Group	Description
A. Amide	____ Currently used only in topical anesthetics
B. Ester	____ Metabolized in blood plasma
	____ Low incidence of allergic reactions
	____ Less effective and shorter acting
	____ Higher incidence of allergic reactions
	____ Less effective and shorter acting
	____ Metabolized by the liver
	____ Causes vasodilation

28. Which ingredient in noninjectable topical anesthetic is most likely to cause an allergic reaction in your patient?

29. Which ingredient in noninjectable topical anesthetic is the most likely to cause a toxic reaction in your patient?

30. In your own words, describe the techniques and armamentarium used for administering noninjectable anesthesia.

31. What techniques can be used to apply topical anesthesia to oral tissues?

32. Identify two vasoconstrictors commonly used in dental anesthetic and indicate the standard concentration of each one.

33. A vasoconstrictor offsets the vasodilating action of the local anesthetic. List reasons for including a vasoconstrictor in local anesthetic solution.

34. What preservative for the vasoconstrictor can cause a potential allergic reaction?

35. What potential drug interactions can cause an adverse reaction when dental anesthetics with vasoconstrictors are used?

36. Name the drug that can be injected to reverse the effects of local anesthetic. What action reverses the effects?

37. What are the sources of information you will use to assess your patient before providing local anesthetic?

38. What patient risk factors will you consider when selecting which local anesthetic solution to use during dental hygiene treatment?

39. What medical conditions indicate the need for patient-specific evaluation and very careful consideration when determining local anesthesia use during dental hygiene treatment?

40. List the armamentarium you will assemble before providing local anesthesia.

41. Why do you position the patient with the head lower than the heart during a local anesthesia injection?

42. What is prevented from happening when you aspirate before injecting local anesthesia solution?

43. In your own words, describe the procedure for aspiration using a conventional anesthetic syringe.

44. The steps for syringe assembly are listed below. Some syringe components are printed in boldface; label each one on Figure 38-2 on the next page.

Step 1: Pull back on the ***thumb ring.***

Step 2: Insert the ***cartridge*** *that contains the selected type of anesthetic. Identify the* ***rubber stopper*** *and the* ***diaphragm end*** *of the cartridge. Identify the* ***volume*** *of solution in the cartridge. Identify the* ***window*** *openings in the syringe that will allow you to view the cartridge during aspiration.*

Step 3: Set the ***harpoon*** *into the appropriate end of the cartridge and test for lock.*

Step 4: Discard the ***safety cap*** *from the* ***cartridge end*** *of the needle.*

Step 5: With your fingers holding the ***needle hub,*** *screw the needle securely onto the end of the syringe. Identify the* ***needle*** *that is used for injection. Indicate the available* ***lengths*** *and* ***diameters*** *of the needles that are used for injecting dental anesthetic.*

In the detail view of the needle tip, identify the ***bevel*** *of the needle and draw a line to indicate where the* ***bone*** *will be relative to the bevel when the needle is inserted for injection.*

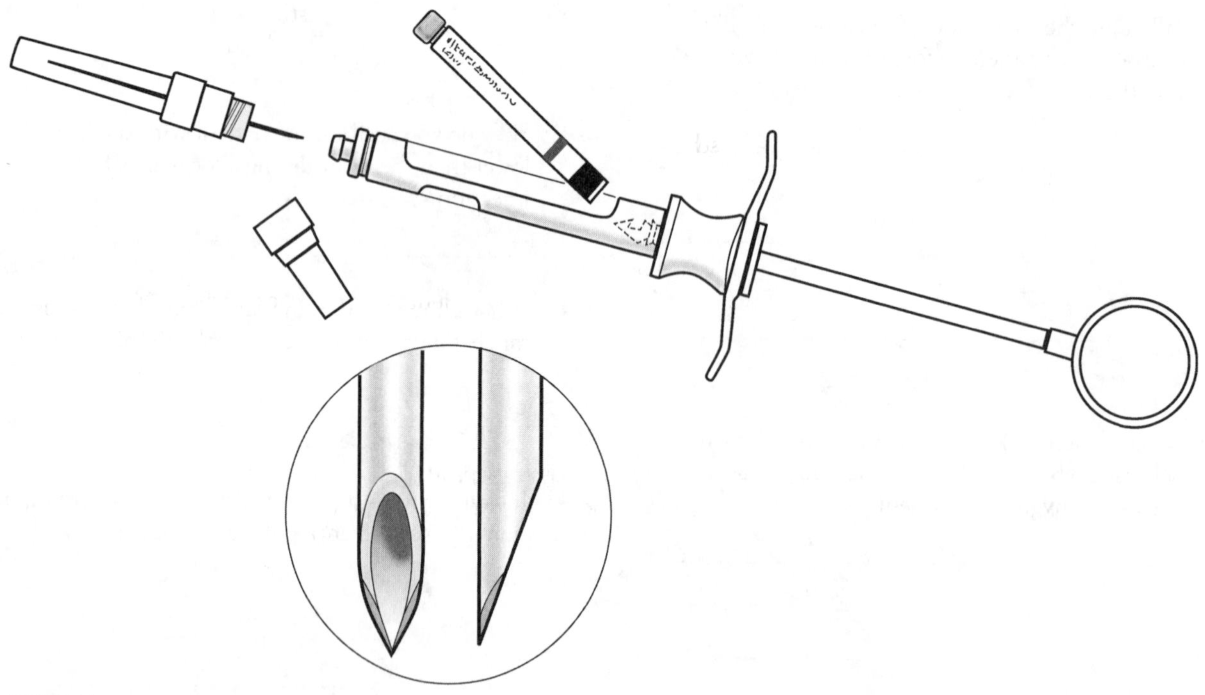

FIGURE 38-2

45. Describe what you will do if you see blood in the anesthetic cartridge when you aspirate while providing local anesthetic for your patient.

46. Identify the proper amount of time for depositing (injecting) a local anesthetic solution. Describe why the local anesthetic solution is deposited slowly.

47. What injections will ensure complete soft and hard tissue anesthesia for your patient when you are providing periodontal treatment for all of the teeth in the mandibular left quadrant.

48. Which injection will be needed to anesthetize the lingual tissue so that complete patient comfort is achieved during dental hygiene procedures in this same area of the mouth?

49. Use a colored pencil to mark Figure 38-3 to identify the areas that are anesthetized after a MSA injection on the right-hand side of the patient's mouth.

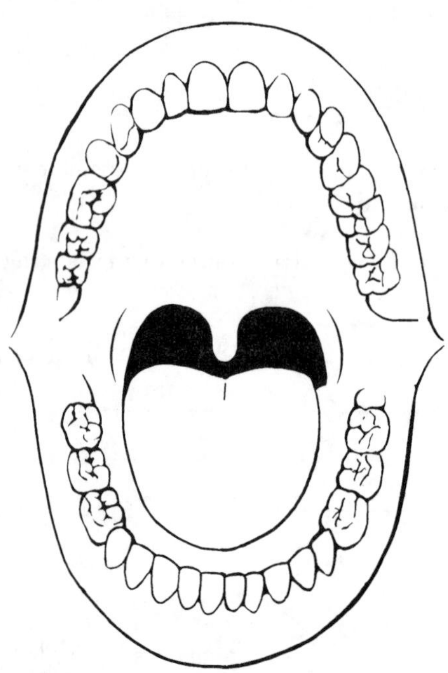

FIGURE 38-3

50. Use a colored pencil to mark Figure 38-3 to identify the area that is anesthetized after the ASA injection on the right-hand side of the patient's mouth.

51. What structure in the molar teeth is not anesthetized after a PSA injection?

____

52. Which injections anesthetize only the terminal nerve endings for one individual tooth?

____

____

____

53. It is imperative to be able to identify the type and the cause of any patient reaction quickly when you are providing local anesthesia. Match each description with the correct symptom. Some symptoms are used more than once; some descriptions apply to more than one type of symptom.

Symptom	Description
A. Adequate anesthesia	____ Anxiety reaction
B. Allergy	____ Can be the result of too rapid absorption of a drug into bloodstream
C. Epithelial desquamation	____ Can indicate that topical anesthetic was left in contact with the tissue for too long
D. Hematoma	____ Can result from reduced ability to eliminate or metabolize the local anesthesia drug
E. Overdose	____ Caused when a vein or artery is opened and leaks blood into the surrounding tissue
F. Paresthesia	____ Experience of a profound effect for the duration of the procedure
G. Psychogenic reaction	____ Extended duration of anesthesia effect
H. Trismus	____ Hypersensitive state that can result in exaggerated response to a subsequent exposure to local anesthesia drug
	____ Onset may range from a few seconds to many hours later
	____ Patients will sometimes report this reaction as an allergy to local anesthesia
	____ Response can range from mild to generalized life-threatening anaphylaxis
	____ Spasm of jaw muscle that restricts opening after injection
	____ Syncope and hyperventilation are the most common responses
	____ Tissue sloughing
	____ Toxic levels of local anesthesia drug are present in the bloodstream
	____ Prevention of these complications relies on the use of excellent injection technique
	____ This response can be made less likely if you use excellent patient communications skills and gentle administration techniques when you are injecting local anesthesia

COMPETENCY EXERCISES

Apply information from the chapter and use critical thinking skills to complete the competency exercises. Write responses on paper or create electronic documents to submit your answers.

1. Today you are presenting your dental hygiene care plan for four-quadrant, initial therapy scaling and root planing to Mr. Shizoka. You will ask the patient to sign an informed consent form before you begin your treatment. Mr. Shizoka does not have much previous dental experience. When you were collecting assessment data for the care plan, he appeared to be very nervous. He asked lots of questions about what you were doing and stopped you frequently when you were trying to probe because he was concerned about whether he would feel pain.

   Mr. Shizoka's medical history indicates that he has iron-deficiency anemia and takes a daily ferrous iron supplement. He has hypertension and takes an antihypertensive medication; however, he tells you that whenever he is highly stressed, he gets a headache. Write a dental hygiene diagnosis statement related to Mr. Shizoka's anxiety about receiving dental hygiene treatment.

2. In the dental hygiene care plan you have developed, you plan to use nitrous oxide–oxygen for pain and anxiety control during Mr. Shizoka's four scaling and root planing appointments. You have already explained to Mr. Shizoka what nitrous oxide–oxygen sedation is and how it works. Explain the advantages and disadvantages so that he can be completely informed about the use of this pain and anxiety control measure.

3. Mr. Shizoka agrees to try the nitrous oxide–oxygen sedation for at least his first dental hygiene appointment to see if he is comfortable with it. Use your institution's guidelines for writing in patient records to document that you have fully informed Mr. Shizoka and that he has agreed to the use of nitrous oxide analgesia during his dental hygiene treatment.

4. At his next appointment, you carefully titrate the nitrous oxide–oxygen combination for Mr. Shizoka, and he shows all the signs of ideal sedation. When you begin the injection of local anesthesia into the area where you will be providing care, Mr. Shizoka becomes agitated and starts moving his arms and legs. His rate of respiration increases significantly, he starts to sweat, and his eyes tear up. You immediately stop injecting the local anesthesia. He says he feels sick to his stomach and wants to sit up. Discuss two possibilities for what is happening in this scenario?
5. What will you do next in the situation that is described in question 4?
6. Use your institution's guidelines for writing in patient records to document what happened today at Mr. Shizoka's dental hygiene appointment.
7. Explain, in patient-appropriate language, how the noninjectable local anesthesia patch is administered.

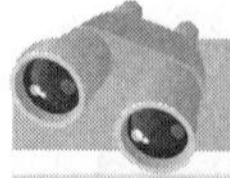

BOX 38-1 MeSH TERMS

Use a combination of MeSH terms and other key words to develop an effective and efficient PubMed literature search strategy.

Anesthesia, dental
Amides
Esters
Bupivacaine
Lidocaine
Mepivacaine
Prilocaine
Vasoconstrictor agents
Epinephrine
Nitrous oxide

EVERYDAY ETHICS

Before completing the learning exercises below, reread and reflect on the Everyday Ethics Scenario and Questions for Consideration in this chapter of the textbook. It may also be useful to review the Dental Hygiene Ethics discussion in Chapter 1, the Ethical Applications in the introduction pages for each section in the textbook, as well as the Codes of Ethics in textbook Appendices I–IV.

Individual Learning Activity

Imagine that you are the dental hygienist in this scenario. Answer each of the questions for consideration at the end of the scenario.

Collaborative Learning Activity

Answer each of the questions for consideration at the end of the scenario in the textbook. Compare what you wrote with answers developed by another classmate and discuss differences/similarities.

Factors To Teach The Patient

This scenario is related to the following factors listed in this chapter of the textbook:

- ▷ Be careful not to bite lip, cheek, or tongue while tissues are without normal sensations. Warn and watch children to prevent injury. Do not test anesthesia by biting the lip.
- ▷ Avoid chewing hard foods and avoid hot food and drinks until normal sensation has returned.

Because a scheduled patient did not arrive and you have some time free, you are asked to spend the time speaking to Miriam's mother. Miriam Carroll is 9 years old. She has many dental problems but is always cooperative during treatment. At Miriam's appointment today, Dr. Steve will extract three primary molar root tips, and both the maxillary and mandibular arches on the left-hand side of her mouth will be anesthetized for the extractions. This is the first time Miriam will experience the effects of local anesthesia.

Using the principles of motivation interviewing (see Appendix D) as a guide, prepare a conversation that you might use to provide postoperative follow-up information to Miriam's mother.

COMPETENCY EXERCISES

Apply information from the chapter and use critical thinking skills to complete the competency exercises.

The only real way to become competent in the skills described in this chapter of the textbook is to practice. It is, of course, difficult to help you do that in a workbook format. But here are some exercises you can do on your own to help you become competent in identifying instruments and practicing the principles of instrumentation. If you'd like, work in small groups with two or three of your student colleagues. Using the information and descriptions in Chapter 39 in the textbook, group members can provide feedback about each person's instrument technique.

1. Gather together a variety of instruments and lay them out on a table in front of you. Examine them carefully and thoroughly, identifying the instrument parts, the types, and the adaptation characteristics (such as the angle of the shank) of each instrument you have available. Then practice picking up the instrument in the modified pen grasp, placing a fulcrum on the tip of the thumb of your nondominant hand, and adapting the blade of the instrument on your fingernail in the correct position for activation.
2. Examine each instrument to determine its characteristics—such as balance, shank length, fabrication materials, and shape and rigidity of the shank. Discuss the purpose and uses of each instrument. Think about area of the mouth the instrument is appropriate for, the technique the instrument is intended for (heavy calculus or root planing, e.g.), and any other indications/contraindications for use that pertain to the instrument's design.
3. Examine each instrument to determine the correct cutting edge and area of the cutting edge most useful for calculus removal.
4. To develop your dexterity, practice each of the strength, stretching, writing, and instrument exercises described in the Dexterity Development section of Chapter 39 in the textbook.
5. Sit comfortably in a chair that has no arms. Practice placing shoulders, arms, elbows, and wrists in a neutral position. While you are sitting there, practice each of the exercises in Figures 39-21–39-23 in the textbook.

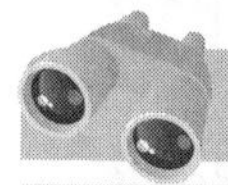

BOX 39-1 MeSH TERMS

Use a combination of MeSH terms and other key words to develop an effective and efficient PubMed literature search strategy.

Dental instruments	Periodontal debridement
Dental prophylaxis	Cumulative trauma disorders
Dental scaling	Carpal tunnel syndrome
Root planing	

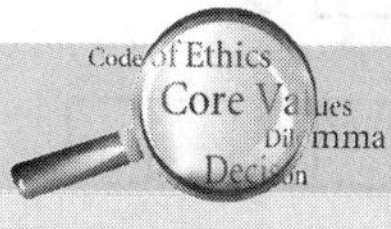

EVERYDAY ETHICS

Before completing the learning exercises below, reread and reflect on the Everyday Ethics Scenario and Questions for Consideration in this chapter of the textbook. It may also be useful to review the Dental Hygiene Ethics discussion in Chapter 1, the Ethical Applications in the introduction pages for each section in the textbook, as well as the Codes of Ethics in textbook Appendices I–IV.

Individual Learning Activity

Imagine that you have observed what happened in the scenario, but are not one of the main characters involved in the situation. Write a reflective journal entry that:

describes how you might have reacted (as an observer—not as a participant),

expresses your personal feelings about what happened,

or

identifies personal values that affect your reaction to the situation.

Discovery Activity

Ask a dental hygienist who has been practicing for a year or more to read the scenario. Provide them with a copy of the Code of Ethics as well. Share the responses you have made to answer each question and ask that person to discuss the situation with you. What insights did you have or what did you learn during this discussion?

Factors To Teach The Patient

This scenario is related to the following factors listed in this chapter of the textbook:

▷ Why it is necessary to use a variety of instruments for scaling.

Today is your first scaling and root-planing appointment with Mr. Nicholas Diamond. When you open your sterilized instruments and line them up on the tray, Mr. Diamond expresses amazement at the number of them and comments on their different shapes.

Write a statement explaining to Mr. Diamond why you have so many different instruments on your tray. Use the conversation you create to educate a patient or friend who is not a student colleague.

Crossword Puzzle

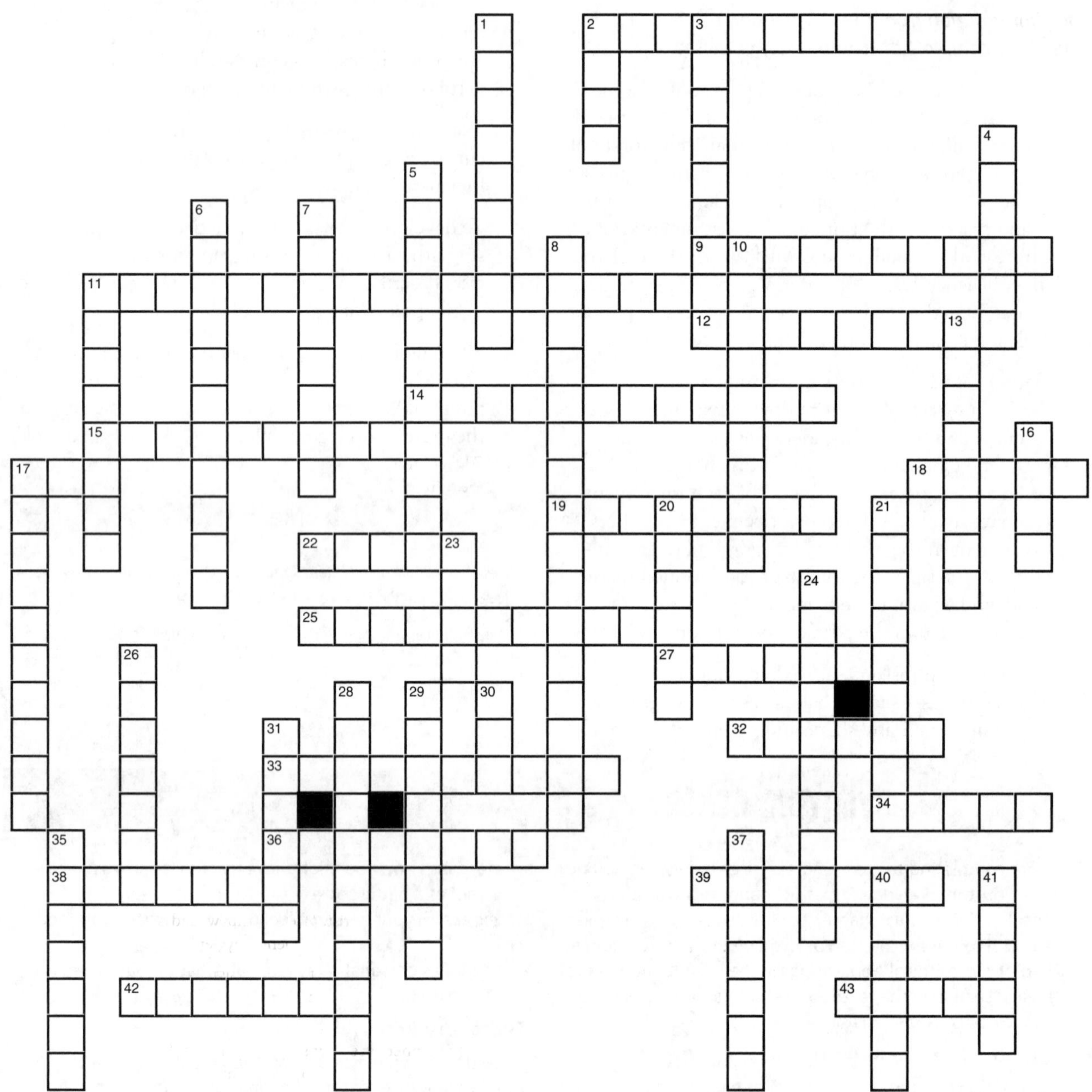

Puzzle Clues

Across

2. A light pressure stroke that disrupts dental biofilm from the root surface of a previously root-planed tooth surface.
9. Relationship between the working end of the instrument and the tooth surface being treated.
11. Area of the tooth where treatment is indicated and the stroke of the dental instrument is applied (two words).
12. This type of lateral pressure can result in gouging of the root surface, patient discomfort, and clinician fatigue.
14. This type of lateral pressure when scaling contributes to burnishing of calculus.
15. The finger that establishes a fulcrum when using a modified pen grasp during instrumentation (two words).
17. A type of scaling instrument that has a single straight cutting edge that is turned at a 99° angle to the shank.
18. The thick, stronger, less flexible instrument shank needed for the removal of heavy calculus deposits.
19. Refers to the size of the instrument handle; usually available in four sizes.
22. Term used to describe the cutting edge of an instrument that is a fine line, has no width, and does not reflect light.
25. This type of instrument has paired working ends that may be either mirror image or complementary (two words).
27. The pressure that is required of an instrument against the tooth during a scaling procedure.
32. This instrument is used to dislodge heavy calculus by pushing horizontally from facial to lingual on the proximal surface of teeth.
33. Provides stabilization and control during instrumentation (two words).
34. Connects the handle and the working end of a dental instrument.
36. This type of instrument shank indicates the instrument is primarily used in anterior teeth.
38. One of three types of strokes that can be applied against the tooth surface with an instrument; a diagonal stroke.
39. To smooth and polish the surface of calculus (usually with an instrument that is not sharp) instead of removing it completely with a well-sharpened instrument.
42. The combined push-and-pull stroke commonly used to activate a periodontal probe.
43. Sharpened working end of a dental instrument.

Down

1. The two cutting edges of this instrument meet at the point of the tip.
2. Term used to describe the cutting edge of an instrument that visually presents a rounded, shiny surface that reflects light.
3. Refers to a stroke that is dependent on the surface texture of the area being instrumented; lighter pressure is applied progressively as strokes continue and the surface becomes smooth (two words).
4. Single, unbroken movement of the instrument as it is applied against the tooth surface.
5. Dental hygiene instrument usually held by the nondominant hand using a modified pen grasp (two words).
6. Refers to the fine line where the face and the lateral surfaces of a well-sharpened dental instrument meet (two words).
7. Refers to the hand that is usually used for holding a scaling instrument during treatment.
8. The hand position that is used to hold a dental instrument (three words).
10. The control, coordination, and strength needed to become proficient in the efficient and effective use of dental instruments.
11. Refers to the use of a mirror to view an area of the mouth.
13. A working stroke parallel with the long axis of the tooth being treated.
16. A type of scaling instrument that has multiple cutting edges lined up on a round, oval, or rectangular base.
17. A working stroke applied parallel with the occlusal surface of the tooth being treated.
20. When you are using the modified pen grasp, the position of the instrument against this finger is extremely important to instrument control.
21. This body part is relaxed and level when working in the neutral position.
23. The type of stroke used when activating most scaling instruments.
24. Refers to the unique area of each instrument used to carry out the purpose and function of that instrument (two words).
26. The position of wrist, forearm, elbow, and shoulder that prevents occupational pain risk for dental hygienists.
28. The type of instrument shank designed to help adapt the instrument to difficult-to-reach areas, such as the distal surfaces of molars (two words).
29. This thinner type of instrument shank may provide more tactile sensitivity and is used to remove fine calculus or for maintenance root debridement.
30. Metal particles removed during sharpening that remain attached to the edge of the instrument.
31. The position of the blade of an area-specific Gracey curet.
35. Stroke that applies definite, well-controlled pressure [illegible]ce of a tooth; refers to instrumentation of a tooth to remove calculus.
37. The support upon which your scaling hand finger rests so force can be exerted during the scaling procedure in order to remove calculus.
40. Refers to any scaling instrument with two cutting edges that meet in a point; can have a curved or straight blade.
41. A scaling instrument with a rounded working end; there are two types: universal and area specific.

40

Instrument Care and Sharpening

LEARNING OBJECTIVES

Upon successful completion of these exercises, you will be able to:

1. Identify and define key terms and concepts related to care and sharpening of dental instruments.
2. Describe and practice basic sharpening techniques for a variety of dental instruments.

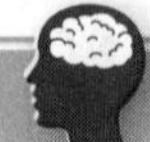

KNOWLEDGE EXERCISES

Write your answers for each question in the space provided.

The following questions help you look at each type of instrument from several perspectives. If possible, have real instruments available to look at as you are doing these exercises so you can thoroughly understand the instruments' similarities and differences and visualize their parts.

1. In your own words, explain the benefits of using carefully sharpened instruments during patient care.

____

____

____

2. Describe the objective and purpose of sharpening the cutting edge of a dental instrument.

____

____

____

____

____

____

3. Two basic sharpening techniques include the moving ____________ and the moving ____________ techniques.

4. When sharpening curets and scalers, the visible angle at which the stone is placed relative to the face of the instrument is ____________ degrees.

5. Without looking at the figure in the textbook, draw a straight line on Figure 40-1 (on the next page) to indicate how the face of the sharpening stone would be placed (and angled) to sharpen *each* of the cutting edges of each instrument shown. After you draw your lines and label each angle, use a protractor to measure those angles. If your diagram is not correct, erase your lines and redraw them using the protractor to help you place the angle of your sharpening stone correctly.

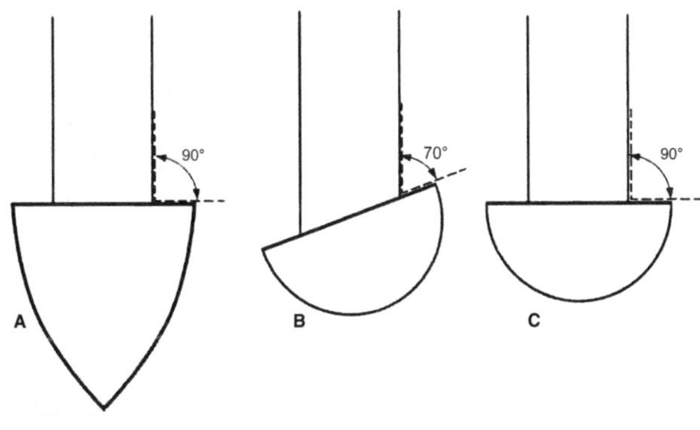

FIGURE 40-1

6. Imagine that you are using the moving-stone technique to sharpen the instruments shown in Figure 40-1. Draw an arrow to indicate the direction of the stroke in which you would apply the most pressure as you move the stone. (*Hint:* This is also the direction you would finish each area as you are sharpening.)

7. In your own words, describe how to care for a flat sharpening stone.

____

____

____

____

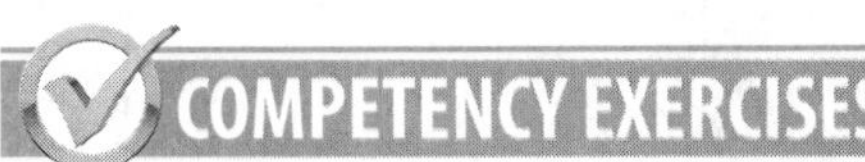

COMPETENCY EXERCISES

Apply information from the chapter and use critical thinking skills to complete the competency exercises.

The only real way to become competent in the skills described in this chapter of the textbook is to practice. It is, of course, difficult to help you do that in a workbook format. However, here are some exercises you can do on your own to help you become competent in identifying instruments and practicing the principles of instrument sharpening. If you'd like, work in small groups with two or three of your student colleagues. Using the information and descriptions in Chapter 40 in the textbook, group members can provide feedback about each person's instrument sharpening technique.

1. Gather together a variety of instruments and lay them out on a table in front of you. Examine them carefully and thoroughly to determine whether the cutting edge is sharp. Practice the correct placement of a sharpening stone to sharpen each instrument.

2. Explain the benefits of telling your patient you always make sure to use a "well-honed" instrument rather than a "sharpened" instrument during patient care.

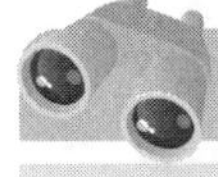

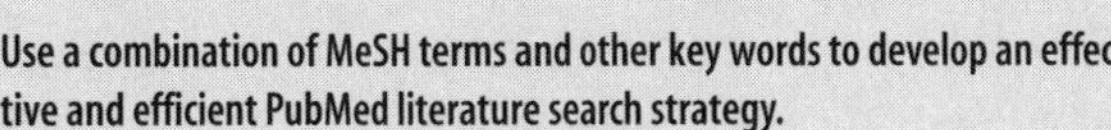

BOX 40-1 MeSH TERMS

Use a combination of MeSH terms and other key words to develop an effective and efficient PubMed literature search strategy.

Dental instruments
Dental scaling
Root planing

EVERYDAY ETHICS

Before completing the learning exercises below, reread and reflect on the Everyday Ethics Scenario and Questions for Consideration in this chapter of the textbook. It may also be useful to review the Dental Hygiene Ethics discussion in Chapter 1, the Ethical Applications in the introduction pages for each section in the textbook, as well as the Codes of Ethics in textbook Appendices I–IV.

Individual Learning Activity

Imagine that you have observed what happened in the scenario, but are not one of the main characters involved in the situation. Write a reflective journal entry that:

describes how you might have reacted (as an observer—not as a participant),

expresses your personal feelings about what happened,

or

identifies personal values that affect your reaction to the situation.

Discovery Activity

Ask a dental hygienist who has been practicing for a year or more to read the scenario. Provide them with a copy of the Code of Ethics as well. Share the responses you have made to answer each question and ask that person to discuss the situation with you. What insights did you have or what did you learn during this discussion?

Factors To Teach The Patient

This scenario is related to the following factors listed in this chapter of the textbook:

- ▷ Benefits of using a finely sharpened instrument for calculus removal.
- ▷ Harmful effects of using dull instruments.

Today is your first scaling and root-planing appointment with Mr. David Crawford. When you begin to check the cutting edges of each instrument before using them, he wants to know what you are looking for.

Write a statement explaining to Mr. Crawford why you always make sure each one of your instruments is well honed before you begin his treatment. Use the conversation you create to educate a patient or friend who is not a student colleague.

Crossword Puzzle

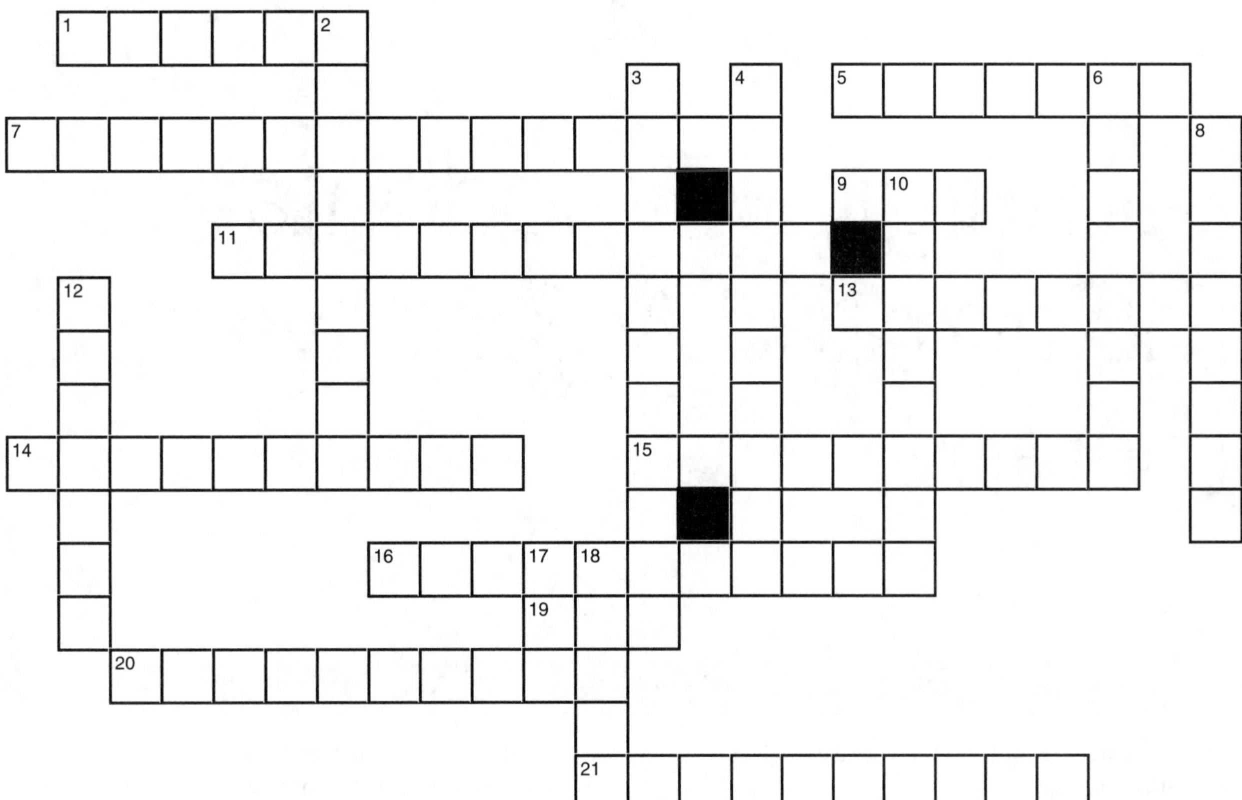

Puzzle Clues

Across

1. A more patient-friendly term for sharpening.
5. A sharpening stone made from quarried mineral stones.
7. Sharpening technique recommended when sharpening with certain quarried stone sharpeners.
9. The number of surfaces to be sharpened on a sickle scaler.
11. Type of curet that is only sharpened on the longer cutting edge (two words).
13. A fine grit natural sharpening stone.
14. Placing the stone at the correct ________________ when sharpening ensures a fine, sharp edge.
15. A file scaler is sharpened with this flat sharpening instrument (two words).
16. The fine line formed between the face and lateral surface of a dental hygiene scaling instrument (two words).
19. The number of surfaces to be sharpened on a hoe scaler.
20. Sharpening stones need to be ______________ prior to use.
21. A ceramic aluminum oxide sharpening stone is this type.

Down

2. Examination of the cutting edge under a light to determine the sharpness of the cutting edge (two words).
3. When using this sharpening technique, the hand holding the instrument is stabilized against an immovable surface (two words).
4. You will feel this when a well-sharpened explorer or scaling instrument is pulled over the surface of a plastic testing stick.
6. Minute particles on a sharpening stone that accomplish the work of grinding the instrument.
8. A sharpening technique that does not use water or a lubricant (two words).
10. Metal particles remaining on the edge of a newly sharpened instrument (two words).
12. This can happen when a dull scaler is passed over tenacious calculus in an attempt to remove the deposit.
17. This rounded portion of the universal curet is sharpened along with the cutting edges on both sides of the face.
18. A natural stone that comes in a variety of grits.

41

Nonsurgical Periodontal Therapy and Adjunctive Therapy

LEARNING OBJECTIVES

Upon successful completion of these exercises, you will be able to:

1. Identify and define key terms and concepts related to nonsurgical periodontal therapy and adjunctive therapy.
2. Define the scope, purpose, and effect of nonsurgical and adjunctive periodontal therapy.
3. Describe appointment preparation and follow-up procedures for nonsurgical and adjunctive periodontal treatment.
4. Identify and describe techniques used for nonsurgical periodontal instrumentation and adjunctive therapy.
5. Describe the types and components of power-driven scalers.
6. Describe and compare delivery methods and types of supplemental antimicrobial therapies for periodontal disease.

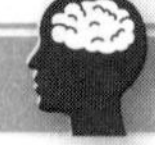

KNOWLEDGE EXERCISES

Write your answers for each question in the space provided.

1. List the components of nonsurgical periodontal therapy.

2. What are the goals of nonsurgical periodontal treatment for the patient with early-to-moderate periodontitis?

3. What are the goals of providing nonsurgical periodontal treatment for the patient with more advanced periodontal conditions?

4. Describe the aims and expected outcomes of providing complete and carefully performed nonsurgical periodontal therapy.

5. Briefly describe the clinical end points that indicate successful nonsurgical periodontal instrumentation?

6. What changes occur in the subgingival microflora after instrumentation procedures during periodontal debridement.

7. List situations that indicate the need to plan multiple appointments for completion of periodontal debridement procedures.

8. In your own words, describe tissue conditioning.

9. If multiple dental hygiene appointments are planned for nonsurgical periodontal therapy, when should you evaluate the success of your initial periodontal debridement?

10. In your own words, briefly describe the process and rationale for a full-mouth disinfection.

11. Describe definitive nonsurgical periodontal therapy.

12. List the steps that will help you formulate your strategy for instrumentation when preparing to provide nonsurgical periodontal instrumentation.

13. What will you look for during a visual examination of your patient's gingival tissues to help you formulate your strategy for instrumentation?

14. Why will you perform a tactile subgingival examination, using a periodontal probe and explorer, before beginning periodontal instrumentation to remove calculus?

15. Why is it important to have your patient's radiographs available for review during scaling and root-planing procedures?

16. What postcare instructions will you provide for your patient following scaling and root-planing procedures?

17. What factors are taken into account when determining a maintenance interval after completion of nonsurgical periodontal treatment?

18. Identify some factors that affect which instruments you will select for calculus removal during an individual patient's nonsurgical care.

19. List the factors and variables that make instrumentation of subgingival surfaces more complex.

20. Some suggested steps for providing manual scaling are listed below. Put the list in the correct order (1 = first step; 10 = last step).

Step Number	Description
_____	Select the correct cutting edge of the instrument.
_____	Stabilize your hand, using a finger rest.
_____	Adapt the toe of the cutting edge of the instrument against the tooth surface.
_____	Use smooth, overlapping, light pressured finishing strokes that provide maximum sensitivity to minute irregularities of the tooth surface.
_____	Apply sufficient (moderate-to-heavy) lateral pressure for calculus removal.
_____	Angle the instrument blade for insertion to the base of the periodontal pocket.
_____	Apply light lateral pressure for instrument insertion and confirmation of soft tissue attachment.
_____	Activate the instrument, maintaining the angulation and adaptation of the cutting edge evenly during the stroke.
_____	Pick up the instrument using a light-modified pen grasp.
_____	Repeat in overlapping, channeled strokes to remove all calculus.

21. What is the purpose of making scaling strokes in overlapping channels during subgingival scaling.

22. In your own words, list some factors or visual cues that will help you ensure the cutting edge of the instrument is correctly adapted on the tooth surface during scaling and root planing.

23. List three factors that will enhance your ability to accomplish successful debridement of a furcation.

24. In your own words, explain endoscope-assisted dental hygiene care.

25. In your own words, explain how a power driven scaler removes calculus and enhances debridement of bacteria in the sulcus or periodontal pocket.

26. Explain cavitation.

27. List the steps used to prepare an ultrasonic unit.

28. Identify important factors to consider when preparing your patient before you use a power-driven scaler.

29. Complete Infomap 41-1 (located on the next page) with information from the textbook to help you compare the different types of power-driven scaling devices.

30. Briefly describe the use of lasers for nonsurgical periodontal therapy.

31. What factors are taken into consideration to determine a continuing care interval once a patient has completed initial therapy?

32. List two ways in which pharmacologic agents are used as adjuncts to scaling and root planing for treatment of periodontal disease.

33. Explain how the appropriate systemically-delivered antibiotic is selected.

INFOMAP 41-1

TYPE	FREQUENCY	MODE OF ACTION	TIP TYPE AND MOVEMENT	WATER USE	CONTRAINDICATIONS, PRECAUTIONS, AND RISK FACTORS FOR USE	PRINCIPLES OF INSTRUMENTATION AND TECHNIQUE FOR USE
Sonic scaler						
Ultrasonic magnetostrictive						
Ultrasonic piezoelectric						

34. List at least four factors that contribute to the success of antimicrobial materials placed directly in an infected periodontal pocket.

35. Describe and compare two antibacterial agents used for direct placement in infected periodontal pockets.

36. Locally delivered antibiotic therapy is contraindicated for patients who are sensitive to ____________________ and for women who are pregnant and breastfeeding.

37. List some potential reasons for recurrence or progression of periodontal disease following treatment.

COMPETENCY EXERCISES

Apply information from the chapter and use critical thinking skills to complete the competency exercises. Write responses on paper or create electronic documents to submit your answers.

The only real way to become competent in the skills described in this chapter of the textbook is to practice. It is, of course, difficult to help you do that in a workbook format. One way to enhance your competency in instrumentation skills is to work with a partner to provide feedback for each other during clinical exercises. Exercise 1 below provides one scenario for you to consider. As you work with student colleagues, you will find many more opportunities to explain and provide feedback on each other's instrumentation skills.

1. You are watching your student colleague, Mary Neely, while she is scaling. You have been designated as her mentor colleague, and your task for today is to give her verbal feedback about all areas of her clinical performance and instrumentation techniques while she is providing patient care. Tomorrow she will observe you providing patient care and will have feedback for you.

   While you are observing Mary, you notice that as she is scaling in the maxillary posterior areas she is having some trouble placing a comfortable fulcrum during her activation stroke. You also observe that as she activates the instrument her wrist motion seems to move the instrument handle from side to side and her hand pivots back and forth on her finger rest.

   Explain what this type of hand motion might indicate about the angle of the blade of the instrument against the surface of the tooth down inside the periodontal pocket. Explain what Mary is doing incorrectly and how she might change the motion of her hand to increase her ability to remove calculus. (*Hint:* You can practice moving your instrument on a typodont or model to help you visualize what you are trying to describe.)

2. Describe how advanced instrumentation strategies can enhance outcomes of treatment for patients with advanced periodontal disease.

3. Explain why it is important to be extremely careful to control the pressure with which you express the liquid when using a cannula to insert antimicrobials into a periodontal pocket.

4. Develop an infomap to help you compare information about the type and amount of active ingredient or agent that is delivered to the sulcus, delivery methods, placement procedures, and care and storage of each of the different types of local delivery antimicrobials.

   To make this a discovery exercise, gather samples of each of the products that are described in the book and use the packaging information to complete the infomap.

   To enhance your ability to make evidence-based decisions for planning patient care, consult Chapter 2 in the textbook and the list of MeSH terms below to help you complete a review of the current literature about one or more of the local delivery systems described in this chapter.

5. You are filling out the patient record for Bruce McDonald after his appointment. Today you placed one cartridge of minocycline in a 6-mm pocket on the mesiolingual surface of tooth #3 and another one in a 7-mm pocket on the mesial surface of tooth #5. You educated Mr. McDonald about the self-care regimens he will follow for the next few days, and you scheduled an appointment for follow-up procedures. Using your institution's guidelines for writing in patient records, document Mr. McDonald's appointment procedures.

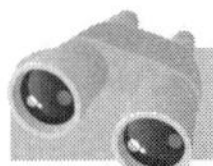

BOX 41-1 MeSH TERMS

Use a combination of MeSH terms and other key words to develop an effective and efficient PubMed literature search strategy.

Periodontal debridement	Chlorhexidine
Root planing	Doxycycline
Subgingival curettage	Minocycline
Dental instruments	Endoscopy
Anti-infective agents	

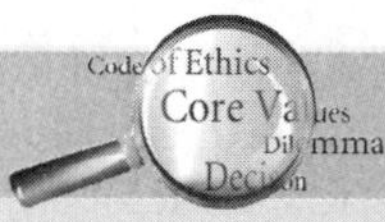

EVERYDAY ETHICS

Before completing the learning exercises below, reread and reflect on the Everyday Ethics Scenario and Questions for Consideration in this chapter of the textbook. It may also be useful to review the Dental Hygiene Ethics discussion in Chapter 1, the Ethical Applications in the introduction pages for each section in the textbook, as well as the Codes of Ethics in textbook Appendices I–IV.

Collaborative Learning Activity

Work with another student colleague to role-play the scenario. The goal of this exercise is for you and your colleague to work though the alternative actions in order to come to consensus on a solution or response that is acceptable to both of you.

Discovery Activity

Ask a dental hygienist who has been practicing for a year or more to read the scenario. Provide them with a copy of the Code of Ethics as well. Share the responses you have made to answer each question and ask that person to discuss the situation with you. What insights did you have or what did you learn during this discussion?

Factors To Teach The Patient

This scenario is related to the following factors listed in this chapter of the textbook:

- ▷ The rationale for re-evaluation following the completion of scaling and root planing.

At the last appointment in a multiple appointment series, during which you have provided quadrant-by-quadrant scaling and root planing for Mr. Davis, you remind him to schedule a treatment evaluation appointment in 3–4 weeks with the front desk manager on his way out. He complains that he really does not want to come to see you one more time this year and he feels that a recall visit 6 months from now will be sufficient.

Use the principles of motivational interviewing (see Appendix D) as a guide to prepare a conversation that you will use to explain the need for final evaluation prior to determining an appropriate recall interval. Use the conversation you create to educate a patient or friend. Then modify your conversation based on what you learned from their feedback.

Crossword Puzzle

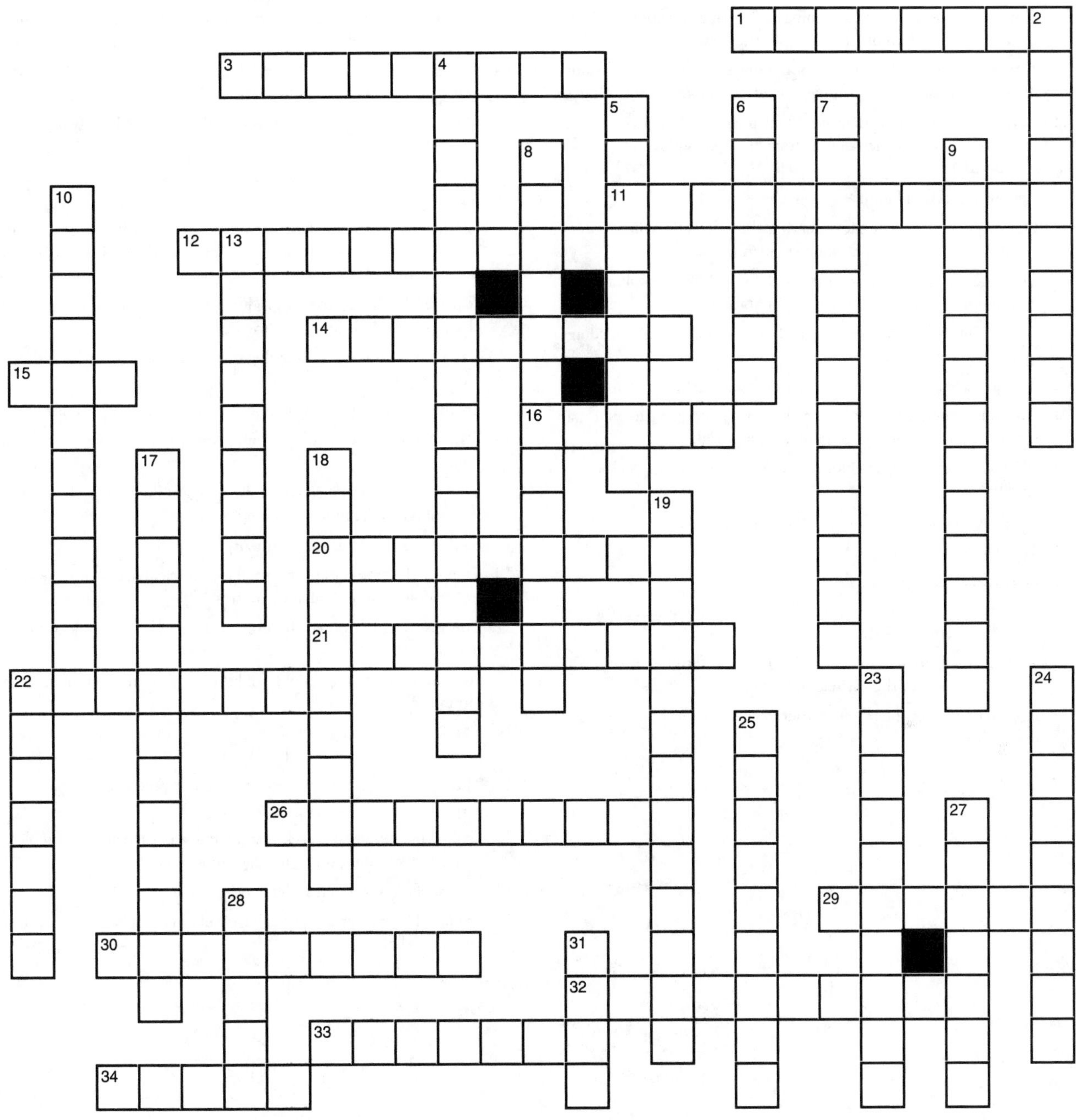

Puzzle Clues

Across

1. Applying pressure and maintaining the cutting edge of the instrument on the tooth in order to remove calculus.
3. A type of area-specific instrument or Gracey curet useful for adapting into concavities and confined furcations during root planing.
11. Definitive periodontal treatment that removes altered cementum or contaminated surface dentin from the root surface of a tooth (two words).
12. Removal of dental biofilm and calculus
14. Lipopolysaccharide complex found in the cell wall of many gram-negative microorganisms; toxic to human tissue.
15. The outermost third of the instrument cutting edge kept in contact with the tooth surface during instrumentation.
16. The amount of lateral pressure used during assessment procedures and instrument insertion.
20. The area between the roots of a multirooted tooth.
21. An agent produced by or obtained from microorganisms that can kill other microorganisms or inhibit their growth.
22. Method of delivering antibiotics to the infected area through blood circulation.
26. A device that converts energy or power from one form to another.
29. Therapeutic washing.
30. kHz; 1,000 cycles per second.
32. The last step of calculus removal in which the clinician uses an explorer to determine the outcome of treatment.
33. Tubular end of an instrument used to introduce antimicrobial medication directly into the periodontal pocket.
34. Another name for the magnetostrictive insert in the handpiece of a power-driven scaler.

Down

2. Type of infection caused by normal flora from the skin, nose, mouth, intestinal, or urogenital tracts.
4. A power-driven scaler that produces tip vibrations by expansion and contraction of a metal stack or rod.
5. Method of delivering minocycline hydrochloride directly into periodontal pocket.
6. Pressure applied during instrumentation.
7. Antimicrobial rinse recommended after nonsurgical periodontal therapy is provided for advanced periodontitis or acute gingival infections; can be used as a preprocedural rinse to reduce microorganisms.
8. A power-driven scaler that produces tip vibrations by dimensional changes in crystals housed in the handpiece.
9. Can be broken down by a biological process, such as by bacterial or enzymatic reaction.
10. Treatment by means of a chemical or pharmaceutical agent.
13. Type of infection caused by acquired organisms that are not normal flora.
17. Type of infection that can occur from organisms not usually harmful if an individual's immune system is impaired or altered.
18. Not responding to usual treatment.
19. Therapy that uses chemical or pharmaceutical agents for the control or destruction of microorganisms.
22. The instrumentation of the crown or root surfaces of a tooth to remove calculus.
23. Formation and collapsing of bubbles in the water surrounding an ultrasonic tip.
24. The speed of movement of the tip of a power-driven scaler; expressed as cycles per second.
25. The distance of tip movement when a power-driven scaler is activated.
27. Scaling technique that uses overlapping strokes to ensure complete removal of calculus from a tooth or root surface.
28. A type of power-driven scaler driven by compressed air.
31. Produced if a power-driven scaler is held in one place on the tooth for a period of time.

42

Acute Periodontal Conditions

LEARNING OBJECTIVES

Upon successful completion of these exercises, you will be able to:

1. Identify and define key terms and concepts related to acute periodontal conditions.
2. Identify the causes, clinical signs and symptoms, and risk factors for acute periodontal infections.
3. Identify the causes, clinical signs and symptoms of PHG.
4. Plan dental hygiene care for a patient with acute periodontal or primary herpetic infections.

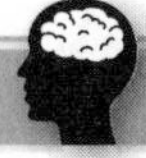

KNOWLEDGE EXERCISES

Write your answers for each question in the space provided.

1. In your own words, explain the difference between an acute and a chronic condition.

2. Describe what you would observe during the examination of a patient diagnosed with necrotizing ulcerative gingivitis.

3. What is a pseudomembrane?

4. Identify and describe the four microscopic layers of the gingival tissue that contain spirochetes in necrotizing lesions.

5. What types of microorganisms are found in greater numbers in necrotizing lesions?

6. What health-related factors can predispose your patient to necrotizing oral conditions?

7. What personal factors predispose an individual to necrotizing oral conditions?

8. What is NUP?

9. Briefly describe necrotizing stomatitis.

10. What is malaise and what additional health-related symptoms may accompany a diagnosis of necrotizing oral conditions?

11. When you are taking the medical history of a patient who presents with signs of necrotizing ulcerative oral lesions, what additional questions will you ask to aid in the diagnosis?

12. In your own words, describe an abscess.

13. What is a fistula?

14. In your own words, define the term *gum boil*.

15. Identify the factors that can cause the formation of a gingival or periodontal abscess.

16. List the classic signs of a periodontal abscess.

17. What are the objectives for immediate treatment if your patient presents with a periodontal abscess?

18. What methods are used to establish drainage of a periodontal abscess?

19. What posttreatment instructions will you give your patient after you have provided dental hygiene care for a periodontal abscess?

20. What is pericoronitis?

21. What is the usual causative agent for PHG and how is it spread?

22. What are the clinical manifestations of PHG?

23. What are the implications of PHG for dental or dental hygiene treatment?

24. What are the oral hygiene concerns during the acute phase of PHG?

COMPENTENCY EXERCISES

Apply information from the chapter and use critical thinking skills to complete the competency exercises. Write responses on paper or create electronic documents to submit your answers.

1. Mr. Rufus is introduced in the Everyday Ethics in Chapter 42 of the textbook. Read about the details of his health history and oral inspection. Then use the Patient-Specific Dental Hygiene Care Plan Template (Appendix B) and the outline for appointments for

acute stage necrotizing infection in Chapter 42 of the textbook to develop a complete care plan for the dental hygiene treatment of Mr. Rufus's condition. Include a plan for follow-up procedures.

2. Develop an infomap or a table that will help you to compare primary gingivostomatitis and NUP. Include information related to signs, symptoms, etiology, oral manifestations, resolution, diagnosis, management, and treatment considerations for each condition.

3. Develop an infomap to compare development, etiology, clinical signs and symptoms, tooth vitality, and radiographic appearances between a periodontal abscess and a pulpal abscess.

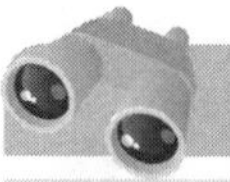

BOX 42-1 MeSH TERMS

Use a combination of MeSH terms and other key words to develop an effective and efficient PubMed literature search strategy.

Periodontal diseases	Gingival diseases
Periodontal cyst	Stomatitis, herpetic
Periapical periodontitis	Gingivitis, necrotizing ulcerative

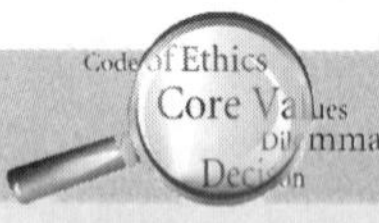

EVERYDAY ETHICS

Before completing the learning exercises below, reread and reflect on the Everyday Ethics Scenario and Questions for Consideration in this chapter of the textbook. It may also be useful to review the Dental Hygiene Ethics discussion in Chapter 1, the Ethical Applications in the introduction pages for each section in the textbook, as well as the Codes of Ethics in textbook Appendices I–IV.

Collaborative Learning Activity

Answer each of the questions for consideration at the end of the scenario in the textbook. Compare what you wrote with answers developed by another classmate and discuss differences/similarities.

Discovery Activity

Ask a dental hygienist who has been practicing for a year or more to read the scenario. Provide them with a copy of the Code of Ethics as well. Share the responses you have made to answer each question and ask that person to discuss the situation with you. What insights did you have or what did you learn during this discussion.

Factors To Teach The Patient

This scenario is related to the following factors listed in this chapter of the textbook:

- ▷ Premature discontinuation of treatment for NUG because acute signs have subsided and can lead to recurrence of the infection.
- ▷ The role of diet, rest, and dental biofilm control in the prevention of NUG.
- ▷ The avoidance of an oral irrigating device in the presence of acute inflammatory conditions. (Microorganisms may be forced into the tissues beneath a pocket, and bacteremia can be produced.)

After you complete the care plan for Mr. Rufus in Competency Exercise question 1, use the details of your plan and the principles of motivational interviewing (see Appendix D) as guides to prepare a conversation educating Mr. Rufus about the condition in his mouth. Explain the dental hygiene interventions you have planned so that Mr. Rufus can give his informed consent for treatment.

43

Sutures and Dressings

LEARNING OBJECTIVES

Upon successful completion of these exercises, you will be able to:

1. Identify and define key terms and concepts related to sutures and periodontal dressings.
2. Identify components/materials used for sutures and periodontal dressings.
3. Explain procedures for placement and removal of sutures and periodontal dressings.
4. Discuss rationale for and provide posttreatment instructions to patients with periodontal dressings.
5. Identify the components of appropriate documentation for surgical treatment, and suture and dressing placement and removal.

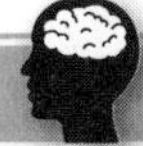

KNOWLEDGE EXERCISES

Write your answers for each question in the space provided.

1. List three functions of postsurgical suture placement.

2. Which type of suture is capable of causing adverse tissue reaction?

3. What type of intraoral sutures must be removed by a dentist or dental hygienist within a specific period of time?

4. Many types of suturing needles are available. What three factors influence selection of a specific type?

5. Which part of the needle is grasped by a needle holder during the suturing procedure?

6. List at least three requirements of an acceptable surgical suture needle.

7. Describe the main reason why suture knots are tied on the facial surface of the alveolar ridge and tied with a 2–3 mm suture tail.

8. How long should removable sutures be left in place?

9. When removing a suture, it is necessary to raise the knot and hold it with a slight tension, slightly depress the tissue with the back of the scissors blade, and cut the suture in the part that was previously buried in the tissue. In your own words, describe why this procedure is followed.

10. Describe the purposes of using a periodontal dressing.

11. Describe the characteristics of an acceptable dressing material.

12. List three disadvantages of zinc oxide with eugenol dressing material.

13. List three advantages of chemical-cured dressings.

14. List the characteristics of a well-placed dressing.

15. Describe the benefit of using a collagen dressing.

16. How long is a surgical dressing typically left in place?

17. Identify a necessary component of the patient dismissal process following the placement of a periodontal dressing.

18. List the components of the detailed documentation required following suture removal.

19. Following the removal of sutures or dressing, when should the return appointment to observe the surgical area be scheduled?

COMPETENCY EXERCISES

Apply information from the chapter and use critical thinking skills to complete the competency exercises. Write responses on paper or create electronic documents to submit your answers.

1. Mrs. Belinda Hawkins had periodontal surgery about 10 days ago. She is scheduled with you this afternoon for suture removal. List and explain the purpose of all the items and instruments you will need to set up in your treatment room to prepare for her postsurgical dressing and suture removal appointment.

2. After you seat Mrs. Hawkins and update her medical history, you examine the surgical areas and find out that the dressing is completely intact on the maxillary arch but that the dressing on the mandibular arch has partly broken off and the sutures are uncovered. One suture appears as though it may be partially imbedded in the dressing material. You note that all areas are fairly free of debris, and the surrounding mucosal tissue looks healthy. Describe the procedure you will use for removing the periodontal dressings.

3. Explain why you need to place each suture on a gauze sponge for postprocedural counting.

4. You gently rinse and examine Mrs. Hawkins' mouth. All areas appear to be healing well, with only slight redness in the area of tooth 30 where the suture had been embedded in the dressing. Explain follow-up bacterial biofilm control procedures to Mrs. Hawkins.

5. Write a progress note to document Mrs. Hawkins' suture removal procedure. Follow your institution's guidelines for writing in patient records.

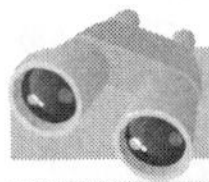

BOX 43-1 MeSH TERMS

Use a combination of MeSH terms and other key words to develop an effective and efficient PubMed literature search strategy.

Periodontal dressings
Eugenol
Sutures

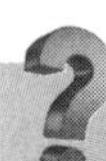

Questions Patients Ask

What sources of information can you identify that will help you answer your patient's questions in this scenario?

When you greet Mrs. Hawkins in the reception room and walk with her back to your treatment room for her suture removal appointment, she is clearly nervous about the impending procedure. She asks, "Will it hurt? Will there be any bleeding?

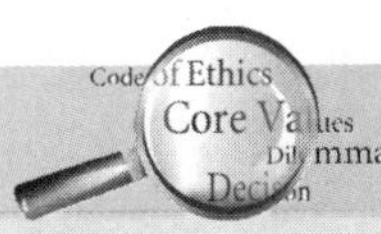

EVERYDAY ETHICS

Before completing the learning exercises below, reread and reflect on the Everyday Ethics Scenario and Questions for Consideration in this chapter of the textbook. It may also be useful to review the Dental Hygiene Ethics discussion in Chapter 1, the Ethical Applications in the introduction pages for each section in the textbook, as well as the Codes of Ethics in textbook Appendices I–IV.

Individual Learning Activity

Imagine that you are the dental hygienist in this scenario. Answer each of the questions for consideration at the end of the scenario.

Discovery Activity

Ask a friend or relative who is not involved in health care to read the scenario and discuss it with you from the perspective of a "patient" who receives services within the healthcare system. Discuss what you learned from the concerns, insights, or difference in perspective that person expressed.

Factors To Teach The Patient

This scenario is related to the following factors listed in this chapter of the textbook:

- ▷ Explanations for the items in Table 43-2 in the textbook.
- ▷ Care of the mouth during the period after surgical treatment while wearing a periodontal dressing.
- ▷ That tobacco use is detrimental and delays healing.

Because you provided initial therapy care for Mr. Bruce Barramundi, you are very interested in observing when he is scheduled for periodontal surgery. After the surgical procedure is complete and the sutures and dressings are placed, you are asked to give him the printed instructions for posttreatment care you created based on Table 43-2 in the textbook.

You know that compliance with recommendations is always better if you provide verbal instructions as well as written. Besides, there are several factors that you think are important to emphasize. You know that Mr. Barramundi is still smoking, even though you have had a conversation about this risk factor. You also know that he has a very vigorous tooth brushing style and is always working very hard to make sure every tiny area of dental biofilm is completely removed.

Use the patient instructions for posttreatment care (Table 43-2 in the textbook) and the principles of motivational interviewing (see Appendix D) as a guide to prepare an outline for a verbal reinforcement of posttreatment instructions for Mr. Barramundi.

Use the conversation you create to role-play this situation with a fellow student. If you are the patient in the role-play, be sure to ask questions. If you are the dental hygienist, try to anticipate questions and answer them in your explanation.

Word Search Puzzle

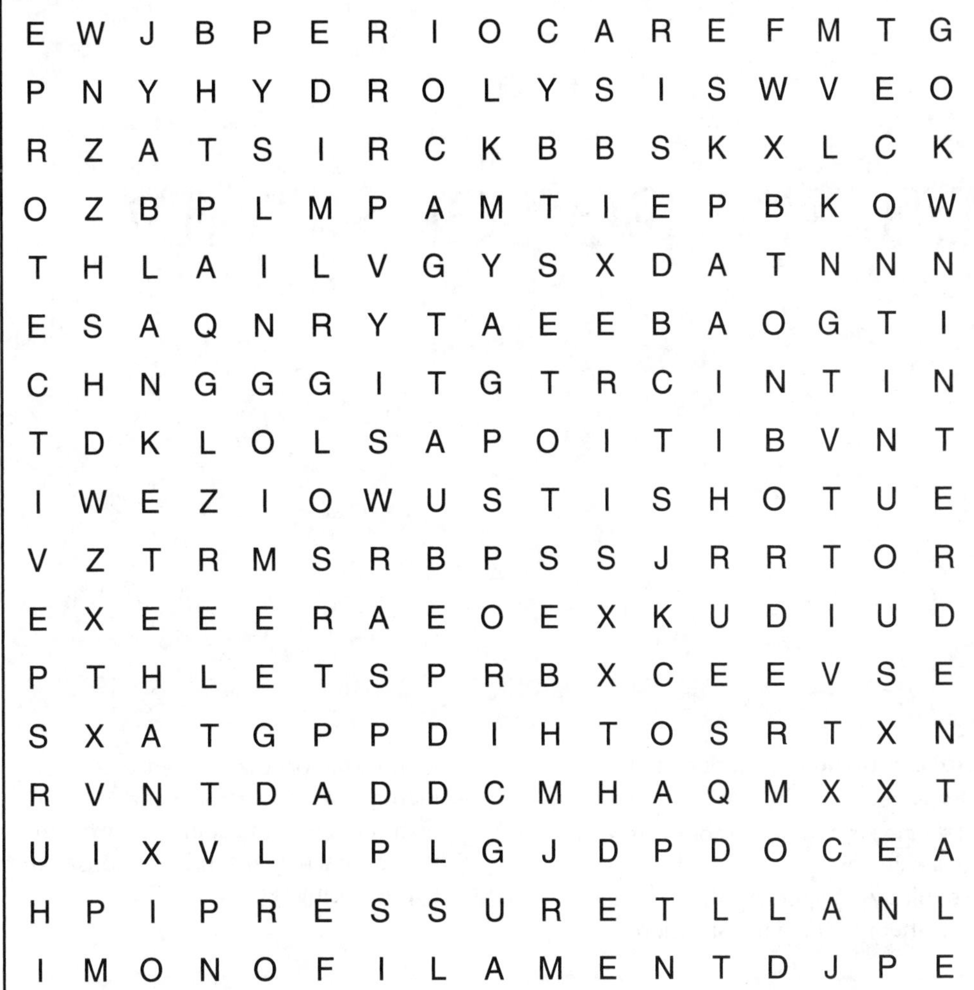

Puzzle Clues

- Suture that is broken down by body enzymes or by water.
- Suturing procedure that forms loops on one side of an incision and a series of stitches directly over the incision; also called a continuous lock.
- Shaping of the peripheries of a dressing by manual manipulation of the tissue adjacent to the borders to duplicate the contour and size of the vestibule (two words).
- Approximate the edges of a wound with no overlap.
- Suture that is an uninterrupted series of stitches tied at one or both ends.
- Material used to cover or protect a wound; also called a pack.
- Termination of bleeding by mechanical or chemical means.
- Process in which water penetrates and causes breakdown of a suture.
- Suture that joins flaps on both the lingual and the facial sides of the dental arch.
- Application of a suture to hold or constrict tissue.
- Single-strand suture.
- Paste–gel type of chemical-cured dressing; a brand name.
- Type of dressing used to control bleeding.
- Type of dressing that shields an area from injury or trauma.
- Suture used when the flap is only one side; also called a suspension suture.
- Important characteristic of a suture or needle for preventing infection.
- Stitch or series of stitches made to secure apposition of the edges of a surgical or traumatic wound.
- Eyeless end of a needle that allows suture material and needle to act as one unit.
- Presence of potentially pathogenic microorganisms.

44

Dentin Hypersensitivity

LEARNING OBJECTIVES

Upon successful completion of these exercises, you will be able to:

1. Identify and define key terms and concepts related to dentin hypersensitivity.
2. Discuss the etiology of hypersensitivity and the hydrodynamic theory of pain transmission.
3. Identify factors that influence desensitization.
4. Identify pain characteristics and determine and document potential differential diagnoses.
5. Plan dental hygiene interventions to manage dentin hypersensitivity.

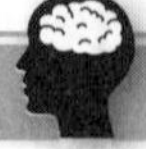

KNOWLEDGE EXERCISES

Write your answers for each question in the space provided.

1. In your own words, define *hypersensitivity*.

 ____

 ____

 ____

 ____

 ____

2. The highest prevalence of hypersensitivity is found in __________. Prevalence and severity usually ____________ in older folks due to the occurrence of natural mechanisms of desensitization.

3. In your own words, list the types of stimuli that can elicit hypersensitivity pain reaction.

 ____

 ____

 ____

 ____

 ____

4. List at least three *patient* behaviors that can trigger a hypersensitivity pain response.

 ____

 ____

 ____

 ____

 ____

5. What condition precedes the development of dentinal hypersensitivity?

6. Describe the role of dentinal tubules in the development of hypersensitivity.

7. There are many, many factors that contribute to gingival recession, subsequent dentin exposure, and potential dentin hypersensitivity. Name as many as you can before looking in the textbook to check your answer.

8. In about __________% of teeth, the enamel and the cementum do not meet, leaving an area of exposed dentin.

9. What factors contribute to erosion on an exposed root surface?

10. In your own words, describe *abfraction*.

11. Which natural desensitization mechanism is related to narrowing of the inside wall of the dentin tubules?

12. A smear layer can reduce dentin sensitivity by blocking the dentin tubules. What causes a smear layer?

13. Explain why a patient may notice sensitivity following the removal of heavy deposits of calculus during a dental hygiene appointment.

14. Pain perception is subjective. What does that statement mean?

15. List the data collected by interview as you assess your patient's dental history of hypersensitivity.

16. Identify two patient response–related diagnostic tests that can be used to determine location and severity of tooth pain.

17. Without looking at the textbook (you won't always have it with you when you are interviewing a patient), identify at least three trigger questions you can ask your patient about tooth pain.

18. You can use a VRS to rate the level of pain your patient is feeling. If your patient describes her

tooth-related pain as a "level 3," what does she mean?

19. Identify the clinical examination techniques and diagnostic tests that can be used to differentiate among the variety of potential causes for dental pain.

20. What are the two basic goals for treatment of dental hypersensitivity?

21. Treatment options offered to the patient should begin with the most ______________ and least ______________ measures.

22. What self-care measures can you suggest to your patient to help reduce dentin hypersensitivity.

23. List at least five factors that you will take into consideration when selecting a desensitizing agent.

24. Briefly explain how the *therapeutic ingredient* in most desensitizing agents work.

25. List as many as you can of the therapeutic ingredients available to improve dental hypersensitivity.

26. Of the agents available for the dental hygienist to recommend for a patient, only ______________ has a substantial body of knowledge validating its usefulness as a desensitizing agent.

27. List two means of physically covering exposed dentinal tubules at the CEJ.

28. How is a laser used to treat hypersensitivity?

29. What dental hygiene procedures can increase potential pain related to hypersensitivity?

COMPETENCY EXERCISES

Apply information from the chapter and use critical thinking skills to complete the competency exercises. Write responses on paper or create electronic documents to submit your answers.

1. Explain how abfraction differs from abrasion.
2. Using patient-appropriate language, describe the hydrodynamic theory.
3. Compare and contrast the two different subjective pain assessment scales (the VAS and the VRS) identified in Box 44-3 in the textbook. Why would you use both of them together for patient assessment?

4. Mr. Mustafa's chief complaint is a frequently occurring, sharply painful sensation on the right-hand side of his mouth. The pain often occurs when he grinds his teeth together during stressful moments at work. He says sometimes that area of his mouth causes pain when he drinks very cold water or chews on cold foods or hard, crunchy foods.

   Dr. Bedron, who is busy with another patient and cannot take time to examine Mr. Mustafa today, asks you to assess Mr. Mustafa's complaint and document your findings and differential diagnosis in the patient record for him to read at the appointment Mr. Mustafa has scheduled with him next week. Your intraoral examination discovers many areas of deep recession along the facial cervical margins, toothbrush abrasion along the facial surfaces of all his molar teeth, and numerous large MOD restorations that were placed a very long time ago. Several of the restorations are beginning to break down, but you do not find any current large carious lesions.

   You know that Dr. Bedron will need to do a very thorough clinical examination and question your patient carefully before he can diagnose the problem. But, using the information you have here and your school's guidelines for writing progress notes, document your differential diagnosis for conditions may potentially be causing Mr. Mustafa's tooth pain? Support your selections using the information in Table 44-1 in the textbook.

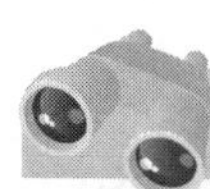

BOX 44-1 MeSH TERMS

Use a combination of MeSH terms and other key words to develop an effective and efficient PubMed literature search strategy.

Dentin	Smear layer
Dentin sensitivity	Pain perception
Dentin Desensitizing Agents	Pain threshold
Fluorides	Pain measurement
Dentin permeability	Tooth abrasion
Dentinal fluid	Gingival recession

Questions Patients Ask

What sources of information can you identify that will help you answer your patient's questions in this scenario?

Some patients express concerns related to a friend's experiences. "My friend bleached her teeth and said that it caused sensitivity. Should I avoid bleaching my teeth?"

A patient may express concern over the diagnosis of hypersensitivity for a specific area. "How do you know that I have sensitivity and not a cavity?"

Many patients will want to understand more completely how the desensitizing agents will work to help their problem. "How soon after I start using sensitivity toothpaste will I notice an improvement in my hypersensitivity? Will I need to use a desensitizing product forever? Will I ever be able to have ice in my summer drinks again? Should I drink my morning orange juice before or after I brush my teeth?"

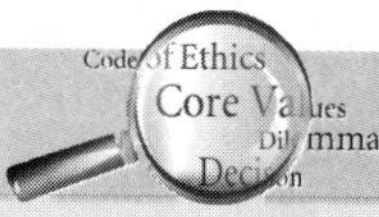

EVERYDAY ETHICS

Before completing the learning exercises below, reread and reflect on the Everyday Ethics Scenario and Questions for Consideration in this chapter of the textbook. It may also be useful to review the Dental Hygiene Ethics discussion in Chapter 1, the Ethical Applications in the introduction pages for each section in the textbook, as well as the Codes of Ethics in textbook Appendices I–IV.

Individual Learning Activities

Imagine that you are the dental hygienist in this scenario. Answer each of the questions for consideration at the end of the scenario.

Imagine the scenario from the patient's perspective. How might the patient's response to the questions following the scenario be different from those of the dental hygienist involved?

Factors To Teach The Patient

This scenario is related to the following factors listed in this chapter of the textbook:

- Contributing factors for dentin hypersensitivity.
- Appropriate oral hygiene self-care techniques, such as using a soft toothbrush and avoiding vigorous brushing, which may contribute to gingival recession and subsequent abrasion of root surface.
- Toothbrushing is not recommended immediately following consumption of acidic foods or beverages.

You are at your desk writing out a dental hygiene care plan for Mrs. Jernigan. Her chief symptom of tooth pain has been diagnosed by Dr. Hockwater as dentin hypersensitivity. Mrs. Jernigan is scheduled with you later this week for education and counseling. This is the first patient you have counseled regarding the management of dentin hypersensitivity, and you want to be thorough.

Use the principles of motivational interviewing (see Appendix D) as a guide to create a conversation and to role-play this situation with a fellow student.

45

Extrinsic Stain Removal

LEARNING OBJECTIVES

Upon successful completion of these exercises, you will be able to:

1. Identify and define key terms and concepts related to removal of extrinsic dental stain.
2. Identify the science, effects, indications, contraindications, precautions, and procedures for selective dental polishing.
3. Describe polishing agents, instruments, and techniques used for removal of extrinsic stains.
4. Identify the components in a progress note that demonstrate documentation of tooth stain removal.

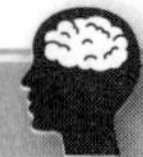

KNOWLEDGE EXERCISES

Write your answers for each question in the space provided.

1. What is the purpose of coronal polishing?

2. List the potential negative effects of polishing.

3. Identify actions you can take and polishing techniques you can use to minimize the negative effects of polishing.

4. Which abrasives commonly used in dental cleaning and polishing agents have a Moh's hardness value that indicates that they are less likely to scratch your patient's exposed tooth surfaces?

5. What characteristics and application principles affect the abrasive action of polishing agents?

   Characteristics of abrasive particles:

   Application principles:

6. In your own words, explain the difference between cleaning and polishing agents.

7. Ultra- or high-speed handpieces rotate between __________ and ___________ revolutions per minute. Low-speed handpieces, typically used for polishing extrinsic stains, rotate between ___________ and ____________ revolutions per minute.

8. Describe the kinds of prophylaxis angle attachments (polishing cups) available for you to use when polishing stain in different areas of the tooth.

9. In your own words, describe the procedure used for applying the polishing agent to an area of stained enamel.

10. How is a bristle brush used?

11. How can stain be removed from proximal surfaces of teeth?

12. What special care is required when using finishing strips to remove stain from proximal surfaces of anterior teeth?

13. How does an air-powder polisher work?

14. List the advantages of air-powder polishing.

15. In your own words, describe the techniques you will use for reducing your exposure to aerosolized spray and for protecting both your patient and yourself when polishing, especially when using an air-powder polisher.

16. What are the indications for polishing?

17. List the clinical findings that indicate you should *not* polish your patient's teeth during the dental hygiene appointment.

18. What is tribiology?

19. What is a three-body abrasive polishing agent?

20. What is the most common cause of aerosol production when using air-powder polishing?

21. Describe potentially negative effects and sequellae of incorrectly directing the handpiece nozzle during air-powder polishing.

22. How can the clinician prevent potential injury while using the air-powder polisher?

COMPETENCY EXERCISES

Apply information from the chapter and use critical thinking skills to complete the competency exercises. Write responses on paper or create electronic documents to submit your answers.

1. What is the difference between polishing and abrasion? In what ways can you produce one but not the other when you remove stain from your patient's teeth?

2. Winston Nottingham always brings you a small packet of tea from England when he comes in for his regular periodontal maintenance appointment. He drinks tea every day, and you usually notice staining on the lingual surfaces of his maxillary and mandibular anterior teeth and on a few lingual proximal surfaces of the lower premolars. He has significant recession, especially on the facial surfaces on his lower molars and the facial and lingual surfaces of his maxillary molars owing to previous history of periodontal infection.

   Write a dental hygiene diagnosis statement identifying Mr. Nottingham's condition in relation to the stain and the recession.

3. What dental hygiene interventions are appropriate for addressing Mr. Nottingham's problem?

4. Using your institution's guidelines for writing in patient records, document the procedure you used to remove the tea stain from Mr. Nottingham's teeth.

5. Mr. Nottingham's son, Will, who is 12 years old, is also your patient. He is in the office for a regularly scheduled 6-month prophylaxis appointment. You are glad he has returned as scheduled, because there are several areas of demineralization that you are monitoring. Will also has significant areas of dental stain because he drinks tea every morning with his parents. You point out the areas of stain to him and you mention that you must polish quite a few areas in his mouth.

   While you are preparing to polish his teeth, Will picks up the container of polishing paste and notices that it contains fluoride. He points that out to you and wants to know why he must also undergo the "icky" fluoride treatment after you finish polishing. He wants to know why you can't just polish all of the areas of his teeth and then skip the regular fluoride treatment completely. Discuss why the use of a fluoride-containing polishing paste is not a replacement for a conventional topical application of fluoride.

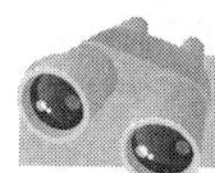

BOX 45-1 MeSH TERMS

Use a combination of MeSH terms and other key words to develop an effective and efficient PubMed literature search strategy.

Dental equipment	Silicon dioxide
Dental polishing	Aerosols
Calcium carbonate	Bacteremia

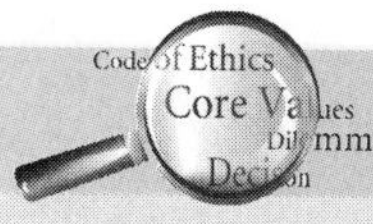

EVERYDAY ETHICS

Before completing the learning exercises below, reread and reflect on the Everyday Ethics Scenario and Questions for Consideration in this chapter of the textbook. It may also be useful to review the Dental Hygiene Ethics discussion in Chapter 1, the Ethical Applications in the introduction pages for each section in the textbook, as well as the Codes of Ethics in textbook Appendices I–IV.

Individual Learning Activity

Identify a situation you have experienced that presents a similar ethical dilemma. Write about what you would do differently now than you did at the time the incident happened—support your discussion with concepts from the dental hygiene codes of ethics.

Discovery Activity

Ask a friend or relative who is not involved in health care to read the scenario and discuss it with you from the perspective of a "patient" who receives services within the healthcare system. Discuss what you learned from the concerns, insights, or difference in perspective that person expressed.

Factors To Teach The Patient

This scenario is related to the following factors listed in this chapter of the textbook:

- ▷ How dental biofilm and stains form on the teeth and their replacements.

As noted in the Everyday Ethics case study for this chapter in the text, Carol explained to Mr. Jackson that colorings from food and drink can stain both natural teeth and the cosmetic restorations he had placed a year ago. Carol encouraged him to cut back on drinking tea, reinforced his role in stain prevention, and stressed the benefits to his appearance of compliance.

Apply the principles of motivational interviewing (see Appendix D) to prepare an outline for a conversation for discussing the concept of stain formation with Mr. Jackson. Use the outline you create as the starting point to educate a patient or friend (not a student colleague) about stain formation.

46

Tooth Bleaching

LEARNING OBJECTIVES

Upon successful completion of these exercises, you will be able to:

1. Identify and define key terms and concepts related to tooth bleaching.
2. Compare types of procedures, and discuss the processes of tooth bleaching systems.
3. Discuss the risks and potential side effects of bleaching.
4. Identify indications and contraindications for dental bleaching treatment.

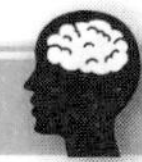

KNOWLEDGE EXERCISES

1. What is the difference between bleaching and whitening?

____

____

____

____

2. External tooth bleaching/whitening procedures can be used for both _________ and ___________ teeth.

3. Describe the process for bleaching nonvital teeth.

____

____

____

4. What ingredients are used for bleaching nonvital teeth?

____

____

5. Describe the mechanism of bleaching vital teeth.

____

____

____

____

____

____

6. Explain the action of each of the two active ingredients used in bleaching systems for vital teeth.

7. Explain the difference in working time for each of the two active ingredients used in bleaching systems for vital teeth.

8. How long does hydrogen peroxide continue to work on the vital tooth after placement?

9. How long does carbamide peroxide continue to work on the vital tooth after placement?

10. List and describe the purpose of additional ingredients used in bleaching systems.

Ingredient(s)	Purpose

11. Identify the safety concerns or effects of bleaching associated with each of the following factors.

Factor	Safety Concerns/Effects of Bleaching
Tooth structure	
Oral soft tissue	
Restorative materials	
Systemic effects	

12. Which vital tooth conditions would respond favorably to tooth bleaching?

13. Which vital tooth conditions do not respond favorably to tooth bleaching?

14. What tooth conditions indicate need for a dental intervention prior to tooth bleaching?

15. Describe effective methods for reducing sensitivity related to bleaching.

16. What factors can influence the final outcome of tooth bleaching treatment?

17. Explain why vital teeth appear whiter immediately after completion of a tooth bleaching procedure.

18. What are the potential *reversible* side effects of bleaching?

19. Identify potential *irreversible* effects of bleaching on tooth structure.

____

____

____

____

20. List methods used for vital tooth bleaching.

____

____

____

____

____

____

COMPETENCY EXERCISES

1. Although many of your patients will desire to have their teeth whitened, each one must be assessed carefully to determine the safety and appropriateness of this dental procedure. Identify contraindications for tooth bleaching. As you answer this question, take into consideration all of the factors you will assess in relation to each of the various types of tooth bleaching systems that are available.

2. Maria Kennedy is a new patient. Right after you seat her in the dental chair, she points to a darkened front tooth and tells you that the tooth had a root canal about 5 years ago. She wants to know why the over-the-counter tooth-whitening product she has applied almost made it look worse. How will you answer her question?

3. As you continue to talk with Maria, you mention that there is a procedure to whiten a nonvital tooth. She gets excited about that possibility and wants to know how the procedure is done. Even though you would like to get started with her complete history assessment and oral exam first, you know that it is important to at least provide a brief answer to her question. How will you explain the procedure to her?

4. During your assessment, you determine there are numerous demineralized areas on the surfaces of Maria's teeth, and you suspect these are probably due to overuse of the whitening products. What interventions will you include in her care plan to address the issue?

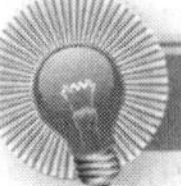

DISCOVERY EXERCISES

Go to the American Dental Association website at http://www.ada.org/ and type the word *whitening* into the search box to find the latest ADA information about whitening products.

Systematic reviews offer the clinician the most reliable research and information. Using the MeSH terms, conduct a literature search by using the following link to PubMed: http://www.ncbi.nlm.nih.gov/pubmed.

Choose clinical queries; then enter the terms in the search box. Learn about the most recent systematic reviews of tooth-whitening products.

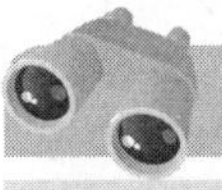

BOX 46-1 MeSH TERMS

Use a combination of MeSH terms and other key words to develop an effective and efficient PubMed literature search strategy.

Esthetics, dental
Tooth bleaching
Tooth bleaching agents
Dentin sensitivity
Enamel microabrasion

Questions Patients Ask

"Which bleaching/whitening method is best?" "How white will my teeth actually get?" "Should I whiten my teeth before or after you place those new fillings in my front teeth?" "Can I have my teeth bleached in the office now and then use an over-the-counter product to keep them white?"

EVERYDAY ETHICS

Before completing the learning exercises below, reread and reflect on the Everyday Ethics Scenario and Questions for Consideration in this chapter of the textbook. It may also be useful to review the Dental Hygiene Ethics discussion in Chapter 1, the Ethical Applications in the introduction pages for each section in the textbook, as well as the Codes of Ethics in textbook Appendices I–IV.

Individual Learning Activity

Imagine that you are the dental hygienist in this scenario. Answer each of the questions for consideration at the end of the scenario.

Discovery Activity

Ask a friend or relative who is not involved in health care to read the scenario and discuss it with you from the perspective of a "patient" who receives services within the health-care system. Discuss what you learned from the concerns, insights, or difference in perspective that person expressed.

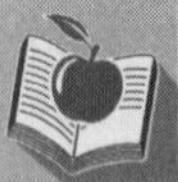

Factors To Teach The Patient

Using the principles of motivational interviewing (Chapter 26) as a guide, write a conversation you could use to obtain informed consent for a light-activated, in-office tooth-bleaching procedure. Use your conversation to educate a patient or a friend, and then modify it based on what you learned from the interaction.

This scenario is related to the following factors:

- ▷ In-office whitening may produce more sensitivity than over-the-counter and at-home products.
- ▷ In most cases, whitening must be periodically repeated to maintain desired tooth color.
- ▷ Existing tooth-colored restorations will not change color, and therefore may not match and may need to be replaced after whitening.

SECTION VII Summary Exercises

Implementation: Treatment

Chapters 38-46

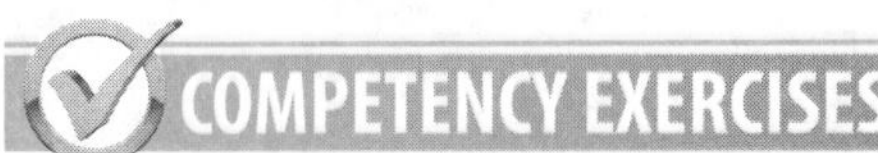

Apply information from the chapters and use critical thinking skills to complete the competency exercises. Write responses on paper or create electronic documents to submit your answers.

<table>
<tr><th colspan="4">SECTION VII – PATIENT ASSESSMENT SUMMARY</th></tr>
<tr><td>Patient Name: Aidan O'Connor

Provider Name: D.H. Student</td><td>Age: 21

Date: Today</td><td>Gender: [M] F</td><td>☑ Initial Therapy
☐ Maintenance
☐ Re-evaluation</td></tr>
<tr><td colspan="4">Chief Complaint:
"I came home from college this weekend and my mother made this appointment for me. I can't believe how much my teeth and gums are hurting. This upper right tooth—I think it is one of the molars—has just been throbbing for the past two weeks. And my mouth tastes terrible, but I can't even brush my teeth because my gums hurt so much!"</td></tr>
<tr><th colspan="4">Assessment Findings</th></tr>
<tr><td colspan="2">Health History
• No medical visits for two years—no current medications.
• High-stress levels related to upcoming end-of-term exams.
• Tobacco use: 1 pack per day for 1 year—mostly while studying.
• Alcohol use: usually only 1 alcoholic drink daily –however, on questioning, he admits to occasional excess in alcohol use as a stress reduction measure.
• ASA classification—I
• ADL level—0</td><td colspan="2">At Risk For:</td></tr>
<tr><td colspan="2">Social and Dental History
• Had regular dental care as a child; most recent visit was 2 years ago.
• Denies neglect of regular daily oral hygiene measures except for the past week or so when mouth has been hurting.
• Sips high sucrose, carbonated beverage while studying.</td><td colspan="2">At Risk For:</td></tr>
</table>

Dental Examination	At Risk For:
• *Generalized visible oral biofilm and debris in all areas of mouth.* • *Generalized visible calculus.* • *Generalized erythematic and sloughing gingival tissue; craterlike defects in lower anterior and lower left premolar area.* • *No visible decay; no restorations; intact dental sealants detectable on #14 and #19. Broken sealant remnants on #3 and #30.*	
Periodontal Diagnosis/Case Type and Status:	**Caries Management Risk Assessment (CAMBRA) Level:** ☐ Low ☐ Moderate ☐ High ☐ Extreme
DENTAL HYGIENE DIAGNOSIS statements related to TREATMENT interventions	
Problem	**Clinical Treatment Interventions**
PLANNED INTERVENTIONS **(to arrest or control disease and regenerate, restore or maintain health)**	
Clinical Treatment Interventions	

Review the Section VII Patient Assessment Summary for Aidan O'Connor to help you answer questions 1–3. The template included with his assessment summary will provide spaces for you to record your answers for these questions.

1. Complete the blank "At Risk For," "Periodontal Diagnosis," and "CAMBRA" sections of the assessment form as best you can with the information in the patient assessment.

2. Write at least three dental hygiene diagnosis statements for Aidan's dental hygiene care plan that are related to clinical treatment interventions that are within the scope of dental hygiene practice.

3. List clinical treatment interventions you will plan to help arrest or control disease and regenerate, restore, or maintain oral health in Aidan's mouth.

4. Describe the dental hygiene instruments and procedures you will select and use when you are providing dental hygiene care for each of the following patients. Discuss the rationale for your selections.
   - Mrs. Louise Gaiter presents with heavy, tenacious ledges of subgingival calculus in all areas of her mouth. In most areas of her mouth, you have recorded 3- to 5-mm pocket probing depths, but in several molar areas, there is calculus to the base of 7- to 9-mm pocket probing depths. Her gingival tissues are keratinized from long-term tobacco use.
   - Mr. Randall Forbes presents with spiny or nodular areas of calculus on surfaces just beneath the proximal contact areas of almost all of his teeth. His gingival tissues were bleeding heavily as you recorded probing depths during your assessment.
   - Mrs. Amelia Pritchert, who has had previous periodontal surgery, presents for her continuing care appointment with some areas of slight calculus and no probing depths deeper than 3 mm. But you have recorded 3–4 mm of gingival recession in most of the areas of her mouth.
   - Ms. Claudia Exeter drinks tea. She has very slight supragingival calculus in a few areas of her mouth but has a generalized moderate extrinsic stain on most of her tooth surfaces.
   - Amal, who is 8 years old, presents with slight lower anterior calculus, generalized dental biofilm, and moderate gingivitis with bleeding on probing in all areas of his mouth.
   - Mr. Robert Galen presents with slight generalized supragingival and subgingival calculus. He has a dental implant to replace tooth 38.

DISCOVERY EXERCISES

1. Spend time searching the Internet to find manufacturer and/or product websites that provide information about instruments and local anesthesia–related products, such as syringes, cartridges, and needle-safety devices. Create a "Webliography" (similar to an annotated bibliography) that contains a list of web addresses (URLs) for sites providing information about specific dental hygiene–related products; include a brief description of the information each website contains.

2. Use the product information you find to compare current dental hygiene instruments in terms of availability, handle size, design, and price.

3. Search the literature to locate the most current evidence to support the use of a specific dental hygiene therapy, such as root planing, selective polishing, ultrasonic scaling, tooth whitening, or placement of local-delivery antibiotics during the treatment of periodontal disease. Write a brief report on your findings.

4. Search the American Dental Hygienists' Association website (www.adha.org) to find information about which states in the United States allow provision of local anesthesia within the scope of dental hygiene practice. Describe how the ability to provide pain control during dental hygiene procedures can affect the success of the patient's treatment.

5. Research to find out which treatment interventions described in this section of the textbook are legal within the dental hygiene scope of practice.

6. Conduct a review of literature to determine:
   - Types of topical anesthesia that can be applied to an abraded or incompletely healed area.
   - Types of water-based gel that can be used to soften crusted sutures.

FOR YOUR PORTFOLIO

1. Include a Webliography you create about any topic related to dental hygiene care (see Discovery Exercise 1).

2. A brief written report (make sure to cite your references accurately) about the information you gathered during your literature search for Discovery Exercise 3 would provide excellent documentation of your ability to use outside sources to find current information about dental hygiene care.

3. Include a variety of patient care plans you have developed to highlight your expertise at planning patient-specific clinical interventions for your patients.

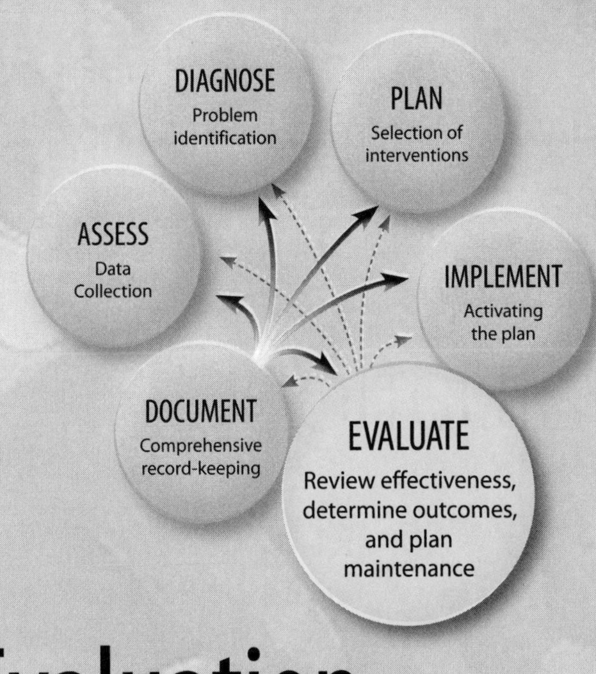

SECTION

VIII

Evaluation

Chapters 47-48

SECTION VIII LEARNING OBJECTIVES

Completing the exercises in this section of the workbook will prepare you to:

1. Identify key concepts in evaluating the outcomes of dental hygiene interventions.
2. Apply outcomes assessment findings to plan maintenance care.
3. Document patient outcomes and recommendations for follow-up and continuing care.

COMPETENCIES FOR THE DENTAL HYGIENIST (Appendix A)

Competencies supported by the learning in Section VIII

Core Competencies: C3, C4, C5, C6, C7, C9, C10, C11, C12, C13

Health Promotion and Disease Prevention: HP2, HP4, HP5, HP6

Patient Care: PC1, PC2, PC3, PC4, PC11, PC12, PC13

47

Principles of Evaluation

LEARNING OBJECTIVES

After studying this chapter, the student will be able to:

1. Identify and define key terms and concepts related to evaluation of dental hygiene interventions.
2. Discuss standards for dental hygiene practice.
3. Identify skills related to self-assessment and reflective dental hygiene practice.

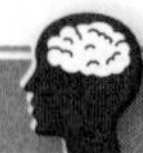

KNOWLEDGE EXERCISES

Write your answers for each question in the space provided.

1. State the purpose of evaluating treatment outcomes at the end of a sequence of dental hygiene interventions.

2. State the purpose of ongoing evaluation during each appointment of a multiappointment treatment sequence.

3. What steps will you take to evaluate the dental hygiene care you provide for each patient?

4. List three ways to evaluate posttreatment outcomes.

5. What is interview evaluation?

6. What is the reason for comparison of pre- and post-treatment assessment findings?

7. List the six categories that provide guidance for adhering to the ADHA standards for clinical dental hygiene practice.

8. List three sources for determining standard of care during a legal dispute.

9. What is the purpose for ongoing self-assessment and personal reflection regarding professional skills and knowledge in dental hygiene practice?

10. Unscramble the following words help you learn about the skills you can develop for reflective dental hygiene practice.

kcabdeef

notiflecer

fwesrsa-lseaen

yanslais (this one is critical)

notleavuai

11. Define three steps that can be used to direct reflective thinking and self-assessment about everyday occurrences related to dental hygiene practice.

COMPETENCY EXERCISES

Apply information from the chapter and use critical thinking skills to complete the competency exercises. Write responses on paper or create electronic documents to submit your answers.

1. Explain the concept of professional standards of care. Discuss the role dental hygiene standards of care can play in ongoing self-assessment and reflective dental hygiene practice.

2. Ms. Olivia Qaba has just moved into your town and is scheduled today as a new patient in your clinic. Dr. Kish briefly examines her, and then you spend the rest of the appointment collecting thorough assessment data and providing the dental hygiene clinical interventions and education required to meet her needs.

   When dental hygiene care is complete, you evaluate treatment outcomes. When you are planning maintenance care for Ms. Qaba (or for any patient), Dr. Kish requires that you consult with him to decide the appropriate continuing care interval for each case. Because Dr. Kish has only briefly examined Ms. Qaba prior to your treatment, he is unlikely to know as much about her as you do after your interaction with her during the series of dental hygiene appointments. What important knowledge do you bring to recommending a continuing care interval for your patient that Dr. Kish may not know after his brief examination? (*Hint*: Think about this question particularly in terms of the indicators you will use to measure the success of your dental hygiene interventions related to health behaviors).

DISCOVERY EXERCISES

Initiate the practice of reflective self-assessment of your professional approach to dental hygiene care by starting a "Critical Incident" journal. Plan to write in the journal at least once every week until you graduate. Each week, select a situation related to your dental hygiene education that poses a question for you, causes you confusion, or is in some way meaningful for your professional development. Follow the three steps and use example questions

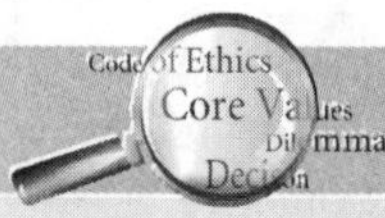

EVERYDAY ETHICS

Before completing the learning exercises below, reread and reflect on the Everyday Ethics Scenario and Questions for Consideration in this chapter of the textbook. It may also be useful to review the Dental Hygiene Ethics discussion in Chapter 1, the Ethical Applications in the introduction pages for each section in the textbook, as well as the Codes of Ethics in textbook Appendices I–IV.

Collaborative Learning Activity

Answer each of the questions for consideration at the end of the scenario in the textbook. Compare what you wrote with answers developed by another classmate and discuss differences/similarities.

Discovery Activity

Ask a dental hygienist who has been practicing for a year or more to read the scenario. Provide them with a copy of the Code of Ethics as well. Share the responses you have made to answer each question and ask that person to discuss the situation with you. What insights did you have or what did you learn during this discussion?

from Table 47-2 in this chapter to write a brief (no more than 1–2 pages) journal entry that describes what happened, analyzes why it was important for your learning or professional practice, and outlines additional learning or next steps that will help you enhance your professionalism, clinical skills, or knowledge.

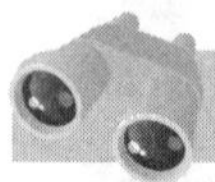

BOX 47-1 MeSH TERMS

Use a combination of MeSH terms and other key words to develop an effective and efficient PubMed literature search strategy.

Outcome assessment (health care)	Self-assessment
Patient outcome assessment	Feedback
Treatment outcome	Standard of care
Data collection	Practice guideline
Analysis	Guideline adherence

Factors To Teach The Patient

This scenario is related to the following factors listed in this chapter of the textbook:

- ▷ The need for evaluation to establish the basis for "next step" treatment and maintenance decisions.
- ▷ How outcomes from dental hygiene interventions are used to determine further treatment needs and maintenance interval.

Salima, the dental hygienist in the Everyday Ethics scenario for this chapter, knows she must educate her patient, Mrs. Midoun, during this appointment about the need to evaluate the outcomes of dental hygiene treatment. Use the motivational interviewing principles found in Appendix D to outline an approach Salima can use as she provides information about the need for outcomes assessment for her patient.

48

Continuing Care

LEARNING OBJECTIVES

Upon successful completion of these exercises, you will be able to:

1. Identify and define key terms and concepts related to the continuing care program in dental hygiene.
2. Identify the purposes, procedures, and methods for planning continuing care.
3. Discuss factors that contribute to recurrence of periodontal infection.

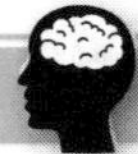

KNOWLEDGE EXERCISES

Write your answers for each question in the space provided.

1. If a disease does not respond to routine therapy, the disease is considered to be resistant, or ________________.

2. The concept of continuing dental hygiene care is introduced to the patient in the initial dental hygiene care plan. Identify the purposes of a periodontal maintenance program for patients who successfully complete initial therapy.

3. List the factors you will consider when deciding upon a continuing care appointment interval that meets your patient's needs.

4. After evaluating the success of your dental hygiene interventions, you will establish your patient's periodontal maintenance interval in consultation with your patient, the attending dentist, and sometimes even the patient's physician. What does the term *consultation* mean?

5. In your own words, define the types or categories of periodontal maintenance therapy.

6. Identify assessment procedures and dental hygiene interventions that are commonly provided during a continuing care dental hygiene appointment.

- Assessment procedures

- Dental hygiene interventions

7. What factors contribute to the recurrence of periodontal disease?

8. You and the attending general dentist will decide together if there is a need to refer your patient to a periodontist for specialized periodontal therapy. Under what conditions might you refer a *new* patient directly to a periodontist?

9. What criteria are used to determine referral when you evaluate treatment outcomes during a periodontal maintenance appointment after you have provided the initial therapy?

10. List factors to consider when scheduling a patient's continuing care interval.

11. A dental clinic continuing care plan can be set up using a card-file system or a computer-assisted approach. Identify two administrative methods for

implementing the scheduling plan and scheduling patient appointments.

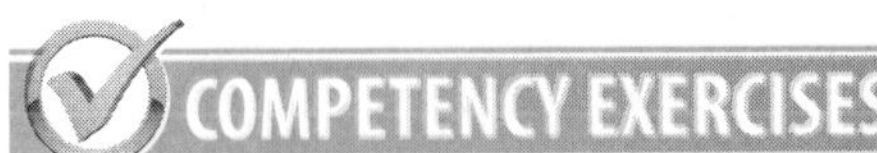

Apply information from the chapter and use critical thinking skills to complete the competency exercises. Write responses on paper or create electronic documents to submit your answers.

1. Many factors contribute to the success of periodontal therapy and the remission or recurrence of periodontal disease.
   - *For which factors are the dental hygienist's actions particularly important in arresting disease?*
   - *How does patient compliance affect the recurrence of periodontal disease?*
   - *What risk factors for recurrence of periodontal disease are not easily modifiable by dental hygiene interventions?*
   - *How do all of these factors interplay when making decisions regarding the frequency of individualized patient maintenance appointments?*

2. Follow your school guidelines to write a progress note documenting maintenance interval recommendations for Mrs. Oaba. (See the Factors to Teach the Patient exercise for this chapter for more information.)

DISCOVERY EXERCISES

Before you do this exercise, take a moment to read Chapter 2 in the textbook. Then read a bit about Ms. Qaba, in the Factors to Teach the Patient exercise below. Develop a PICO question related to determining an appropriate periodontal maintenance interval for Ms. Qaba. Use the PICO question you develop to find evidence in the dental literature to support your maintenance-interval recommendations.

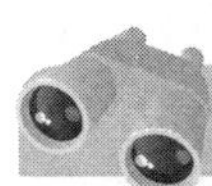

BOX 48-1 MeSH TERMS

Use a combination of MeSH terms and other key words to develop an effective and efficient PubMed literature search strategy.

Comprehensive dental care
Outcome assessment (health care)
Treatment outcome
Treatment failure
Standard of care
Practice guideline
Patient compliance

EVERYDAY ETHICS

Before completing the learning exercises below, reread and reflect on the Everyday Ethics Scenario and Questions for Consideration in this chapter of the textbook. It may also be useful to review the Dental Hygiene Ethics discussion in Chapter 1, the Ethical Applications in the introduction pages for each section in the textbook, as well as the Codes of Ethics in textbook Appendices I–IV.

Individual Learning Activity

Imagine that you are the dental hygienist in this scenario. Answer each of the questions for consideration at the end of the scenario.

Collaborative Learning Activity

Work with another student colleague to role-play the scenario. The goal of this exercise is for you and your colleague to work though the alternative actions in order to come to consensus on a solution or response that is acceptable to both of you.

Factors To Teach The Patient

This scenario is related to the following factors listed in this chapter of the textbook:

- ▷ Purposes of follow-up and continuing care or maintenance appointments.
- ▷ Importance of keeping all maintenance appointments.

Together, you and Dr. Kish decide that a 3-month maintenance interval is appropriate for Ms. Qaba (first introduced in the Competency Exercise in Chapter 47). One reason for this decision is that even though her tissues are healthy right now, she is HIV positive and has a history of significant bone loss from past periodontal infection. You know from her dental history that she has previously been scheduled for 3-month periodontal maintenance, but Ms. Qaba states that she is not sure there is much point to having her teeth cleaned so often. She says that she was really hoping to stretch the interval to 6 months because she no longer has dental insurance.

Use a motivational interviewing approach to write a statement about how you will explain your maintenance-interval recommendation to Ms. Qaba. Make sure to include a discussion of the literature articles you located when you did the aforementioned discovery exercise.

SECTION VIII Summary Exercises

Evaluation

Chapters 47-48

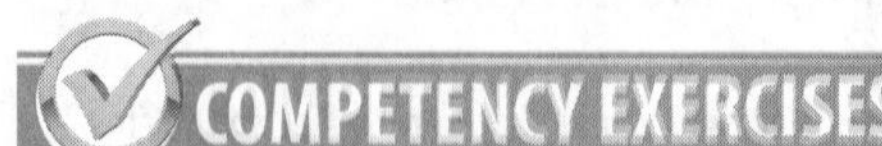

Apply information from the chapter and use critical thinking skills to complete the competency exercises. Write responses on paper or create electronic documents to submit your answers.

Read the Section VIII Patient Assessment Summary to help you answer questions #1 and #2.

SECTION VIII – PATIENT ASSESSMENT SUMMARY			
Patient Name: *Charen Woodmacher*	Age: *15*	Gender: M F	☐ Initial Therapy ☐ Maintenance
Provider Name: *D.H. Student*	Date: *Today*		☑ Re-evaluation

Chief Complaint:
Pt presents for re-evaluation following the completion of a series of quadrant scaling and root planing appointments with significant oral health educational interventions provided at each appointment.

RE-EVALUATION FINDINGS

Retreat ☐ **Refer** ☑ **Continuing care interval:** *6 months recall appointment (in general practice office)*

Description of posttreatment outcomes:
Resolution of carious lesion on tooth #30 (root canal completed, appointment for crown scheduled within 1 month). Patient appears to be more motivated in self-care practices and biofilm levels are significantly reduced. Generalized probing depths are reduced to 3 mm and tissue health improved: reduction in erythema, bulbuous appearance, and generalized bleeding. However, 6–8 mm pockets, with bleeding on probing, have not resolved in lower anterior sextant and in molar areas.

Referral *to physician for complete medical work-up*

Referral *to periodontist for assessment of specialized periodontal treatment needs.*

ASSESSMENT FINDINGS FROM CHAREN WOODMACHER'S PRETREATMENT ASSESSMENT
Provided here for Additional Information

Findings	At Risk For
Health History • *Recent diagnosis of bulimia—currently undergoing psychological assessment and treatment* • *Iron-deficiency anemia* • *Contraceptive pills* • *Daily iron supplement* • *ASA classification: II* • *ADL level: 0*	**At Risk For:** • *Enamel erosion* • *Increased susceptibility to dental caries* • *Increased gingival response to oral biofilm*
Social and Dental History • *Regular dental care until 2 years ago when she started refusing to come to the dentist* • *Good general knowledge, but admits to recent general neglect of oral hygiene* • *Had orthodontic bands until 6 months ago, but all appliances were removed and treatment discontinued*	**At Risk For:** • *Increased susceptibility to dental caries* • *Demineralization* • *Periodontal infection*
Dental Examination • *Deep caries no. 30 with abscess visible on radiograph* • *Evidence of lingual erosion on maxillary incisors* • *General biofilm accumulation* • *Heavy calculus in all areas* • *Generalized erythema, bulbous papilla, and bleeding on probing* • *Generalized 4 mm with 6–8-mm pockets in mandibular anterior sextant and on #3 mesial, #14 mesial and distal, and #18 mesial*	**At Risk For:** • *Oral pain* • *Dental caries* • *Gingival or periodontal infection/abscess*

1. According to the documentation in her re-evaluation section of her care plan, Charen Woodmacher has been referred to the periodontist for specialized care, even though her tissue health has improved because of the dental hygiene treatment she received. Explain why.

2. Even though Charen has been referred to the periodontist, the care plan recommends that a 6-month continuing care appointment is scheduled with the general practice dentist. Explain why. (*Hint:* It may be helpful to look at the pretreatment assessment data as you think about this question.)

DISCOVERY EXERCISES

Investigate and describe the recall system used in your school clinic. What is your role as a student in making the system work and for making sure that complete oral health continuing care is scheduled and delivered as needed for the patients you provide care for in your clinic?

As an exercise in self-evaluation, imagine that you are a clinical instructor assigned to evaluate your patient care and provide feedback at the end of a patient appointment. Take a few moments at the end of one or more patient appointments to complete the same evaluation form your instructor would use to evaluate your progress. Compare your own self-evaluation score with the score and feedback that is actually provided by your instructor for the same patient. How will differences you discover between the two evaluations redirect future self-evaluation of your clinical skills?

FOR YOUR PORTFOLIO

Maintain a reflective journal by writing "critical incident" entries related to patient care experiences over several weeks or months during your education. Organize the individual journal entries by broad topic areas; for example, ethical issues, healthcare knowledge, clinical skills, evaluating patient care, motivating patient behavior change, etc. When you have collected several journal entries related to one topic, you can "reflect on your reflection." This action can enhance your understanding of your professional self and your ability to self-evaluate by analyzing and reflecting about what you have learned over time.

Summary Puzzle Clues

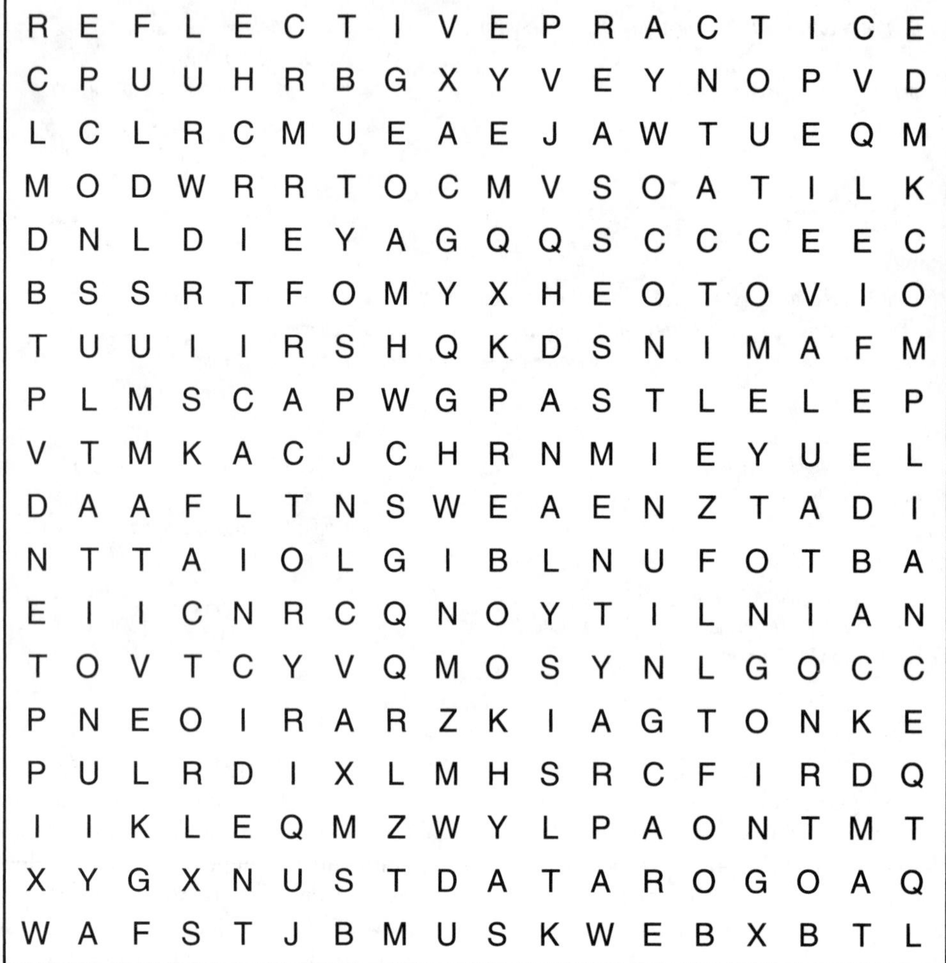

1. Standard #5 in the ADHA Standards for Clinical Dental Hygiene Practice.
2. A reflective-practice journaling approach that is useful in guiding clinicians to assess and to document learning from their actions and responses during clinical situations (two words).
3. A characteristic, habit, or predisposing condition taken into consideration when planning for the patient's maintenance interval following the evaluation of initial treatment outcomes (two words).
4. Information collected during the evaluation procedure.
5. Long-term maintenance phase of dental hygiene care (two words).
6. Evaluated following the completion of dental hygiene treatment and patient education.
7. Providing communication about the outcome of dental hygiene treatment.
8. The "so what" component of reflection and self-assessment.
9. Perceptive self-awareness, judgment, critical analysis and synthesis of information, and application of new knowledge are key skills practitioners need for (two words).
10. This step in the dental hygiene process of care has many of the same components as the evaluation step.
11. A joint deliveration between two or more healthcare providers regarding a particular patient.
12. The method of administering a patient's a maintenance plan by scheduling the next appointment before a patient leaves the current appointment.
13. Refers to the patient's health behavior actions that are in accordance with the clinician's recommendations.
14. Type of evaluation; determines whether goals stated in the patient's care plan have been met.
15. Not responding to therapy.
16. Type of evaluation; provided at all appointments during a patient's treatment sequence.
17. Type of evaluation; checking of root surfaces with an explorer to assess for residual calculus or other iatrogenic factors.

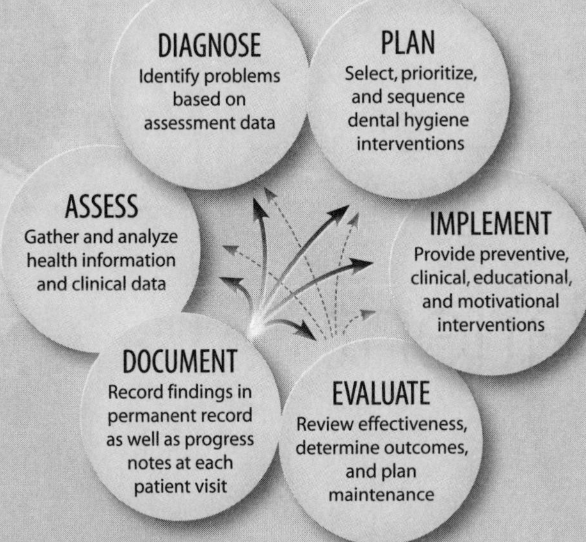

SECTION IX

Patients with Special Health Needs

Chapters 49-69

SECTION IX LEARNING OBJECTIVES

Completing the exercises in this section of the workbook will prepare you to:

1. Identify treatment and education modifications necessary to meet the needs of individuals with physical, mental, and medical conditions or limitations.
2. Plan and provide dental hygiene care for individuals with special needs in both traditional and nontraditional practice settings.
3. Document all aspects of dental hygiene care.

COMPETENCIES FOR THE DENTAL HYGIENIST

All competencies listed in the *ADEA Competencies for Entry into the Profession of Dental Hygiene* (Appendix A) are supported by the learning in Section IX.

49

The Pregnant Patient and Infant

LEARNING OBJECTIVES

Upon successful completion of these exercises, you will be able to:

1. Identify and define key terms and concepts to related oral care for the pregnant patient and infant.
2. Discuss the oral/facial development timetable in relationship to overall fetal development.
3. Describe oral findings common in pregnancy.
4. Describe patient examination, oral care, and anticipatory guidance considerations for the infant patient.
5. Plan and document dental hygiene care that addresses the unique physical, oral, and emotional considerations of the pregnant patient and infant.

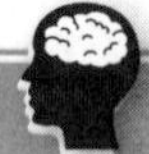

KNOWLEDGE EXERCISES

Write your answers for each question in the space provided.

1. Dental hygiene care is an integral and essential part of your pregnant patient's ________________ care.
2. One-third of a pregnancy, a 3-month period, is referred to as ________________.
3. A factor that can cause disease or malformation during fetal development.

____

4. An antibiotic that has the well-known effect of staining the infant's teeth if taken by the pregnant mother after 4 months of gestation.

____

5. List three oral findings common during pregnancy.

____

____

____

6. In your own words, describe the clinical appearance and significance of a pregnancy epulis.

____

____

____

____

____

____

7. What recommendations can the dental hygienist provide for the patient with a pregnancy-related condition that is a risk factor for demineralization and acid erosion of teeth?

8. Identify reasons why some women have more problems with gingivitis during pregnancy.

9. List three signs you might observe in your pregnant patient that would make you suspect depression.

10. Visualizing a timeline can often help put information into perspective. Use the timeline to identify the oral/facial feature developing in the fetus during the approximate time indicated by each of the lettered segments.

a.

b.

c.

d.

e. By this time (8th week) a ________________ is apparent in the developing fetus.

f. By this time (12th week) a________________ is apparent in the developing fetus.

11. What are the possible adverse effects on the fetus when a woman uses tobacco, alcohol, or other substances of abuse during pregnancy?

12. What is supine hypotensive syndrome?

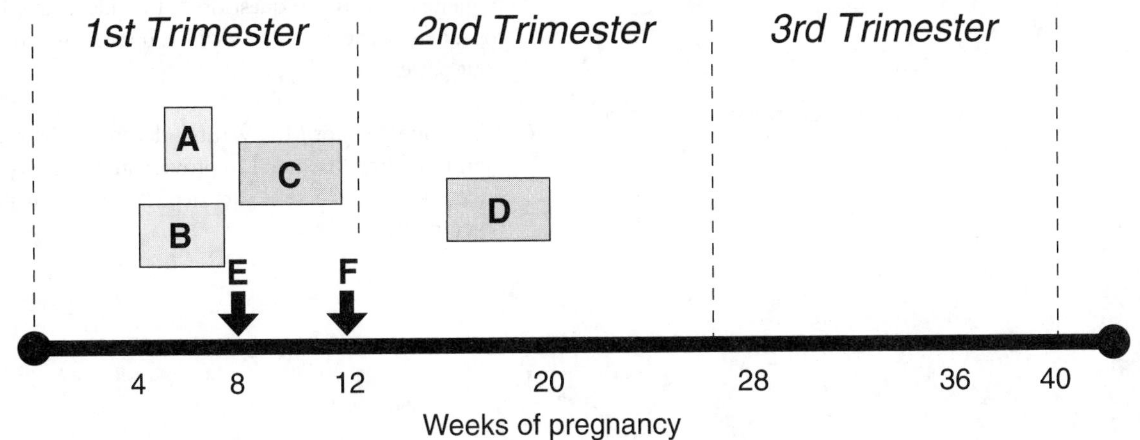

13. List the symptoms of supine hypotensive syndrome.

14. What preventive measure will you provide for a pregnant patient to prevent the symptoms of supine hypotensive syndrome?

15. As it gets closer to the time your patient's baby will be born, the focus of your oral health education will likely be toward ________________ guidance so she can know what to expect and be able to prevent oral problems for her infant.

16. List as many topics as you can think of that are appropriate to include in oral health the education you provide for a patient who is a new mother or mother-to-be.

17. Describe the position that provides the most effective visual access for examining an infant's oral tissues.

COMPETENCY EXERCISES

Apply information from the chapter and use critical thinking skills to complete the competency exercises. Write responses on paper or create electronic documents to submit your answers.

1. Mrs. Jill Mason, who is in her late second trimester of a healthy pregnancy, presents for her dental hygiene appointment with a toothache and a swelling on the right-hand side of her mandible. The dentist orders a single periapical radiograph of the area. Mrs. Mason is concerned about the effect of the radiation on her developing baby. Using all the information available to you in Chapters 49 and 13 describe the educational approach, protective measures, and radiographic techniques you will use to relieve her fears and maximize safety for her and the baby.

2. Using the format for writing progress notes that is used in your school, document the patient position adaption used during Mrs. Mason's treatment.

Read the Chapter 49 Patient Assessment Summary for Mrs. White to help you answer questions the following questions.

3. Mrs. White mentions she frequently experiences nausea, gagging, and vomiting, followed by an unpleasant taste. You realize from looking at the patient assessment data collected during her previous appointment that she is at risk for several additional oral problems. Identify the possible oral problems, and provide three self-care measures that will minimize their oral effects.

4. Using the dental hygiene diagnosis format, identify a cause or factor that could result in increased risk for dental caries during the course of Mrs. White's pregnancy.

5. Write a goal for the problem identified in the dental hygiene diagnosis in question 4. Include a time frame for meeting the goal. How will you measure whether your patient met the goal?

6. Write one goal for Mrs. White's dental hygiene care plan to address the need to provide anticipatory guidance related to the oral care needs of her soon-to-be-born infant.

Questions Patients Ask

What sources of information can you identify to help you answer your patient's questions in this scenario?

"Because of my nausea, I have to eat frequent small snacks. I usually nibble on granola bars—those are healthy snacks, aren't they?" "I heard that pregnancy takes calcium away from my teeth, so is that why I seem to be getting more cavities?" "Should I just wait until after the baby is born to have my fillings done?" "Is it safe to use a mouthwash while I am pregnant?"

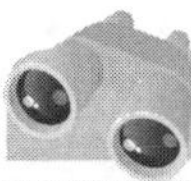

BOX 49-1 MeSH TERMS

Use a combination of MeSH terms and other key words to develop an effective and efficient PubMed literature search strategy.

Pregnancy	Infant, newborn
Pregnancy trimester, first	Breast feeding
Pregnancy trimester, second	Bottle feeding
Pregnancy trimester, third	Natal teeth
Pregnancy outcomes	Tooth, deciduous
Dental care for children	Tooth eruption
Infant	

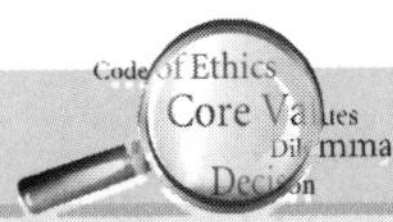

EVERYDAY ETHICS

Before completing the learning exercises below, reread and reflect on the Everyday Ethics Scenario and Questions for Consideration in this chapter of the textbook. It may also be useful to review the Dental Hygiene Ethics discussion in Chapter 1, the Ethical Applications in the introduction pages for each section in the textbook, as well as the Codes of Ethics in textbook Appendices I–IV.

Collaborative Learning Activity

Answer each of the questions for consideration at the end of the scenario in the textbook. Compare what you wrote with answers developed by another classmate and discuss differences/similarities.

Discovery Activity

Ask a friend or relative who is not involved in health care to read the scenario and discuss it with you from the perspective of a "patient" who receives services within the health-care system. Discuss what you learned from the concerns, insights, or difference in perspective that person expressed.

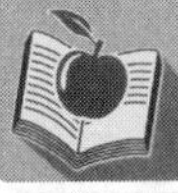

Factors To Teach The Patient

This scenario is related to the following factors listed in this chapter of the textbook:

- ▷ The relationship of oral health of the mother to the general health of the fetus and newborn.
- ▷ The serious effects of tobacco and other drugs on the health of the fetus, the infant, and the child.
- ▷ Reasons for limiting fermentable carbohydrate intake and maintaining a healthy diet from the fruit, vegetable, grain, meat, and meat alternatives, and dairy food groups.

Using the example Patient Assessment Summary for Mrs. White, your answers to the questions about her in the competency exercises for this chapter, and the principles of motivational interviewing (see Appendix D) as a guide, prepare an outline for a conversation that you might use to educate Mrs. White regarding one of the problems identified in the dental hygiene diagnosis. Use the conversation to educate a patient or friend, and then modify it based on what you learned by using the outline.

CHAPTER 49 – PATIENT ASSESSMENT SUMMARY

Patient Name: *Mrs. Diane White* Age: *27* Gender: M [F]

☐ Initial Therapy
☑ Maintenance
☐ Re-evaluation

Provider Name: *D.H. Student* Date: *Today*

Chief Complaint:
Presents for routine maintenance appointment. Gum tissues bleed when brushing and flossing.

Assessment Findings

Health History

- *First trimester of first pregnancy; experiences significant nausea daily and occasional morning vomiting*
- *Husband smokes cigarettes in house and car; patient does not smoke.*
- *ASA Classification - II and ADL level - 0*

At Risk For:

- *Enamel erosion and increased dental caries risk*
- *Infant at risk for second-hand smoke exposure*

Social and Dental History

- *9 months since previous recall appointment; missed her 6-month appointment.*
- *Infrequent flossing*
- *Uses bottled water with no fluoride content; smell of fluoridated toothpaste makes her feel nauseated.*
- *Frequent high-carbohydrate snacks (graham crackers) to help control nausea*

At Risk For:

- *Increased risk for periodontal disease*
- *Increased caries risk and risk for enamel erosion*
- *Increased caries risk*

Dental Examination

- *No current cavitated lesions; a small number of occlusal surface restorations are all in good repair.*
- *Moderate biofilm along cervical margins and on proximal surfaces*
- *Generalized 4 mm probing depths; no radiographic indication of bone loss*
- *Generalized red, bulbous tissue and generalized bleeding on probing*

At Risk For:

- *Increased risk for caries and periodontal infection*
- *Oral infection, increased risk for periodontal/gingival infection*
- *Increased risk for periodontal/gingival infection and pyogenic granuloma*

Periodontal Diagnosis/Case Type and Status

- *Gingivitis*

Caries Management Risk Assessment (CAMBRA) Level:

☐ Low ☑ Moderate ☐ High ☐ Extreme

50

The Pediatric Patient

LEARNING OBJECTIVES

Upon successful completion of these exercises, you will be able to:

1. Identify and define key terms and concepts related to pediatric oral health care.
2. Discuss the role of the dental hygienist in providing early oral care intervention.
3. Identify risk factors for oral disease in children and adolescents.
4. Discuss anticipatory guidance for parents of pediatric patients.
5. Explain tooth development and eruption patterns.
6. Discuss specific oral health issues, child management techniques, caries management by risk assessment, and clinical procedures required to plan dental hygiene care and oral health education for children and their parents.

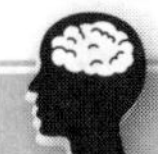

KNOWLEDGE EXERCISES

Write your answers for each question in the space provided.

1. Match each characteristic on the right (as described in this chapter of the textbook) with the most appropriate age category on thew left. Each age category can be matched to more than one characteristic.

Age Category	Characteristic
A. Toddler	____ Lift the lip to examine anterior teeth.
B. Preschool child	____ All permanent dentition.
C. School age child	____ Avoid using negative words.
D. Adolescent	____ Usually have mixed dentition.
	____ Able to become an active, cooperative participant during the dental visit.
	____ Conversations become more mature and links past actions to present events.
	____ Increased need for privacy and desire for independence.
	____ Can dress self and begin to brush own teeth with supervision.
	____ First dental visit.
	____ Risk taking behaviors more likely to begin.
	____ Most are capable of sitting in the dental chair.
	____ Use tiny "smear" of toothpaste on brush.
	____ Begin use of pea-sized amount of toothpaste spread across surface of brush.
	____ Crying during oral examination is normal.
	____ Important to begin periodontal assessment at this age.
	____ Reliance on friends and in influenced by peers.

2. In your own words, briefly describe why it is imperative to establish a dental home and a regular schedule of preventive visits for a child patient.

____

____

____

____

3. Excellent ______________ communication skills will aid in gaining the confidence and cooperation of a child patient.

4. Explain how child-friendly dental terms are used during dental hygiene treatment for a young child.

____

____

____

5. In your own words, describe the best way for a dental hygienist to access and examine the oral cavity of child patient who is not old enough or cooperative enough to sit in the dental chair for an oral examination.

____

____

____

____

6. Why is a periodontal assessment necessary for the school age through adolescent child patient?

____

____

7. ______________ fluctuations can increase the adolescent patient's risk for biofilm-induced gingivitis.

8. The type of dental hygiene services provided for a child patient depends on the child's ________ and________________.

9. The need to take dental radiographs of the pediatric dental patient is determined by the _____________ guidelines and the dentist's professional judgment about the patient's needs.

10. A recommendation for fluoride supplementation is considered when the child's exposure to fluoride is ________________.

11. Dental sealants are recommended for the child patient when __________________ or _______________________ are noted during caries risk assessment.

12. Syrup, gum, or lozenges with ________________ can be recommended for the child with a moderate or high caries risk.

13. Briefly list the four principles of caries risk assessment.

____

____

____

____

____

____

14. In your own words, briefly explain the balance of risk factors and protective factors in determining a child's level of caries risk.

____

____

____

____

15. List the criteria used to determine a high caries risk classification for a child patient.

____

____

____

____

____

16. _________________________lesions, as well as cavitated carious lesions, are considered indicative of ECC or S-ECC.

17. Identify the two most important factors that predispose to ECC.

____

____

18. How much toothpaste is appropriate for parents to place on the toothbrush of a 4 year old?

____

____

19. Identify at least three topic areas appropriate to address during anticipatory guidance educational interventions for the parents of a 4 year old.

____

____

____

20. Identify at least three topic areas appropriate to address during anticipatory guidance educational interventions for a 13-year-old patient and parents.

____

____

____

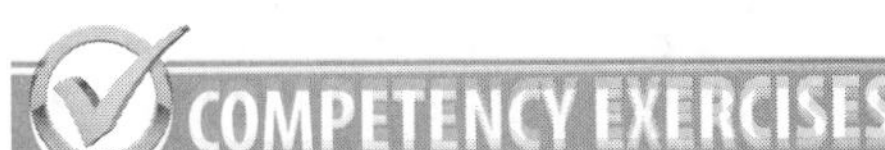

COMPETENCY EXERCISES

Apply information from the chapter and use critical thinking skills to complete the competency exercises. Write responses on paper or create electronic documents to submit your answers.

1. You are conducting an oral health education class for a mother's group at the community center near your house as part of a community service project. The mother of a darling 18-month-old girl asks you how many more teeth her child will get. Explain the development and eruption patterns of primary teeth.

2. Explain to this young mother why healthy primary teeth are important for the growth and development of a healthy permanent dentition.

3. In your own words, define *early childhood caries* as if you were explaining the concept to a parent.

4. Select one of the pediatric age groups identified in the chapter. Explain how knowledge of expected developmental milestones and the child's actual developmental level can assist you to provide dental hygiene care or self-care instruction for that child.

5. Make up three terms/names for dental equipment or instruments (different from those mentioned in the textbook) that you might use to explain what is happening during a dental visit to an anxious preschooler. For extra fun, share your names with those of your student colleagues.

6. Angela Flores, 3 years old, sits quietly in the dental chair for several minutes while you speak with her mother. She allows you to tilt the chair into a supine position but begins to cry as soon as you approach her mouth with your mirror and explorer. She continues to cry and reach for her mother even after you explain all the fun games you will play together while you count her teeth. Outline an appropriate response to this situation.

7. Describe some ways in which a parent might prevent the transfer *Streptococcus mutans* from her mouth to her child's mouth.

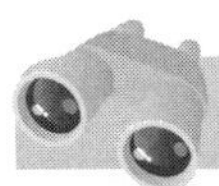

BOX 50-1 MeSH TERMS

Use a combination of MeSH terms and other key words to develop an effective and efficient PubMed literature search strategy.

Dental care for children	Tooth eruption
Pediatric dentistry	Tooth, deciduous
Child	Dentition, mixed
Adolescent	Dentition, permanent

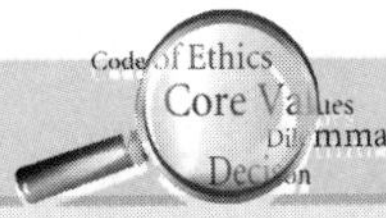

EVERYDAY ETHICS

Before completing the learning exercises below, reread and reflect on the Everyday Ethics Scenario and Questions for Consideration in this chapter of the textbook. It may also be useful to review the Dental Hygiene Ethics discussion in Chapter 1, the Ethical Applications in the introduction pages for each section in the textbook, as well as the Codes of Ethics in textbook Appendices I–IV.

Individual Learning Activity

Imagine that you have observed what happened in the scenario, but are not one of the main characters involved in the situation. Write a reflective journal entry that:

describes how you might have reacted (as an observer—not as a participant),

expresses your personal feelings about what happened,

or

identifies personal values that affect your reaction to the situation.

Discovery Activity

Ask a dental hygienist who has been practicing for a year or more to read the scenario. Provide them with a copy of the Code of Ethics as well. Share the responses you have made to answer each question and ask that person to discuss the situation with you. What insights did you have or what did you learn during this discussion?

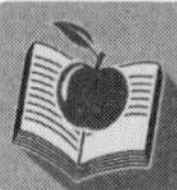

Factors To Teach The Patient

This scenario is related to the following factors:

- ▷ How the bacteria that cause dental caries can be transferred to a baby's mouth from parents or other family members.
- ▷ How fluoride makes enamel stronger and more resistant to the bacteria that cause dental caries.
- ▷ Methods to prevent dental caries from developing in a young child's mouth.
- ▷ How feeding methods and snacking patterns can contribute to dental caries.
- ▷ How the parent can examine the infant/child's mouth and what to look for during the examination.

Mr. and Mrs. Jacobson are in your treatment room with their son, Eric, who is 2.5 years old. The dentist has diagnosed incipient early childhood caries based on observations made during her examination. You have been asked to educate these very concerned parents about how and why this is happening to their son and what can be done to arrest the decay process and prevent further problems.

Use the principles of motivational interviewing (see Appendix D) as a guide to outline a conversation you might have with the Jacobson's. Compare your conversation with a student colleague's to identify any missing information.

51

The Patient with a Cleft Lip and/or Palate

LEARNING OBJECTIVES

Upon successful completion of these exercises, you will be able to:

1. Identify and define key terms and concepts related to oral/facial clefts.
2. Identify prenatal risk factors and developmental time frame for oral/facial clefts.
3. Describe treatment for oral/facial clefts.
4. Use knowledge of the oral, physical, and personal characteristics of the patient to plan and document dental hygiene care and oral hygiene instructions.

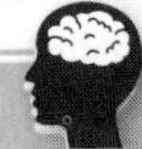

KNOWLEDGE EXERCISES

Write your answers for each question in the space provided.

1. Describe the direction of the formation/fusion of the lip and palatal structures during development.

2. During which embryonic weeks does the palate develop?

3. Which class of cleft is identified as a submucous, imperfect muscle union cleft across the soft palate, producing an incomplete closure of the pharynx?

4. How is a class 3 craniofacial cleft defined?

5. Which classes of facial cleft involve lack of fusion in the premaxilla?

6. List three environmental risk factors for craniofacial clefts.

7. List three common characteristics that can affect the *teeth* of a patient with a craniofacial cleft.

8. List the three categories of professionals who contribute to the treatment of an individual with cleft lip and/or palate.

____

____

____

9. The dental hygienist is a member of the ________________ team of specialists who care for individuals with a cleft lip and/or palate.

10. Select one of the dental specialties in which clinicians may provide care for a patient with a cleft and describe that practitioner's role in the treatment of the patient.

____

____

____

____

11. Ideally, treatment of a craniofacial cleft is begun before the infant is 6 months old. What is the purpose for such early intervention?

____

____

____

____

12. What are the goals of surgical treatment for cleft lip and palate?

____

____

____

____

____

____

13. In your own words, describe the benefits a dental prosthesis can provide for a patient with a cleft lip and palate.

____

____

____

____

____

____

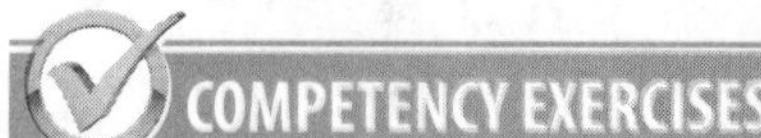

COMPETENCY EXERCISES

Apply information from the chapter and use critical thinking skills to complete the competency exercises. Write responses on paper or create electronic documents to submit your answers.

1. Discuss why lack of prenatal care is considered a risk factor for cleft lip and/or palate.

2. Describe characteristics that may make it difficult to communicate with an individual who has an incomplete palatal closure.

3. Adam Horconcitos, a 12 year old, has recently come to America from Honduras to live with Mr. and Mrs. Mehlisch, his American adoptive parents. Adam has a class 5 unilateral (left side) facial cleft that was not treated when he was an infant. He is scheduled for his first surgical procedure in about 3 weeks. You are a member of Adam's care team, and you are seeing him today for the first time to evaluate his oral status.

   The only dental visits Adam has had previously were about 2 years ago with a prosthodontist in Honduras. The doctor fabricated an appliance to provide for some closure of the palatal opening to enhance Adam's ability to swallow and speak.

   When you talk with Adam and the Mehlisches before the boy's examination, you find that Adam speaks fairly good English, because he went to an American school in his own country. He is a handsome, personable, and likable young man; however, he is really very shy and frequently hides his mouth and nose behind his hand as he speaks to you. His voice has a kind of nasal sound, but his hearing is normal, and with a bit of concentration, you can understand him fairly well. Adam does not have any major health problems, except for a susceptibility to frequent sore throats and ear infections.

   Adam did not enjoy a good dental experience during the fabrication of his prosthesis or during his recent visits with the oral surgeon to plan his surgical care. He is extremely fearful of anyone or anything that comes near his mouth. In spite of that, he is wearing the prosthetic appliance every day, and it seems to be working well for him.

   You are successful in using all of your most comforting patient management techniques, and you convince Adam to allow his mouth to be examined. During your examination, you discover that he has a mixed dentition with five primary molars still being retained, significant malocclusions, and two missing anterior teeth in the area of the cleft. His level of dental caries is fortunately quite low—only one small cavity in a deciduous molar that is already loose. You conclude, from a discussion with Mrs. Mehlisch, that Adam's snacking habits are not highly cariogenic.

His gingival health, however, is another matter. He won't usually let anyone touch his mouth, and he doesn't like to have a toothbrush near his mouth even when he does it himself. You find extensive biofilm accumulation on his teeth, gums, and tongue as well as on the prosthodontic appliance he wears. His mother complains that his breath is often very bad. His gums bleed extremely easily when they are touched.

Using the information in the case description above and a copy of the Dental Hygiene Care Plan template in Appendix B of the workbook, write an individualized dental hygiene care plan for Adam.

4. Using your school's format for writing progress notes, document the assessment visit for Adam's permanent record.

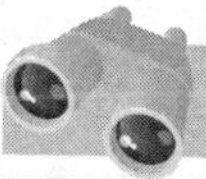

BOX 51-1 MeSH TERMS

Use a combination of MeSH terms and other key words to develop an effective and efficient PubMed literature search strategy.

- Cleft lip
- Cleft palate
- Cleft soft palate
- Palatal obturators

EVERYDAY ETHICS

Before completing the learning exercises below, reread and reflect on the Everyday Ethics Scenario and Questions for Consideration in this chapter of the textbook. It may also be useful to review the Dental Hygiene Ethics discussion in Chapter 1, the Ethical Applications in the introduction pages for each section in the textbook, as well as the Codes of Ethics in textbook Appendices I–IV.

Individual Learning Activities

Imagine that you are the dental hygienist in this scenario. Answer each of the questions for consideration at the end of the scenario.

Identify a situation you have experienced that presents a similar ethical dilemma. Write about what you would do differently now than you did at the time the incident happened—support your discussion with concepts from the dental hygiene codes of ethics.

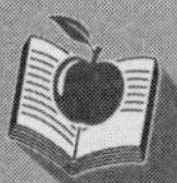

Factors To Teach The Patient

This scenario is related to the following factors listed in this chapter of the textbook:

▷ Parental anticipatory guidance (Tables 49-3 and 50-7 in Chapters 49 and 50 of the textbook).

Today your patient is Mrs. Diane White. You have been providing dental hygiene care for her since she was in her first trimester of pregnancy. About 3 months ago, her little girl was born with a class 3 cleft palate. Although the child is well cared for by an interdisciplinary team of healthcare workers at the local hospital, Mrs. White notes that there is no dental hygienist on the team. She asks you for advice in providing oral care for her child as she grows.

Use information about cleft palate (Chapter 51 in the textbook) and what you have learned about parental anticipatory guidance (in Chapters 49 and 50 in the textbook) and the motivational interviewing approach (Appendix D) to role-play this situation with a fellow student. If you are Mrs. White in the role-play, be sure to ask questions. If you are the dental hygienist, try to anticipate questions and answer them in your explanation.

Crossword Puzzle

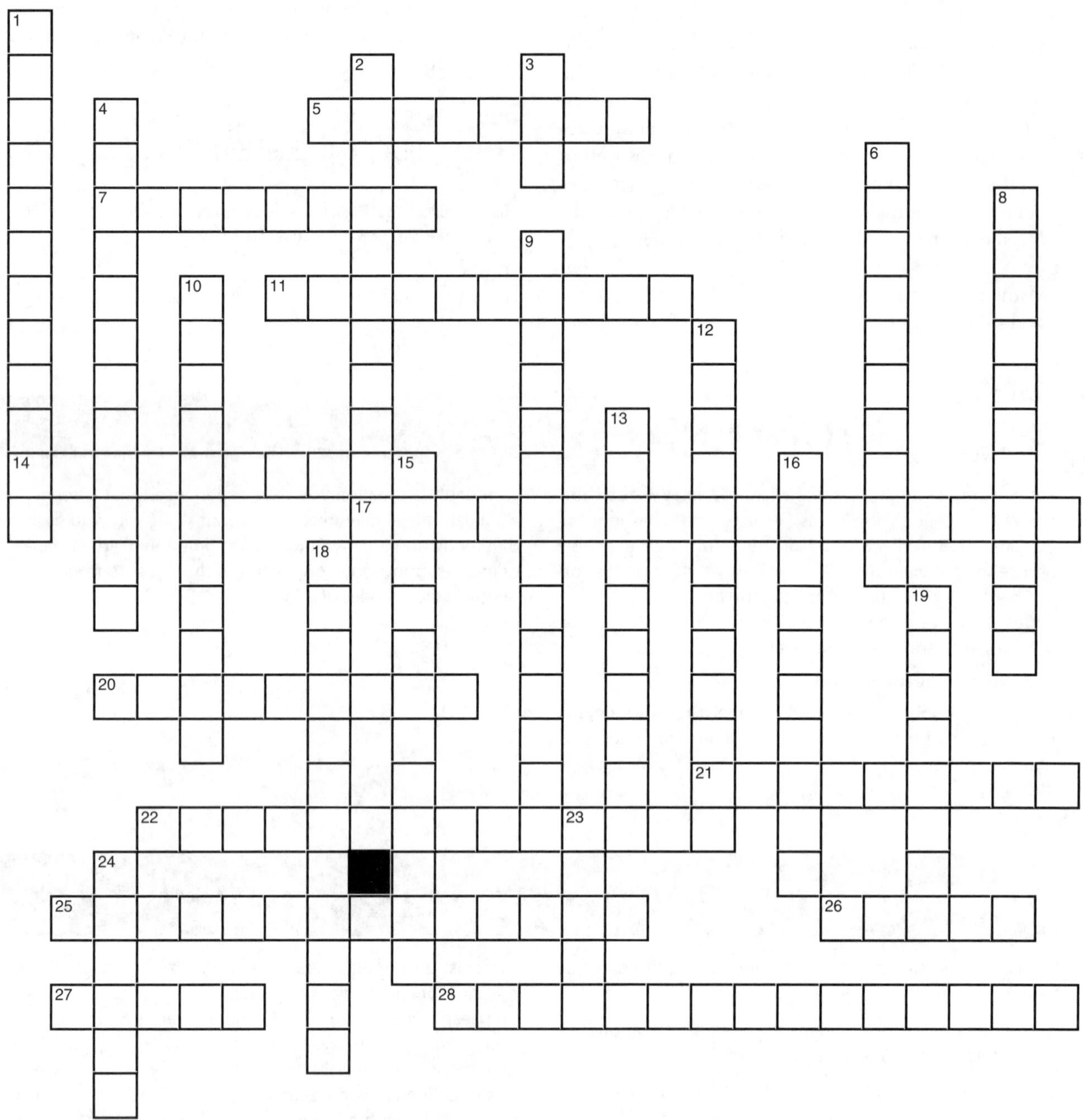

Puzzle Clues

Across

5. Genetic transmission of traits from parents to offspring.
7. A type of graft placed before the eruption of maxillary teeth at a cleft site to create a normal architecture through which the teeth can erupt.
11. Replaces or improves function of any absent part of the human body.
14. Pertaining to the function of the skeletal system and its associated functions.
17. Plastic surgery of nose and lip.
20. A prosthesis designed to cover the cleft of a hard palate.
21. A graft transferred from one part of the patient's body to another part.
22. This insufficiency affects closure of the opening between the mouth and nose in speech, resulting in a nasal-sounding voice.
25. Pertaining to or arising through the action of many factors.
26. A unilateral or bilateral congenital facial fissure.
27. A term describing a cleft of the uvula.
28. One important member of the interdisciplinary team who will treat the patient with a cleft lip and/or palate (two words).

Down

1. The process of acquiring fitness for the first time; associated with persons who have acquired disabilities.
2. An agent, such as drugs of abuse during the first trimester of a pregnancy, that can increase risk for cleft lip and palate.
3. One source of the bone used for an autogenous bone graft.
4. Insertion of an indwelling tube to facilitate passage of air or evacuation of secretions.
6. Bilateral cleft lip separates this from its normal fusion with the entire maxilla.
8. Type of surgical procedure that repositions parts of the maxilla or mandible.
9. The process of restoring a person's abilities to the maximum possible fitness.
10. Plastic surgery of the nose.
12. Pertaining to the part of the skull that encloses the brain and the face.
13. Hereditary material contained within the ovum and the sperm.
15. A surgical repair of a lip defect.
16. Present at and existing from the time of birth.
18. Plastic reconstruction of the palate.
19. Combination of symptoms commonly occurring together.
23. Tissue transplanted and expected to become a part of the host tissue.
24. When this normal process does not happen during development, a facial cleft can result.

52

The Patient with an Endocrine Disorder or Hormonal Change

LEARNING OBJECTIVES

Upon successful completion of these exercises, you will be able to:

1. Identify and define key terms and concepts related to hormonal function and hormone disorders.
2. Identify the major endocrine glands and describe the function of each.
3. Identify signs, symptoms, and potential oral manifestations of endocrine gland disorders.
4. Identify and describe physical, mental, emotional, and oral health factors commonly associated with puberty, menses, contraceptives, and menopause.

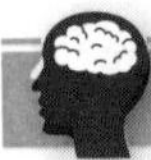

KNOWLEDGE EXERCISES

Write your answers for each question in the space provided.

1. Hormones, which together with the nervous system maintain body homeostasis, are excreted by ________________ and transported to body cells or other glands by ________________.
2. In your own words, describe the purpose of the endocrine system.

____

____

3. In your own words, describe a hormone.

____

____

____

4. List the vital functions that hormones regulate.

____

____

____

____

____

5. List the major endocrine glands and briefly describe the function of each.

____

____

____

____

____

____

6. Both ____________ and ____________ of a hormone can affect a patient's physical and mental status.

7. Cyclic menstruation is regulated by fluctuations in estrogen and progesterone and, with some variations and irregularities, is usually about 28 days in length. In your own words, explain how the levels of each of these two hormones vary relative to menstruation and ovulation during the menstrual cycle. (*Hint*: Describe Figure 52-2 in the textbook.)

8. Some women experience discomfort for several days preceding the beginning of their menstrual flow. If your patient mentions that she is feeling the effects of premenstrual symptoms, what is she likely to be experiencing?

9. If your patient is experiencing irregularity or other problems with her menstrual cycle, a careful assessment and review of her health history is imperative, because she can also be experiencing other __________ problems.

10. List the side effects of oral contraceptives that will be of concern when you are providing dental hygiene care for your patient.

11. Summarize the effects of puberty-linked hormone increases on the physical development of both males and females.

12. Match the statement (first column) with the gland (second column). Letters representing glands may be used more than once.

Statement	Gland
____ The anterior lobe serves as the master gland of the body.	A. Adrenals
____ These glands are located on the kidneys.	B. Gonads
____ Levothyroxine is a medication used to treat disorders of this gland.	C. Hypothalamus
____ The hormone of this gland regulates calcium, phosphorus, and vitamin D levels in the blood and bone.	D. Pancreas
____ Cushing's syndrome is caused by an increase in cortisol secreted by this gland.	E. Parathyroid
____ Humoral factors hormones are produced by this gland.	F. Pineal
____ The hormone of this gland regulates blood glucose.	G. Pituitary
____ Grave's disease is associated with this gland.	H. Thymus
____ This gland secretes melatonin.	I. Thyroid
____ The hormones of these glands influence puberty.	
____ An adenoma is the most common form of tumor of this gland.	
____ This gland controls hormone production in the pituitary gland.	
____ A lack of hormone produced by this gland is related to Hashimoto's disease.	
____ Addison's disease is associated with this gland.	

13. Most adverse oral changes related to menopause can be prevented or diminished with adequate nutrition and thorough daily oral hygiene care. List the oral changes that can be associated with menopause.

14. Too high or too low of a hormone level can cause a variety of uncomfortable signs and symptoms. Contrast and compare the general characteristics of hypothyroidism and hyperthyroidism. In other words, what are the differences between the signs and symptoms of hypothyroidism as compared to hyperthyroidism?

Hypothyroidism	Hyperthyroidism

15. An adrenal crisis is associated with ____________.

16. List the signs and symptoms of adrenal crisis.

17. Which gland is associated with myxedema?

18. What is the cause of myxedema?

19. What are the signs of myxedema?

20. List the patient management considerations for a patient who presents with hypoadrenalism.

COMPETENCY EXERCISES

Apply information from the chapter and use critical thinking skills to complete the competency exercises. Write responses on paper or create electronic documents to submit your answers.

Georgina Steele, a woman in her late 40s, was last seen 6 months ago. Today, when you entered the reception area, you noticed that Georgina's appearance seemed different. She was significantly heavier than you remembered and appeared flustered. You made a mental note to investigate the weight gain during the health history update. She also was wearing a heavy winter sweater even though it was August.

As you escorted her to the treatment room, you offered to hang her sweater, but she preferred to keep it on due to the air conditioning. It was too cold for her, even though the office temperature was 72 degrees. Her last visit with her physician was 13 months ago. Georgina expressed concern and frustration with her recent weight gain over the last few months. She didn't think her eating patterns had changed significantly and was now being extra diligent about her eating habits. She mentioned to you that she felt tired all the time and suffered from muscle cramps and even pain most days, regardless of her level of physical activity. She told you that at work she often is feeling confused and overwhelmed by the work project, something that had never happened before. She was not taking any prescription medication, but occasionally took 200 mg of ibuprofen because of the pain in her legs and arms. But this provided little relief, so she was coping the best she could by trying to stay busy. Vital signs were taken. Her BP, temperature, and respirations were normal, but her pulse rate was 55.

As you began the extraoral examination, you noticed that the facial skin appeared rather dry. Georgina stated that she had been trying different moisturizers with little improvement. As you palpated the neck/throat region, you sensed an enlargement in her thyroid gland which was not present 6 months ago. It was not tender. All other extraoral findings were normal.

Intraorally, the tissues seemed dry. Most of the left buccal mucosa had a pattern of lacy white lines covering the tissue. Georgina reported no discomfort in the tissues, other than the dryness. Her periodontal status remained unchanged (slight localized gingivitis) and no new areas of decay were evident.

1. What are the adverse medical and oral signs and symptoms discovered during the examination?
2. Based on the findings of your examination and interview with the patient, what do you suspect could be causing these changes in appearance and behavior? What are the differential diagnoses based on the findings of this exam?
3. What are your recommendations for Georgina?
4. In outline form, devise a plan for discussing the findings with Georgina.

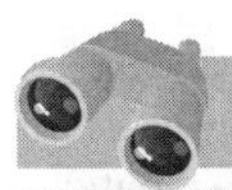

BOX 52-1 MeSH TERMS

Use a combination of MeSH terms and other key words to develop an effective and efficient PubMed literature search strategy.

Endocrine system	Adrenal glands
Endocrine glands	Hormones
Pineal gland	Menstruation
Pituitary gland	Menopause
Thyroid gland	Premenstrual syndrome
Parathyroid glands	Puberty
Thymus gland	Oral contraceptives
Pancreas	

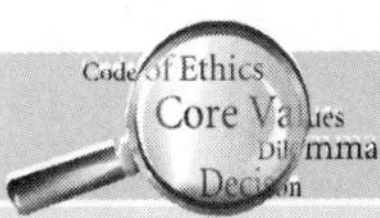

EVERYDAY ETHICS

Before completing the learning exercises below, reread and reflect on the Everyday Ethics Scenario and Questions for Consideration in this chapter of the textbook. It may also be useful to review the Dental Hygiene Ethics discussion in Chapter 1, the Ethical Applications in the introduction pages for each section in the textbook, as well as the Codes of Ethics in textbook Appendices I–IV.

Individual Learning Activity

Imagine that you are the dental hygienist in this scenario. Answer each of the questions for consideration at the end of the scenario.

Collaborative Learning Activity

Work with another student colleague to role-play the scenario. The goal of this exercise is for you and your colleague to work though the alternative actions in order to come to consensus on a solution or response that is acceptable to both of you.

Factors To Teach The Patient

This scenario is related to the following factors listed in this chapter of the textbook:

- ▷ The impact of menopause on oral health.
- ▷ The benefits of fluoride throughout life.
- ▷ The importance of nutrition, exercise, and sleep for good health.

Today is the first time you are providing dental hygiene care for Rosalee Ayers, age 55 years. She arrives late and mentions that because she is under high stress these days and hasn't been eating or sleeping very well; she overslept this morning. Rosalee is a high-powered businesswoman who takes great pride in her youthful appearance and her healthy lifestyle. As you update her health history, you note that she has received regular dental hygiene care for the last 15 years. Her general health status is very good, and she takes no medications. A notation in her record states that she is in menopause; her menses ceased 1 year ago.

When you begin your oral examination, Rosalee mentions that because of the oral hygiene instruction she has received at this clinic, she has always brushed and flossed every day. Lately, however, she has noticed that her mouth frequently feels really dry, and sometimes she feels a burning sensation on her tongue, palate, and inside her lips.

Your assessment findings indicate that her biofilm levels are very low, there are very few dental restorations, and there are no current carious lesions.

Her oral tissues are generally very healthy looking. Periodontal pocket depths are all <3 mm. Past periodontal charts have recorded generalized 2- to 3-mm recession in all premolar and molar areas, but there are no changes in the level of recession when you do your periodontal charting today.

After your assessment is complete, you write a brief care plan and, because of your patient's increased risk for root caries, you include a recommendation for fluoride treatment.

When you discuss your care plan with Rosalee, she chuckles and says, "Look, I'm not a kid any more. What on earth do I need a fluoride treatment for?"

Use a motivational interviewing approach found in Appendix D as a guide to develop a conversation to use when you are talking with Rosalee about the value of fluoride treatments.

Word Search

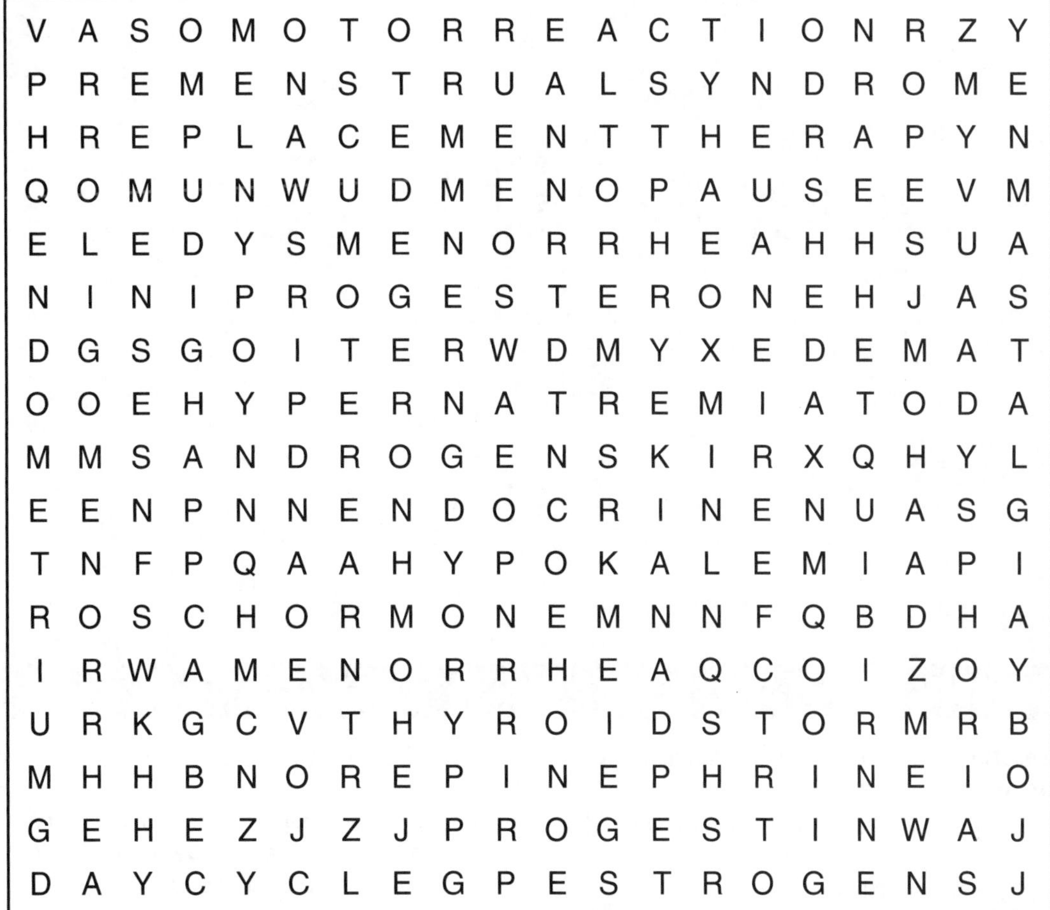

V A S O M O T O R R E A C T I O N R Z Y
P R E M E N S T R U A L S Y N D R O M E
H R E P L A C E M E N T T H E R A P Y N
Q O M U N W U D M E N O P A U S E E V M
E L E D Y S M E N O R R H E A H H S U A
N I N I P R O G E S T E R O N E H J A S
D G S G O I T E R W D M Y X E D E M A T
O O E H Y P E R N A T R E M I A T O D A
M M S A N D R O G E N S K I R X Q H Y L
E E N P N N E N D O C R I N E N U A S G
T N F P Q A A H Y P O K A L E M I A P I
R O S C H O R M O N E M N N F Q B D H A
I R W A M E N O R R H E A Q C O I Z O Y
U R K G C V T H Y R O I D S T O R M R B
M H H B N O R E P I N E P H R I N E I O
G E H E Z J Z J P R O G E S T I N W A J
D A Y C Y C L E G P E S T R O G E N S J

Puzzle Clues

- Absence of spontaneous menstrual cycles during the reproductive years.
- A collective name for the hormones produced by the testes; responsible for development of male characteristics.
- Difficult and painful menstruation.
- Feeling unwell, unhappy, or depressed.
- Pertaining to secretion of a substance directly into blood or lymph rather than into a duct; the opposite of exocrine.
- The lining of the uterus.
- A collective name for the hormones produced by the ovaries; responsible for development of female characteristics.
- Enlargement of the thyroid gland, may indicate Grave's disease or Hashimoto's thyroiditis.
- A chemical produced by the human body that has a specific regulatory function on other body cells or organs.
- A prescription of purified or synthetic hormone to correct or prevent undesirable symptoms of menopause (two words).
- An elevated level of sodium in the bloodstream.
- A lower than normal level of potassium in the bloodstream.
- A feeling of fullness, soreness, or pain in the breast.
- A normal condition of aging in which there is complete and permanent cessation of menstrual flow.
- A term referring to menstruation.
- Thickening of the skin, blunting of the senses and intellect, labored speech associated with hypothyroidism.
- A catecholamine that transmits signals from one neuron to another or to a muscle cell.
- Menstrual intervals greater than 45 days.
- A cluster of behavioral, somatic, affective, and cognitive disorders that appear in the luteal phase of the menstrual cycle and resolve rapidly with the onset of menses (two words).
- A hormone that, along with estrogen, is present at various levels during the female menstrual cycle.
- A synthetic hormone contained, either as a combination with estrogen or as a single preparation, in oral contraceptives.
- When the thyroid suddenly releases large amounts of thyroid hormone (two words).
- The period of time from the beginning of one menstrual flow to the beginning of the next menstrual flow.
- Physiologic reaction that causes the hot flashes and night sweats characteristic of menopause (two words).

53

The Older Adult Patient

LEARNING OBJECTIVES

Upon successful completion of these exercises, you will be able to:

1. Identify and define key terms and concepts related to aging.
2. Identify physical, general health, and oral health changes that are characteristic of aging.
3. Describe the effects of age-related chronic conditions on oral health status.
4. Plan and document dental hygiene interventions and health education approaches that enhance the oral health of the older adult patient.

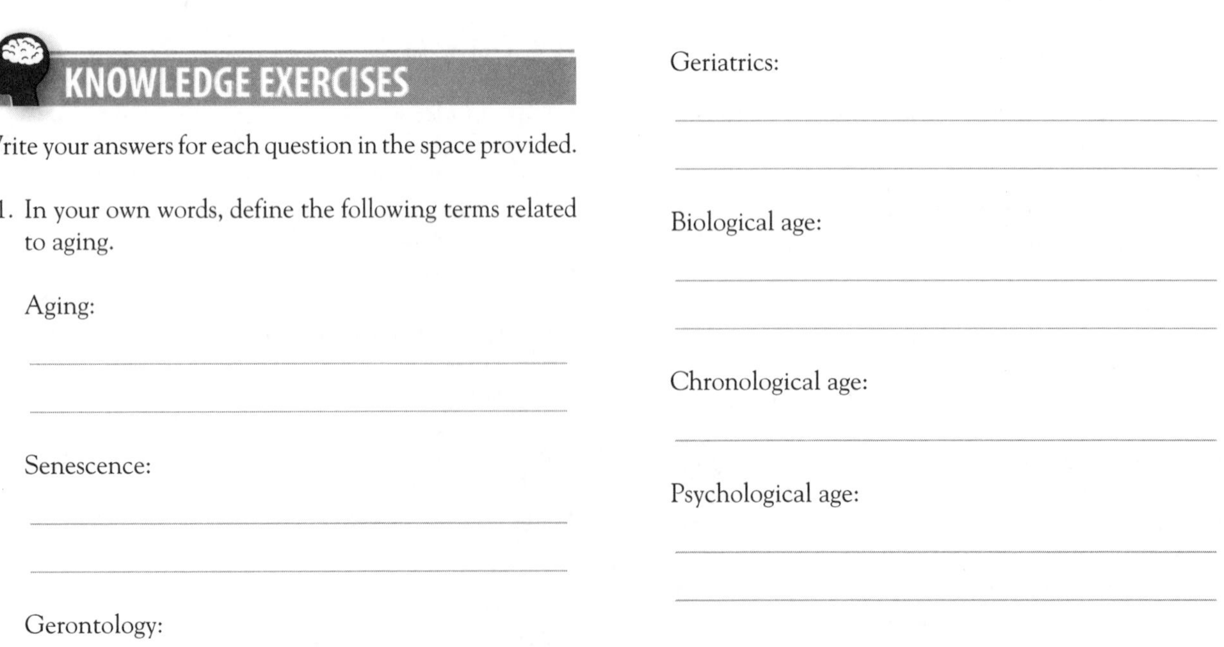

KNOWLEDGE EXERCISES

Write your answers for each question in the space provided.

1. In your own words, define the following terms related to aging.

   Aging:

   Senescence:

   Gerontology:

   Geriatrics:

   Biological age:

   Chronological age:

   Psychological age:

Life expectancy:

2. There are two common classifications used to define individuals from older adult populations: age related and function related. These two systems used together can help provide an accurate description of your aging patients. List the categories for each of these classifications.

Age-related classifications

Function-related classifications:

3. Differentiate between the terms *primary aging* and *secondary aging*.

4. For each of the following body systems, describe at least two changes that occur due to primary aging.

Musculoskeletal system:

Cardiovascular system:

Respiratory system:

Gastrointestinal system:

Central nervous system:

Peripheral nervous system:

Sensory system:

Endocrine system:

Immune system:

5. An older adult may react differently to disease than your younger patients. Identify the differences mentioned in the textbook.

6. What risk factor related to chronic diseases is associated with increased risk for dental caries in older adult patients?

7. List some of the most common chronic diseases associated with aging.

8. Identify two psychosocial conditions that can be of concern when treating older adult patients.

9. In your own words, define the term dementia.

10. In your own words, briefly summarize what you learned about Alzheimer's disease.

11. List the two types of Alzheimer's disease.

12. What is osteoarthritis?

13. List the risk factors for osteoporosis.

14. Your older patient with osteoporosis is considered to be at greater risk for periodontal bone loss. List the factors and risk factors that relate osteoporosis to periodontal disease.

15. What medication, commonly prescribed for individuals with osteoporosis, is a contraindication for dental surgery?

16. Identify the age-associated oral conditions described by each of the following statements.

Difficulty swallowing:

Oral lesion that appears as skinfolds with fissuring at the corner of the mouth; not specifically an age-related lesion but is frequently seen among older persons:

Burning, smooth, shiny, bald tongue with atrophied papillae; related to nutritional deficiencies:

Deep red or bluish nodular masses commonly found during an intraoral examination of older individuals on either side of the midline on the ventral surface of the tongue:

Oral condition often noted in older adults related to pathologic states, drug-induced changes, or radiation-induced degeneration of salivary glands:

Dental disease occurring in older folks related to cementum exposed by periodontal infections and often to xerostomia:

17. A dry, purse-string opening of your older patient's lips may make wide opening difficult during dental hygiene treatment. What causes this condition?

18. In your own words, describe common age-related atrophic changes to oral mucosa.

19. In your own words, briefly explain the oral effects of xerostomia.

20. Identify the risk factors for oral candidiasis that may be present in your older patient.

21. Identify risk factors that may contribute to root caries in older adults.

22. Periodontal findings reflect the patterns of health and disease over the years of your older patient's life. Describe the range of tissue changes that may be noted when examining an older patient.

23. Identify barriers that can negatively impact access to dental hygiene care for an older individual.

24. Older patients often use more prescription drugs and more over-the-counter medications than other age groups. List the ways you can be sure you know what drugs your patient is taking so you make appropriate decisions when you plan dental hygiene care.

25. List factors likely to occur in your older patient that can contribute to accumulation and retention of dental biofilm and increased difficulty in removal.

26. Describe specific biofilm removal methods and techniques you can recommend for an older patient.

27. What factors can contribute to dietary and nutritional deficiencies in your older patients?

COMPETENCY EXERCISES

Apply information from the chapter and use critical thinking skills to complete the competency exercises. Write responses on paper or create electronic documents to submit your answers.

1. Explain why an older patient's slowness to master new oral hygiene techniques does not necessarily mean an inability to learn.

2. Develop an infomap (table) that briefly describes the characteristics of each of the progressive stages of Alzheimer's disease and make a list of the types of patient care modifications or dental hygiene management considerations appropriate for each stage.

3. Today your patient is Marie Tonawonda, age 89 years. Refer to her patient assessment summary as you complete the following exercises.

   Ms. Tonawonda has been a patient in your clinic for many, many years, and she comes in every 4 months, like clockwork, for her periodontal maintenance appointments. Her father was a dentist, and she was his dental assistant when she was a young girl, so she loves to talk about the changes she has observed in dentistry.

   As her nephew, Stan, escorts her slowly into your treatment room, you notice that, although she greets you cheerfully as usual, she is becoming increasingly frail. As Stan helps with a health history update, he mentions that his aunt has recently been placed on an antidepressant by her physician. Stan visits his aunt in her home nearly daily and recently noticed that she hasn't been eating regular meals. There has been other evidence that Ms. Tonawonda has been decreasingly able to provide her own daily self-care, and Stan says that, even when he reminds her, she does not always remember to brush her teeth or comb her hair every day.

   Stan states that he will continue to bring her in for her regular dental care and that Ms. Tonawonda's insurance will continue to cover the cost of any dental needs she has.

   While your dental assistant is taking radiographs of Ms. Tonawonda's teeth, you begin to jot down notes for her dental hygiene care plan. You suddenly remember the OSCAR assessment approach to identifying the needs of older individuals (see Table 24-2 in the textbook). Complete an OSCAR assessment to identify factors of concern for Ms. Tonawonda.

4. Using the assessment data from Ms. Tonawonda's patient assessment summary, your OSCAR assessment notes, and the information in Chapter 53 of the textbook, write three dental hygiene diagnoses statements for Ms. Tonawonda's care plan.

5. Because Ms. Tonawonda's cognitive abilities are declining, her need for education and oral hygiene instruction are very different from that of most of

CHAPTER 53 – PATIENT ASSESSMENT SUMMARY

Patient Name: *Marie Tonawonda* Age: *89* Gender: M [F]

☐ Initial Therapy
☑ Maintenance
☐ Re-evaluation

Provider Name: *D.H. Student* Date: *Today*

Chief Complaint:
Her nephew states: "I brought her in today for her regular cleaning appointment."

Assessment Findings

Health History
- *Taking calcium-channel blocker for hypertension and sublingual nitroglycerine tablet as needed for occasional angina*
- *Recent antidepressant prescription*
- *Osteoporosis – exhibits curvature of upper back*
- *Increasing mental confusion and cognitive disability*
- *Decreased visual acuity even when corrected with glasses*
- *Wears a hearing aid*
- *ASA Classification - II and ADL level - 2*

At Risk For:

Social and Dental History
- *History of dental visits every 4 months*
- *Recent increase in sucrose intake (described by nephew)*
- *High dental literacy—but recent cognitive decrease*
- *Assisted with daily care by her nephew who has little dental knowledge*

At Risk For:

Dental Examination
- *Xerostomia*
- *Generalized recession: 3 – 5 mm.*
- *Generalized 3 – 4 mm probing depths; generalized slight bleeding at gingival margins*
- *Several class 1 and class II furcations in molar areas*
- *Very few restorations—all in good condition*

At Risk For:

Periodontal Diagnosis/Case Type and Status
- *History of generalized, controlled chronic periodontitis with recent increase in marginal gingivitis*

Caries Management Risk Assessment (CAMBRA) Level:
☐ Low ☑ Moderate ☐ High ☐ Extreme

your other patients. Ms. Tonawonda will need ways to receive reminders for daily oral care. Using your school's format for writing progress notes, document the education and home care instructions you will provide during today's appointment.

Questions Patients Ask

What sources of information can you identify that will help you answer your patient's question in this scenario?

A healthy, functionally independent 70-year-old patient asks you if, at her age, she should consider dental implants for the molar teeth that were recently extracted. How will you respond?

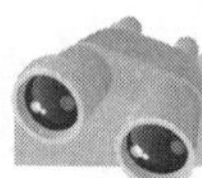

BOX 53-1 MeSH TERMS

Use a combination of MeSH terms and other key words to develop an effective and efficient PubMed literature search strategy.

Dental care for aged	Aged
Health services for the aged	Aged, 80 and over
Geriatric dentistry	Frail elderly
Geriatrics	Aging
	Ageism

EVERYDAY ETHICS

Before completing the learning exercises below, reread and reflect on the Everyday Ethics Scenario and Questions for Consideration in this chapter of the textbook. It may also be useful to review the Dental Hygiene Ethics discussion in Chapter 1, the Ethical Applications in the introduction pages for each section in the textbook, as well as the Codes of Ethics in textbook Appendices I–IV.

Collaborative Learning Activity

Work with another student colleague to role-play the scenario. The goal of this exercise is for you and your colleague to work though the alternative actions in order to come to consensus on a solution or response that is acceptable to both of you.

Discovery Activity

Ask a friend or relative who is not involved in health care to read the scenario and discuss it with you from the perspective of a "patient" who receives services within the health-care system. Discuss what you learned from the concerns, insights, or difference in perspective that person expressed.

Factors To Teach The Patient

This scenario is related to the following factors listed in this chapter of the textbook:

- ▷ That dentition can last a lifetime.
- ▷ The value of a well-balanced diet.
- ▷ Importance of drinking fluoridated water.

You have recently learned that Marie Tonawonda (introduced in the Competency Exercises) has been moved to an extended-care facility. Her nephew, Stan, comes in for his regular appointment and thanks you again for all the information you provided when Ms. Tonawonda was in for her appointment. He reaffirms his commitment to maintaining his aunt's oral health.

He mentions his concern about your instructions to limit Ms. Tonawonda's exposure to high-sucrose foods. In order to increase nutritional intake, the residents at the Sunshine Residence Home seem to have access to food at any time they desire and, unfortunately, that includes availability of cookies all the time. Stan has encouraged the staff to provide support for his aunt's efforts at limiting sweets and conducting daily brushing and flossing, but he isn't sure his wishes are being met.

You decide that you will investigate the possibility of volunteering to provide staff in-service presentations about oral health to the caregivers at the extended-care facility. Develop an outline of the topics you would cover in these presentations.

54

The Edentulous Patient

LEARNING OBJECTIVES

Upon successful completion of these exercises, you will be able to:

1. Identify and define key terms and concepts related to an edentulous patient.
2. Identify potential adverse effects of dental prostheses on oral tissues.
3. Plan and document dental hygiene interventions that address patient needs before and after insertion of a denture.
4. Identify criteria and procedures for marking dentures.

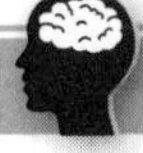

KNOWLEDGE EXERCISES

Write your answers for each question in the space provided.

1. Identify reasons for wearing a denture to replace the missing teeth in an edentulous arch.

2. List three reasons why a denture may be constructed to replace primary dentition for a child patient.

3. What is the purpose of a provisional or interim dental prosthesis?

4. Why is it often necessary to reline or remake an immediate denture approximately 6 months after initial placement?

5. As a dental hygienist, you may provide counseling and education for your patient both before and after

he or she receives a new denture. Explain the purpose of predelivery patient counseling.

____

____

6. When a denture is placed immediately after extractions, you instruct your patient to leave the denture in place for ________________ without removing it, to aid in control of bleeding and swelling.

7. Because adjustments can be expected when a new denture is placed over healed ridges, you instruct your patient to return within ______________; you then make reappointments as needed.

8. What is the purpose of a postinsertion appointment with the dental hygienist after a new denture is placed? (*Hint:* The dentist will adjust the new denture, if needed, not the dental hygienist.)

____

____

9. List the potential effects of alveolar ridge remodeling after placement of a complete denture.

____

____

____

____

____

10. Your patient may resort to ________________ remedies to counter the effects of alveolar remodeling or poor denture fit, but you will counsel him or her to seek dental care if there are any problems, because other remedies are ________________ if used improperly or over time.

11. List factors that contribute to the varying tissue reactions experienced by patients who wear dentures.

____

____

____

____

____

____

12. Xerostomia can adversely affect denture ____________ and tissue ________________.

13. List two negative oral effects related to the sensory changes that may be experienced by your patient who wears complete dentures.

____

____

14. For most of your patients who wear complete dentures, a ________________ continuing care appointment frequency is adequate, unless they are experiencing problems.

15. At dental hygiene appointments, it is important to thoroughly examine the oral tissues of a patient who wears complete dentures. In your own words, describe the tension test for examining the mouth of your edentulous patient.

____

____

____

____

16. List the three *most common* causes of oral lesions under a dental prosthesis.

____

____

____

17. What is the effect of xerostomia for your patient who wears dentures?

____

____

____

____

18. What is an epulis fissuratum?

____

____

____

____

19. Name the common fungal infection that can result in denture stomatitis.

____

20. List three factors that can contribute to angular cheilitis in your patient who wears dentures.

____

21. If you observe a localized ulcerated lesion related to an overextended denture border that persists longer than normal healing times, you should bring the situation to the attention of the dentist so that the lesion can be ______________.

22. List the topics to include when you are educating your patient about ways to prevent damage to oral tissues related to wearing dentures.

23. List three reasons to mark your patient's denture with identifying information.

24. In your own words, briefly summarize the criteria for an adequate denture-marking system relative to the following issues.

    The denture:

    The material used:

    The procedure used:

25. List two areas in which identification information can be incorporated as a denture is fabricated.

26. Where should an inclusion identification marker be placed on an existing denture that was not previously labeled?

    Maxillary denture:

    Mandibular denture:

27. Identify two methods for marking identification information on the surface of a denture.

28. What information is included when marking the denture of a patient who is in a long-term care nursing home?

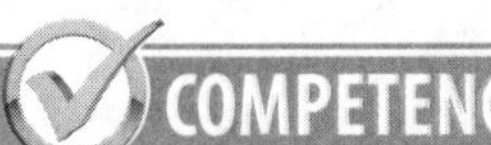

COMPETENCY EXERCISES

Apply information from the chapter and use critical thinking skills to complete the competency exercises. Write responses on paper or create electronic documents to submit your answers.

1. Explain why regular dental hygiene maintenance care is important for edentulous patients, whether or not they are wearing complete dentures.

2. Explain why caries-control methods are important to teach your patient who wears an overdenture.

3. After discussing several alternate treatment plans with the dentist, Mr. Bruehner has decided to have all of his remaining natural teeth extracted and immediate maxillary and mandibular dentures placed. He is very concerned, because his mother wore dentures and had lots of problems with them over the years. He has confided to Dr. Joseph that his mother's dentures didn't look like they belonged to her face and mouth, that she couldn't eat what she wanted to, that the dentures were not comfortable, and—worst of all—that his mother always had what he calls "dragon breath."

   Mr. Bruehner has an appointment with you today to begin preinsertion patient counseling before he schedules the extraction appointment. You are developing a dental hygiene care plan before he arrives.

When you read the assessment data in his patient record, you learn that Mr. Bruehner has been receiving his dental treatment in this practice for a bit longer than 1 year. His general health status is relatively good, and he is currently taking one medication for hypertension that contributes to xerostomia. He has a history of periodontal disease for which the original prognosis was rated as poor. He has a fairly high dental IQ because of education provided by the previous dental hygienist, but the counseling he received was focused on his periodontal status and the attempt to arrest the progress of oral disease.

Use a copy of the Patient-Specific Dental Hygiene Care Plan Template in Appendix B and the information in Table 54-1 in the textbook to develop a dental hygiene care plan for a series of preinsertion and postinsertion appointments for Mr. Bruehner. Be sure to include at least one preinsertion appointment (more if you think he might need them), an appointment for instructions the day of his extractions, and a postinsertion appointment for instructions after he receives his dentures.

4. Use your school's format for writing progress notes to document dental hygiene education provided during a preinsertion appointment for Mr. Bruehner.

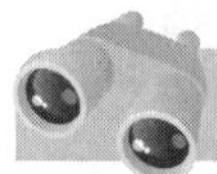

BOX 54-1 MeSH TERMS

Use a combination of MeSH terms and other key words to develop an effective and efficient PubMed literature search strategy.

Mouth, edentulous
Alveolar bone loss
Dental prosthesis
Dentures
Stomatitis, denture

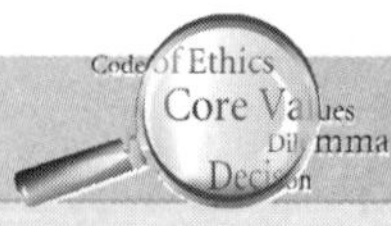

EVERYDAY ETHICS

Before completing the learning exercises below, reread and reflect on the Everyday Ethics Scenario and Questions for Consideration in this chapter of the textbook. It may also be useful to review the Dental Hygiene Ethics discussion in Chapter 1, the Ethical Applications in the introduction pages for each section in the textbook, as well as the Codes of Ethics in textbook Appendices I–IV.

Individual Learning Activities

Identify a situation you have experienced that presents a similar ethical dilemma. Write about what you would do differently now than you did at the time the incident happened—support your discussion with concepts from the dental hygiene codes of ethics.

Identify a situation in which you have resolved a similar ethical dilemma and share the story with a classmate. Discuss how that person might have acted differently to resolve the situation.

Factors To Teach The Patient

This scenario is related to the following factors listed in this chapter of the textbook:

- Dentures and tissues must be examined at least once a year for care of the tissue-supported removable prosthesis; implant-supported dentures require more frequent examination. The frequency of maintenance appointments is geared to the individual, depending in part on that patient's ability to clean the dentures and to keep them free from biofilm, stain, and calculus.
- Dentures may need periodic replacement. Tissues under the dentures change.
- Avoid the use of drugstore remedies, reliners, and other home-applied materials unless the dentist has provided specific instructions.
- There are specific methods of care for dentures.
- Leave the dentures out of the mouth overnight in accord with the dentist's directions.

Mr. Bruehner (introduced in the Competency Exercises in this chapter) received his immediate denture 2 days ago. This morning he is scheduled with Dr. Joseph for a postinsertion appointment to check healing at the extraction sites; then he has an appointment with you for postinsertion education and counseling.

Use the patient-specific dental-hygiene care plan you created for Mr. Bruehner and the motivational interviewing approach (see Appendix D) as guides to prepare an outline for a conversation that you will have with Mr. Bruehner during this appointment.

Word Search Puzzle

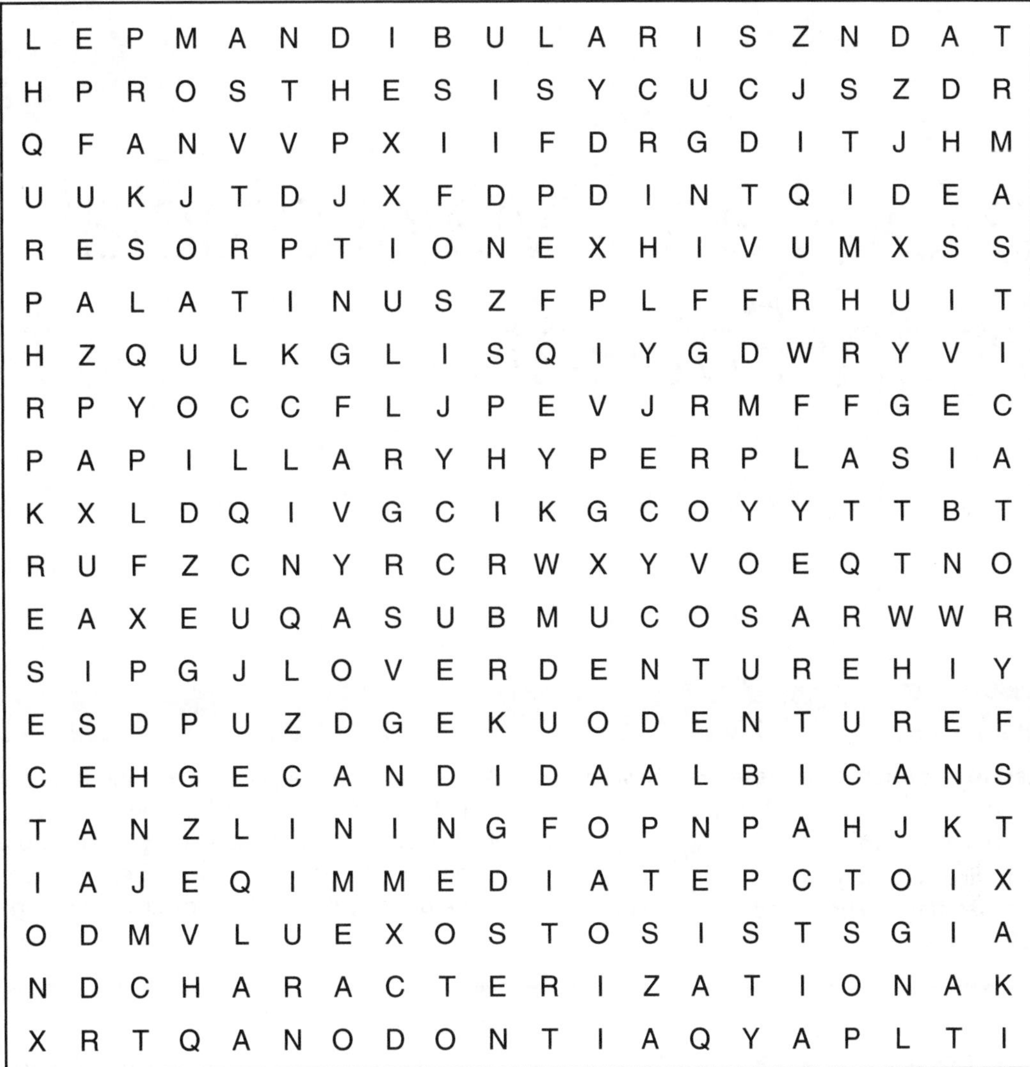

Word Search Clues

- Term for an artificial replacement of one or more teeth and associated oral structures.
- Term for an artificial substitute for missing natural teeth.
- Type of complete denture fabricated for placement directly after the removal of natural teeth or surgical preparation of dental arches.
- Removable prosthesis that covers remaining teeth, roots, or implants.
- Modification of the form and color of the denture base and teeth to produce a more lifelike appearance.
- The mucosa that covers the floor of the mouth, vestibules, and cheeks.
- Type of mucosa that covers the edentulous ridge and hard palate.
- The cushion of connective tissue, vessels, nerves, adipose tissue, and glands between mucosa and bone on the edentulous ridge.
- Excision of a segment of any part (e.g., of the jawbone) or removal of articular ends of bones forming a joint.
- The tori usually removed from the lingual premolar area before fabrication of a denture.
- Bony enlargement (torus) that is surgically removed before fabrication of a maxillary denture.
- Bony changes in the alveolar ridge over time that can lead to loss of denture support, changes in facial structure, and changes in oral functioning.
- Material used to adhere a denture to the oral mucosa; should not be used long term to compensate for poorly designed, constructed, or ill-fitting dentures.
- Fissuring at the corners of the mouth of a patient who wears dentures (two words).
- This condition can cause a generalized redness on the tissues that support a denture; your patient may experience a burning sensation (two words).
- Red, pebble-shaped, edematous lesions on the palate that are related to ill-fitting dentures, poor oral hygiene, and possible *Candida albicans* infection (two words).
- Congenital absence of teeth that may require construction of dentures for a child patient.
- Bony protuberance located on the buccal aspect of the alveolar ridge.
- Mucosa that covers the dorsal surface of the tongue and contains filiform papillae.

55

The Oral and Maxillofacial Surgery Patient

LEARNING OBJECTIVES

Upon successful completion of these exercises, you will be able to:

1. Identify and define key terms and concepts related to oral and maxillofacial surgery.
2. Identify causes, classifications, and treatment options for facial fractures.
3. Discuss dental hygiene interventions for patients before and after general surgery.
4. Plan and document dental hygiene care, oral health education, and dietary recommendations for patients before and after oral and maxillofacial surgery.

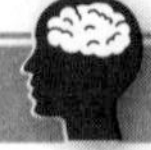

KNOWLEDGE EXERCISES

Write your answers for each question in the space provided.

1. What is orthognathic surgery?

2. In your own words, define *intermaxillary fixation*.

3. Define *exodontics*.

4. List at least three reasons why it is important to provide dental hygiene care for a patient before oral and maxillofacial surgery, even when all of the patient's teeth will be removed during the surgical procedure.

5. List three personal factors that can affect communication with your patient when you are providing oral hygiene instructions to him or her before oral surgery.

6. List at least three types of printed instructions you would provide as part of your presurgical patient education.

7. Identify specific components to include in instructions you provide your patient immediately after a surgical procedure.

8. List postsurgical procedures you may be asked to participate in during follow-up care for your patient.

9. Identify two possible causes of a fractured jaw.

10. List three clinical signs that can aid in recognition of a fractured jaw.

11. Describe a comminuted fracture.

12. Which type of fractured jaw is more likely to occur in a small child?

13. Describe an arch bar and explain how it immobilizes the mandibular jaw.

14. Identify three advantages for using IMF after surgical reduction of a fracture.

15. List three contraindications for using an IMF.

16. List three types of systems/materials used for immobilization after open surgical reduction of a skeletal fracture.

17. List factors that make maxillary fractures more difficult to manage than mandibular fractures.

18. Describe a maxillary alveolar process fracture. (*Hint:* Draw a diagram of what you are trying to describe.) List the components of treatment provided for the patient with this type of fracture.

19. Identify reasons a healthy liquid or soft diet is difficult to plan for a postsurgical patient.

20. List two vitamins that are essential in the diet of a patient who is healing after an oral/maxillofacial surgical procedure.

21. Provide three examples of feeding methods used for patients after a surgical fixation procedure.

22. List at least three foods that can supply needed nutrients as part of a soft diet prepared for a patient with only a single-jaw fixation appliance.

23. When is personal oral care and thorough biofilm removal by the patient resumed after an oral surgical procedure?

24. List three factors that may compromise the patient's own postsurgical biofilm removal or the provision of dental hygiene.

COMPETENCY EXERCISES

Apply information from the chapter and use critical thinking skills to complete the competency exercises. Write responses on paper or create electronic documents to submit your answers.

1. Compare open and closed reduction procedures used for the treatment of a facial fracture.

2. You are asked to provide a presurgical dental hygiene prophylaxis for Mr. Bright, who is scheduled in 2 weeks for oral surgery to remove all of his remaining maxillary teeth and receive an immediate denture. His patient record contains assessment data indicating that teeth 1, 3, 6–9, 13, and 16 are missing; tooth 2 is extremely sensitive owing to a carious lesion; teeth 4 and 5 are mobile; and his gingival tissue is sensitive and bleeds profusely. There is visible calculus and a high level of biofilm on all the remaining teeth. He has not had any regular dental care or oral hygiene instructions for many years. Create an infomap or table that will help you organize the following information.
   - Identify factors from this case scenario that can affect instrumentation techniques when you are providing presurgical scaling for Mr. Bright.
   - Identify why these factors are a problem.
   - Suggest procedures you might use to overcome each problem.
   - Use the format required in your school clinic to write a progress note for an imaginary patient visit that documents the use of one of the potential modifications you have described.

3. Your patient, Alicia Wentworth, is upset today when she comes to the office for her dental hygiene appointment. She tells you that her good friend, David, was recently injured in an automobile accident. She asks you to explain what a simple fracture of the mandible is and what a Le Fort II midfacial fracture is. Draw diagrams you can use to educate Alicia.

4. A week later, Alicia calls and leaves a message on the office voice mail. She says that David is coming home from the hospital and she has agreed to provide meals for him every day. His fracture has been treated using an IMF appliance and he must receive all his nutrition using a straw or a spoon-feeding technique. He is restricted to a full-liquid diet. She asks you to call her back and recommend foods and preparation methods. She wants to know about how he can keep his mouth clean after he eats.

   Make notes that you can refer to when you call her back to give her the information she is asking for.

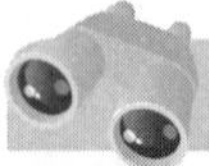

BOX 55-1 MeSH TERMS

Use a combination of MeSH terms and other key words to develop an effective and efficient PubMed literature search strategy.

Oral surgical procedures
Orthognathic surgical procedures
Maxillofacial injuries

Jaw fractures
- Mandibular fractures
- Maxillary fractures

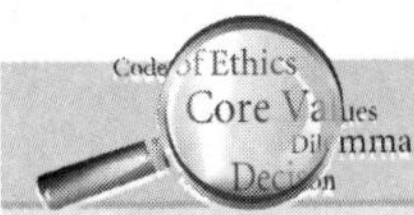

EVERYDAY ETHICS

Before completing the learning exercises below, reread and reflect on the Everyday Ethics Scenario and Questions for Consideration in this chapter of the textbook. It may also be useful to review the Dental Hygiene Ethics discussion in Chapter 1, the Ethical Applications in the introduction pages for each section in the textbook, as well as the Codes of Ethics in textbook Appendices I–IV.

Individual Learning Activity

Imagine that you have observed what happened in the scenario, but are not one of the main characters involved in the situation. Write a reflective journal entry that:

describes how you might have reacted (as an observer—not as a participant),

expresses your personal feelings about what happened,

or

identifies personal values that affect your reaction to the situation.

Discovery Activity

Ask a friend or relative who is not involved in health care to read the scenario and discuss it with you from the perspective of a "patient" who receives services within the healthcare system. Discuss what you learned from the concerns, insights, or difference in perspective that person expressed.

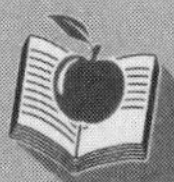

Factors To Teach The Patient

This scenario is related to the following factors listed in this chapter of the textbook:

- ▷ Significance of a clean mouth during general anesthesia.

Mr. Brown is scheduled in about 2 weeks for some very serious surgery that is part of his treatment for pancreatic cancer. His physician has recommended that Mr. Brown visit his dental hygienist for a complete dental assessment before the surgery. As you go over his health history, you discover that he is very confused about why dental hygiene interventions are necessary in his case—after all, his illness has nothing to do with his mouth!

Use the information in Chapter 55 of the textbook and the principles of motivational interviewing (see Appendix D) as a guide to write a statement explaining to Mr. Brown why this dental-hygiene appointment is such an important component of his total health and well-being.

56

The Patient with Cancer

LEARNING OBJECTIVES

Upon successful completion of these exercises, you will be able to:

1. Identify and define key terms and concepts related to the patient with cancer.
2. Identify risk factors for oral cancer.
3. Identify standard cancer treatments and the oral effects of each.
4. Plan and document dental hygiene care for the cancer patient before, during, and after therapy.

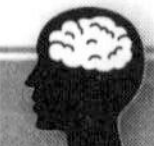

KNOWLEDGE EXERCISES

Write your answers for each question in the space provided.

1. Match the following terms related to the physical and oral effects of cancer treatment with the correct description.

Term	Description of Effect
____ Mucositis	A. Diminishment or abatement of the symptoms of a disease
____ Dysgeusia	B. Recurrence of a disease after its apparent cessation
____ Neurotoxicity	C. Treatment that provides relief of symptoms but is not intended to cure
____ Alopecia	D. A loss of hair
____ Palliative	E. Virus that can cause oral infection during or after radiation therapy
____ Herpes simplex	F. Distortion of the sense of taste
____ *Candida albicans*	G. Limited jaw opening because of spasm or fibrosis of muscles or joint; may occur 3–6 months after radiation treatment to the head and neck
____ Trismus	H. Fungus that commonly causes oral infection related to treatment for cancer
____ Immunosuppression	I. Inhibition of antibody responses resulting from leucopenia related to chemotherapy treatments
____ Relapse	J. Inflammation of the oral mucosa
____ Remission	K. Can cause a bilateral feeling of toothache related to chemotherapy treatments for cancer

2. What is cancer?

3. How are cancers classified and described?

4. What are the risk factors for developing cancer?

5. Why is it important to plan comprehensive and coordinated dental hygiene care for your patient before, during, and after treatment for cancer?

6. Identify the dental hygiene interventions you will most likely provide for your patient before the medical treatment for cancer begins.

7. List oral complications that are commonly the result of any of the various types of treatment for cancer.

8. What are the systemic side effects of chemotherapy cancer treatment?

9. List types of oral infections common during and after treatment for cancer.

10. In your own words, briefly describe a hematopoietic cell transplantation.

11. Describe graft-versus-host disease and list significant oral complications found in affected individuals.

12. ____________ is a destructive blood vessel compromise and necrosis of bone that can occur after high-dose radiation treatment in the head and neck area. This condition results in a decreased ability to heal and increased susceptibility to infection.

13. What oral changes can influence/restrict nutritional intake and further compromise the health status of a patient who is undergoing cancer therapy?

14. List the symptoms you would expect to observe in all five levels of the World Health Organization Oral Mucositis Scale.

Level	Clinical Symptoms

15. List personal care recommendations you can make to help the patient who is undergoing treatment for cancer to reduce the risk for mucositis or to increase ability to maintain daily oral hygiene measures when mucositis is already a problem.

16. Identify measures that could help prevent dental caries in a patient with xerostomia related to cancer treatment.

17. What patient factors can influence your patient's ability to attend to and comply with the counseling and oral hygiene instructions that you provide before, during, and after treatment for cancer?

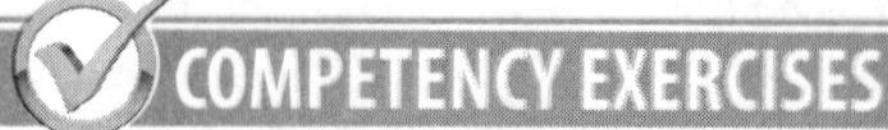

COMPETENCY EXERCISES

Apply information from the chapter and use critical thinking skills to complete the competency exercises. Write responses on paper or create electronic documents to submit your answers.

Mrs. Marge Henley is scheduled today in the hospital dental clinic as an emergency patient. After he examines her, Dr. Singh completes the assessment findings component of a patient care plan form and then calls you in to consult with him. Mrs. Henley is currently undergoing chemotherapy for cancer treatment and is experiencing severe oral symptoms related to the treatment. Dr. Singh has already written a prescription to treat the oral candidiasis. He asks you to counsel Mrs. Henley about daily oral care and to write a dental hygiene care plan for her continuing care during the cancer treatment.

When you carefully examine her, you discover that Mrs. Henley's oral tissues are heartbreakingly inflamed, blistered, and dry. She tells you that she has been feeling a bit guilty because her mouth has been so sore that she cannot brush and floss as often or as thoroughly as she used to do. Her sense of humor has remained intact, though, and she tells you with a twinkle in her eye that she eats vanilla pudding for breakfast, lunch, and dinner every day. She asks for any suggestions you have to help her get through this difficult time.

1. What areas of risk are associated with the assessment findings recorded for Mrs. Henley?

2. Write at least two dental hygiene diagnosis statements to include in Mrs. Henley's written care plan.

3. Write a goal for each of the problems identified in the dental hygiene diagnosis statements you wrote for question 2. Include a time frame for meeting each goal. How will you measure whether your patient met the goal?

4. Using your institution's guidelines for writing in patient records, document Mrs. Henley's visit and write a statement regarding her next visit.

DISCOVERY EXERCISES

1. The National Oral Health Information Clearinghouse (NOHIC) is a resource center for oral health information geared to patients with special needs and the healthcare providers who serve them. Visit their website (www.nohic.nidcr.nih.gov) to discover a wonderful series of education pamphlets about oral cancer and the oral complications of cancer treatment.

2. Investigate the medical and dental literature using a PubMed search to discover which types of cancer

may be treated with drugs, such as bisphosphonates, that can have a long-term effect on oral tissues. (Idea: This topic would make an excellent table clinic presentation.)

Questions Patients Ask

What sources of information can you identify that will help you answer your patient's questions in this scenario?

"How can I possibly keep my mouth clean when it is so sore and/or dry that it hurts to use the toothbrush? And why is that so important anyway?" "When is the best time to have my teeth worked on while I am undergoing treatment for my cancer?" "How soon after my radiation treatment can I get my new dentures and/or partial dentures?" "Will the kind of cancer treatment I am receiving now affect my ability to receive dental care, such as having implants placed, later on?"

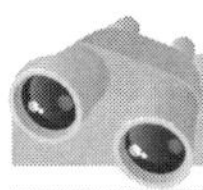

BOX 56-1 MeSH TERMS

Use a combination of MeSH terms and other key words to develop an effective and efficient PubMed literature search strategy.

Neoplasms	Trismus
Neoplasm staging	Xerostomia
Neoplasm metastasis	Mucositis
Antineoplastic agents	Stomatitis
Osteonecrosis	Candidiasis, oral

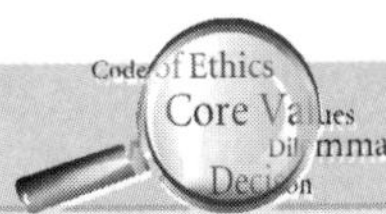

EVERYDAY ETHICS

Before completing the learning exercises below, reread and reflect on the Everyday Ethics Scenario and Questions for Consideration in this chapter of the textbook. It may also be useful to review the Dental Hygiene Ethics discussion in Chapter 1, the Ethical Applications in the introduction pages for each section in the textbook, as well as the Codes of Ethics in textbook Appendices I–IV.

Discovery Activities

Investigate the practice act in your state to determine the legal issues involved as the dental hygienist in this scenario contemplates what action to take.

Ask a dental hygienist who has been practicing for a year or more to read the scenario. Provide them with a copy of the Code of Ethics as well. Share the responses you have made to answer each question and ask that person to discuss the situation with you. What insights did you have or what did you learn during this discussion?

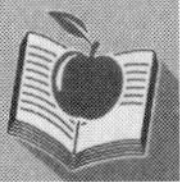

Factors To Teach The Patient

This scenario is related to the following factors listed in this chapter of the textbook:

- ▷ Why the dental hygienist needs to conduct an oral soft-tissue screening and complete oral examination at regular, frequent intervals.
- ▷ How and when to use dental biofilm control methods, gel-tray application, use of saliva substitute, and all other details of personal care to reduce oral side effects caused by the disease and/or cancer treatment.
- ▷ Ideas for remembering to follow the instructions to keep the mouth healthier and more comfortable during cancer treatment.
- ▷ The reasons why a routine schedule of preventive periodontal scaling, fluoride application, and oral hygiene assessment done by a dental hygienist contributes to the success of cancer treatment.

George Murphy, a 45-year-old construction worker, has recently been diagnosed with parotid gland cancer that has spread into his left neck. He will be having surgery to remove the left parotid gland with a left neck dissection, followed by radiation therapy. He is scheduled today for a pretreatment dental examination. Mr. Murphy has not seen a dentist in more than 10 years and has dental caries lesions, moderately advanced periodontal disease, and very poor oral hygiene. You are asked to prepare a dental hygiene care plan to address Mr. Murphy's oral care needs during and after the radiation treatment.

Mr. Murphy tells you that he hates dentists because they always hurt him and that is why he never comes to see one. The only reason he is here today is because he was told that he could not proceed with his cancer treatment unless he gets his mouth into better shape.

Use the information in the Personal Factors section of Chapter 56 of the textbook and the principles of motivational interviewing (see Appendix D) as guides to prepare an outline for a conversation you will use to counsel Mr. Murphy regarding his oral condition.

Crossword Puzzle

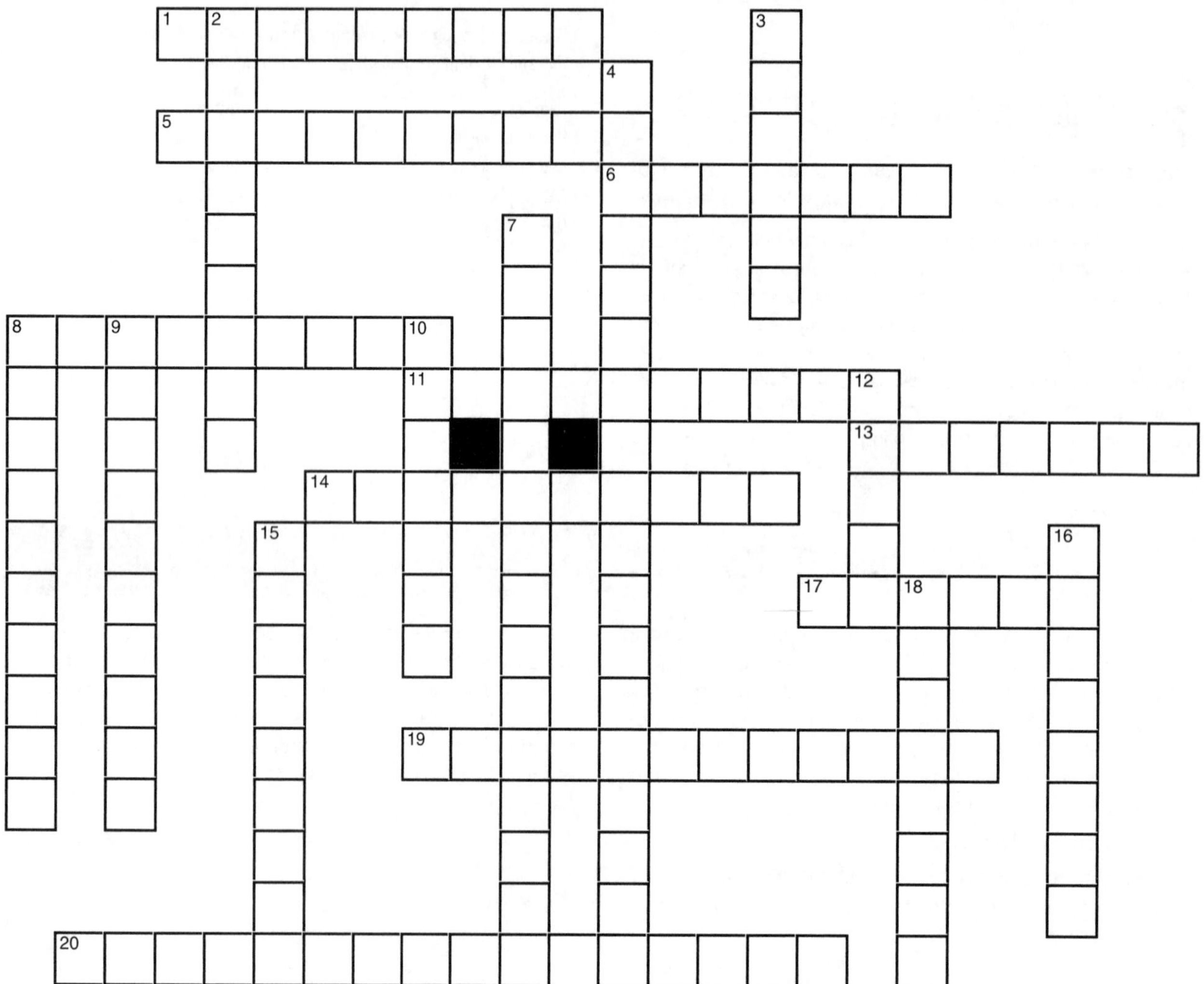

Puzzle Clues

Across

1. Type of tumor that grows at a rapid rate, gains access to blood and lymph channels to metastasize into other areas of the body, and usually causes death unless growth can be controlled.
5. Intervention to provide relief for symptoms.
6. The __________ oncologist is the member of the cancer care team who manages the patient's chemotherapy treatments.
8. Inflammation of oral tissues.
11. Donor for this type of bone marrow transplant is the patient.
13. This condition can limit the patient's ability to open mouth during dental hygiene treatment.
14. The radiation __________ is the member of the cancer care team who is responsible for planning, delivery, and follow-up of radiation therapy.
17. Type of tumor that grows slowly by expansion and does not infiltrate surrounding tissue, does not spread by metastasis, and does not usually cause death unless its location interferes with vital functions.
19. Treatment of an illness by using drugs.
20. Treatment of disease with ionizing radiation (two words).

Down

2. The irreversible alteration in adult cells toward embryonic cell types, characteristic of tumor cells.
3. Confined to the site of origin (two words)
4. Analysis of blood and blood-forming tissues for normal blood values (two words)
7. The __________ is a member of the cancer care team with an important role in identifying and managing oral manifestations related to the patient's cancer treatments (two words).
8. The spread of cancer cells from one body tissue or organ to others through blood and lymph systems.
9. A chemical, physical, or biologic agent that may cause cancer.
10. Tumor composed of cells derived from connective tissue.
12. Clinical classification of a tumor; consists of three components.
15. Malignant tumor of epithelial origin.
16. The study of tumors.
18. Any new and abnormal growth; can be benign or malignant.

57

The Patient with a Disability

LEARNING OBJECTIVES

Upon successful completion of these exercises, you will be able to:

1. Identify and define key terms and concepts related to individuals with disabilities.
2. Identify oral conditions caused by or resulting from disabling conditions.
3. Describe procedures and factors that contribute to safe and successful dental-hygiene treatment for individuals with disabilities.
4. Describe factors that enhance the prevention of oral disease for individuals with disabilities and their caregivers.

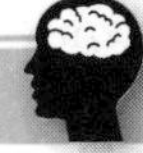

KNOWLEDGE EXERCISES

Write your answers for each question in the space provided.

1. Briefly describe the components included in the two main sections of the World Health Organization International Classifications of Functioning, Disability, and Health.

   Part 1: Functioning and disability

   Part 2: Contextual factors

2. In your own words, define a barrier-free dental treatment facility.

3. How wide must outdoor walkways and indoor passageways be to accommodate a wheelchair?

4. An appropriately constructed wheelchair ramp entrance has a handrail and a gentle slope that rises ____________ for every ____________ in length.

5. Lightweight doors with lever handles must open at least ____________ wide for a wheelchair to pass through.

6. A dental chair that is accessible for wheelchair transfers can be lowered to at least ____________ from the floor.

7. List three areas of risk assessment to consider when treating a patient with a disability.

8. List common oral findings in patients with a disability that can be a source of increased risk for oral disease.

9. List common oral effects related to drug therapies used to treat patients with disabilities.

10. List the components of an oral disease prevention and control program for a patient with a disability.

11. To plan oral hygiene instructions for your patient with a disability, it is important for you to understand the ability of your patient to perform daily living and self-care skills such as toothbrushing. Briefly describe the functioning ability for each ADL/IADL level.

ADL/IADL level 0

ADL/IADL levels 1 and 2

ADL/IADL level 3

12. What is the dental hygienist's role in providing oral hygiene instructions for an individual who is identified as having a moderate- or low-functioning level?

13. When should you recommend that the use of a dentifrice be limited or eliminated from the oral care regimen of a patient with a disability?

14. What recommendations can you make so a patient who cannot use a dentifrice receives the benefits of fluoride?

15. Self-care aids can make a difference in the ability of a patient or caregiver to maximize effectiveness of oral care. List the general prerequisites of a good oral self-care aid.

16. Identify three general modifications that can be made to a toothbrush handle to enhance the ability of a patient with a disability to provide oral self-care.

17. What factors will you take into consideration when recommending the use of a power-assisted toothbrush for a patient with a disability?

18. Briefly describe modifications that can be made to help a patient with a disability care for a removable dental prosthesis.

19. In your own words, describe the position a caregiver can use to be most effective when providing daily oral care for a person with disabilities.

20. List factors to take into consideration when planning dietary recommendations for your patient with a disability.

21. In your own words, summarize precautions you can take and patient care modifications you can make to ensure safety and comfort for your patient with a disability.

22. Unless an extreme cognitive impairment has been identified, communication related to dental-hygiene care is always addressed first to ____________.

23. For you to plan dental hygiene care that takes all of the needs of your patient with a disability into consideration, it is essential to gather as much information as possible before the first appointment. Identify three individuals (or groups) who can provide the needed information.

24. List factors to consider when scheduling appointments for an individual with a disability.

25. List factors that contribute to safety and comfortable positioning or stabilization of your patient with a disability while he or she is in the dental chair.

26. What precautions are required if protective stabilization is considered?

27. Describe a technique for safely stabilizing a patient's head during dental-hygiene treatment.

28. List the types of aids that can be used to stabilize the patient's mouth while providing dental-hygiene treatment or during daily oral care provided by caregivers.

29. List precautions to observe if you are using a mouth prop.

30. List three basic types of wheelchair transfers.

31. What is the first thing you should do before starting a wheelchair transfer?

32. Who can give you advice in how best to help during a wheelchair transfer?

33. List three factors that take special consideration during a wheelchair transfer.

34. Describe the position of the wheelchair with respect to the position of the dental chair when transferring your patient from the wheelchair to the dental chair.

Mobile transfer

Immobile transfer

Sliding board transfer

35. It makes sense, when transferring your patient back to the wheelchair after treatment, to position the seat of the dental chair slightly ____________ than the seat of the wheelchair.

36. If you are helping your patient with a mobile transfer from a wheelchair to the dental chair, where are your patient's arms and hands?

37. Describe the position of the first aide's hands/arms when two people are helping with an immobile patient transfer.

38. What is the responsibility of the second assistant during an immobile patient transfer?

39. What is your role when seating a patient with a walker, crutches, or a cane in the dental chair?

40. What are the best ways to evaluate the success of an in-service program?

41. What topics are included during an in-service presentation that teaches caregivers how to examine oral tissues?

____

____

____

____

____

____

42. List at least four additional oral care/disease prevention topics or techniques to teach during staff in-service training.

____

____

____

____

____

____

COMPETENCY EXERCISES

Apply information from the chapter and use critical thinking skills to complete the competency exercises. Write responses on paper or create electronic documents to submit your answers.

1. In your own words, explain the relationship between the terms *impairment*, *disability*, and *handicap*.

2. To avoid confusion, it is imperative to ask direct questions concerning the type and severity of your patient's disability. In your own words, list some basic categories of information to obtain from a patient with a disability or the caregiver that will assist in patient management.

3. In your own words, identify at least three objectives for providing quality dental and dental-hygiene care for individuals with disabilities.

4. Steve McKnight is your patient with cerebral palsy. He is charming and witty. He works for a company that develops voice technology for computers. He has significant physical impairments associated with his condition and moves about with difficulty, using crutches and special leg braces to walk. He is fiercely independent, preferring to manage as many tasks as possible on his own.

   Steve moves his hands with difficulty and cannot grasp small objects very well. He feeds himself using specially adapted utensils. When you talk to him about his daily oral care, he mentions that he used a power-driven toothbrush for a while but that it was heavy and, when it started to vibrate, he could barely hold it up to his mouth. He sighs and says that he really wishes he could find a regular toothbrush that he could hold on to without dropping it in the sink all the time.

   Find appropriate materials and make a device to adapt a toothbrush and floss handle that would help Steve continue to be independent in his daily oral care. Share your design with your classmates. Does your design meet the general prerequisites for a self-care aid as described in the textbook?

DISCOVERY EXERCISE

Explore the Americans with Disabilities Act website at http://www.ada.gov.

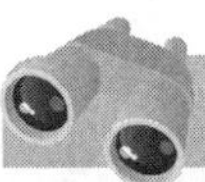

BOX 57-1 MeSH TERMS

Use a combination of MeSH terms and other key words to develop an effective and efficient PubMed literature search strategy.

Dental care for disabled
Developmental disabilities
Intellectual disability
Disabled persons
Amputees
Disabled children
Hearing impaired persons
Mentally disabled persons
Mentally ill persons
Visually impaired persons
Self-help devices
Communication aids for disabled
Wheelchairs

EVERYDAY ETHICS

Before completing the learning exercises below, reread and reflect on the Everyday Ethics Scenario and Questions for Consideration in this chapter of the textbook. It may also be useful to review the Dental Hygiene Ethics discussion in Chapter 1, the Ethical Applications in the introduction pages for each section in the textbook, as well as the Codes of Ethics in textbook Appendices I–IV.

Individual Learning Activity

Imagine that you are the dental hygienist in this scenario. Answer each of the questions for consideration at the end of the scenario.

Collaborative Activity

Answer each of the questions for consideration at the end of the scenario in the textbook. Compare what you wrote with answers developed by another classmate and discuss differences/similarities.

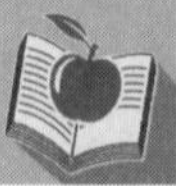

Factors To Teach The Patient

This scenario is related to the following factors listed in this chapter of the textbook:

- ▷ Practice a healthy lifestyle, including a healthy diet.

Use the information about a healthy diet in Chapter 35, the principles of anticipatory guidance (Chapter 50), and a motivational interviewing approach (see Appendix D) to write a conversation educating the mother of a 4-year-old child who has a disability about the general concepts of maintaining a tooth-healthy diet.

Word Search Puzzle

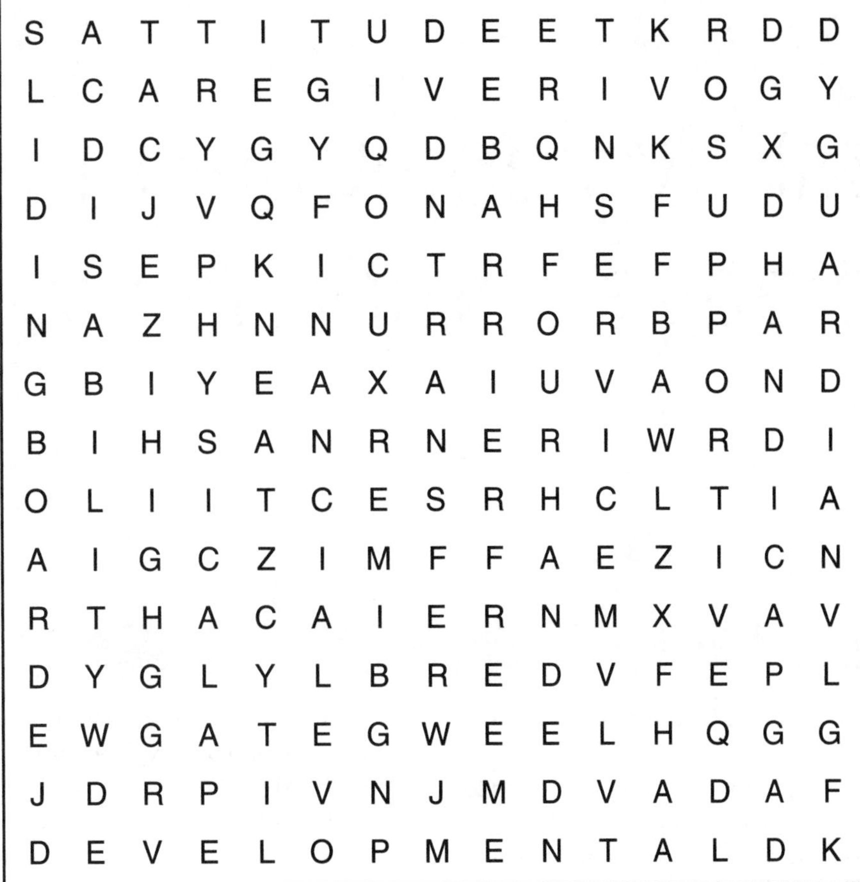

Puzzle Clues

- An aid that can be used to help transfer an individual from a wheelchair to the dental chair and back again (two words).
- Refers to the disadvantage that can limit fulfillment of a normal role for a person with an impairment.
- A dental treatment room that is not wheelchair accessible is an example of this kind of barrier that can hinder access to oral care.
- Person who performs or helps to perform daily life activities.
- The need for longer appointment time—and the dental professional's need to be reimbursed for providing that time—can constitute this type of barrier that limits oral-care options for an individual with a disability.
- Dental professionals who do not feel adequately trained to provide safe treatment is an example of this type of barrier to care for individuals with a disability.
- Refers to a disability of indefinite duration with an onset before the age of 18.
- The individual responsible for making decisions if a person is declared incapacitated in a legal process; requires written proof for decision making.
- Refers to the restriction that results from an impairment.
- Accessible; obstacles to passage or communication have been removed.
- A term that refers to several techniques for moving a person from a wheelchair to a dental chair and back.
- Refers to dental hygiene care delivered with the help of a dental assistant (two words).
- Education program about some specific topic, such as oral care for individuals with disabilities, that is provided for parents, teachers, volunteers, nurses, or other health professionals (without the hyphen).
- The Americans with Disabilities Act, *not* the American Dental Association!
- Padding and other body stabilization methods used to facilitate patient comfort and safety.
- Level of function identified by an ADL/IADL level of 0.

58

Dental Hygiene Care in Alternative Settings

LEARNING OBJECTIVES

Upon successful completion of these exercises, you will be able to:

1. Identify and define key terms and concepts related to dental hygiene practice in alternative settings.
2. Prepare materials necessary for visiting a patient in an alternative practice setting.
3. Plan and document adaptations to dental hygiene care plans and oral-hygiene instructions for the patient who is homebound, bedridden, unconscious, or terminally ill.

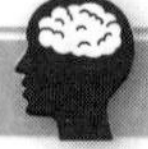

KNOWLEDGE EXERCISES

Write your answers for each question in the space provided.

1. What characteristics help identify a person who may not be able to access dental hygiene care in a traditional private practice office setting?

2. What barriers can prevent an individual from receiving oral health they need?

3. How might dental hygienists address the needs of individuals who experience barriers to accessing traditional private practice–based oral care?

4. In your own words, define direct access dental hygiene care.

5. List objectives of providing dental hygiene care in alternative practice settings for individuals who cannot access the traditional dental practice setting.

6. Identify three unique objects or implements, not usually associated with providing care in a dental office, to include when planning to provide care in alternative practice settings.

7. List three factors that can influence scheduling an appointment time to provide dental hygiene care for a residence-bound patient.

8. Identify unhealthy personal factors that may be associated with inactivity or a monotonous existence of a residence-bound patient.

9. Identify communication and personal approaches that help build a successful relationship with an individual who is relatively helpless, disabled, or ill.

10. When is a firm pillow useful for patient positioning during dental hygiene care?

11. Describe a patient who is comatose.

12. In your own words, define the concept of hospice care.

13. Identify three objectives for providing dental hygiene care for a patient who is critically or terminally ill.

14. Define *palliative care*.

15. What common oral infection is often found in a patient with a terminal illness?

____

____

16. What one item is documented in the patient record when the care is provided an alternative practice setting that is not usually documented for care provided in a traditional dental practice setting?

____

____

COMPETENCY EXERCISES

Apply information from the chapter and use critical thinking skills to complete the competency exercises. Write responses on paper or create electronic documents to submit your answers.

1. You are one of the dental hygienists on a dental care team that visits the Nightingale Long Term Care Center each month to provide oral care for residents. Your first patient of the day is Bruce Wilkerson, a handsome 29 year old who has been in a coma since a diving accident 8 years ago. After looking at the information in Bruce's medical record, you enter his room and greet him. As you prepare your armamentarium, position him for oral care, and place towels under his chin, you keep up a cheerful one-sided conversation. Explain why it is important to talk with this patient even though he will definitely not respond to your remarks.

2. Mrs. Malcolm has been a patient in your clinic for about 15 years. She has always had fairly good oral hygiene and a healthy mouth has been important to her. You haven't seen her in quite a while, though, because Mrs. Malcolm has spent a lot of time in the hospital over the last year. You recently heard that she has been receiving hospice care in her home.

   Dr. Gable, the dentist in your clinic, has agreed to provide some basic comfort care at home for Mrs. Malcolm, and she suggests that you accompany her. When you arrive, you find that Mrs. Malcolm, although very weak, is awake and able to speak with you. She complains of having a very dry mouth and you notice that her lips are coated with a dry looking, crusty material. She mentions that her lower partial denture does not fit very well anymore and often slips around whenever she tries to eat. It is rubbing on her left cheek. She says her mouth feels and tastes bad and that her gums were bleeding when her daughter tried to help her brush her teeth a couple of days ago.

   Write at least three dental hygiene diagnosis statements for Mrs. Malcolm's care plan.

3. Write a goal and evaluation method for one of the diagnosis statements you identified in the question above. Include a time frame for meeting that goal.

4. Describe ways that you can arrange your working situation for providing dental hygiene care to Mrs. Malcolm in her the bedroom of her home.

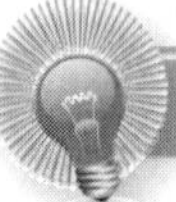

DISCOVERY EXERCISES

1. Use the information in Boxes 58-3 and 58-4 in the textbook as well as additional information from dental supply catalogs and websites to put together a plan and a budget for everything you would need to implement a portable dental hygiene practice.

2. Contact a nearby nursing home or senior residence center and ask to talk to someone on the staff about interprofessional collaborative practice. Explain the value of adding a dental hygienist to their patient care team.

Questions Patients Ask

What sources of information can you identify that will help you answer your patient's questions in this scenario?

"There are so many agencies now that offer health and personal-care services to homebound individuals—why don't they have someone who can come to my house/nursing home so that I could get my teeth cleaned?" "Is there a dentist around here who will make house calls?" "Why doesn't the staff in my mother's nursing home help her brush her teeth every day?" "Can you come to my mother's house to clean her teeth?"

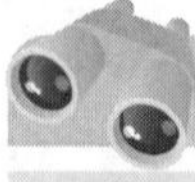

BOX 58-1 MeSH TERMS

Use a combination of MeSH terms and other key words to develop an effective and efficient PubMed literature search strategy.

Homebound persons	Dental care for chronically ill
Terminally ill	Dental care for disabled
Hospice care	Interdisciplinary communication
Dental care for aged	

EVERYDAY ETHICS

Before completing the learning exercises below, reread and reflect on the Everyday Ethics Scenario and Questions for Consideration in this chapter of the textbook. It may also be useful to review the Dental Hygiene Ethics discussion in Chapter 1, the Ethical Applications in the introduction pages for each section in the textbook, as well as the Codes of Ethics in textbook Appendices I–IV.

Individual Learning Activities

Imagine that you are the dental hygienist in this scenario. Answer each of the questions for consideration at the end of the scenario.

Imagine that you have observed what happened in the scenario, but are not one of the main characters involved in the situation. Write a reflective journal entry that:

describes how you might have reacted (as an observer-not as a participant),

expresses your personal feelings about what happened,

or

identifies personal values that affect your reaction to the situation.

Factors To Teach The Patient/Caregiver

This scenario is related to the following factors listed in this chapter of the textbook:

- ▷ The contribution of good oral health to general health.
- ▷ How a clean mouth can contribute to wellness and quality-of-life factors.
- ▷ How to care for the patient's natural teeth: toothbrushing, flossing, rinsing, and other personal needs.
- ▷ How to use a suction toothbrush, power brush, or other device to provide oral care for the patient.

Today you are giving hands-on training in providing daily oral care for a group of nurse's aides at the Nightingale Long Term Care Center. You have set up a suction toothbrush at the bedside of Bruce Wilkerson (introduced in Competency Exercises question 1). Besides showing and telling the nurse's aides how to brush someone else's teeth and care for the suction toothbrush afterward, you also want to explain the reasons for providing daily oral cleansing for all of the residents/patients in the center.

Use a motivational interviewing approach (see Appendix D) as a guide to write an outline of information you need to present to the group of nurse's aides.

Use the conversation you create to role-play this situation with several fellow students. If you are a nurse's aide in the role-play, be sure to ask questions. If you are the dental hygienist, try to anticipate questions and answer them in your explanation.

59

The Patient with a Physical Impairment

LEARNING OBJECTIVES

Upon successful completion of these exercises, you will be able to:

1. Identify and define key terms and concepts related to physical impairment.
2. Describe the characteristics, complications, occurrence, and medical treatment of a variety of physical impairments.
3. Identify oral factors and findings related to physical impairments.
4. Plan and document modifications for dental hygiene care based on assessment of needs that are specific to a patient's physical impairment.

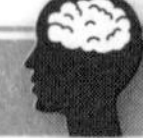

KNOWLEDGE EXERCISES

Write your answers for each question in the space provided.

1. For each definition provided below, identify the correct term or concept related to movement or sensory-motor impairment.
   a. Any disease of the muscle: ____________
   b. Absence or loss of the power of voluntary motion: ____________
   c. Irregularity or failure of muscle action—manifests in loss of equilibrium or coordination: ____________
   d. Impairment of the ability to control movement: ____________
   e. Involuntary muscle quivering: ____________
   f. Condition characterized by constant, involuntary, unorganized movement: ____________
   g. Abnormal slowness of movement: ____________
   h. Flabby, weak muscles: ____________
   i. Stiff (muscles) and resistance to movement: ____________
   j. Muscle spasm reflex: ____________
   k. Wasting or decrease in size of muscle due to disuse, loss of blood supply, or severed nerve connection: ____________
   l. Loss or impairment of motor function: ____________
   m. Slight or incomplete paralysis: ____________
   n. Paralysis on one side of the body: ____________
   o. Paralysis of like parts on either side of the body: ____________

p. Paralysis of three limbs: ___________

q. Paralysis in lower extremities: ___________

r. Paralysis of all four limbs: ___________

s. Another term for paralysis of all four limbs: ___________

t. Difficulty in swallowing: ___________

u. Immobility due to direct union—as in union of bone with bone: ___________

v. Spinal curvature: ___________

w. Convex curvature of the spine as viewed from the side; humpback: ___________

x. With an abdominal protuberance; characteristic of Duchenne muscular dystrophy; swayback: ___________

y. Induration or hardening: ___________

z. Arthritis (inflammation) involvement in many joints: ___________

aa. Appliance or apparatus that improves the function of some part of the body: ___________

2. List three types of neurological disorders associated with physical disability.

3. Describe the sensorimotor effects of the following lesions.

   Complete spinal cord injury lesion:

   Incomplete spinal cord injury lesion:

4. Identify the appropriate descriptive term and the number of vertebrae associated with each of the following letters.

   C: ___________ ___________

   T: ___________ ___________

   L: ___________ ___________

5. A patient's level of disability depends on the level of the spinal cord injury. Paralysis occurs in the limbs and muscle groups innervated by nerve fibers extending at and below the injured vertebrae. Individuals who are most likely to need adaptive measures for daily oral health care procedures are those with a spinal cord injury above ___________

6. Paralysis of limbs, the need for wheelchair use, and potential complications associated with a high spinal cord injury can require that you be prepared to modify standard patient care techniques. Identify modifications you might make during dental hygiene treatment to accommodate your patient's comfort and safety.

7. What causes a decubitus ulcer and how can you help prevent this condition during dental hygiene treatment of a patient with paralysis?

8. Describe the correct response to hyperreflexia?

9. Mouth-held appliances can aid many patients who have upper body disabilities in performing a variety of basic procedures that contribute to independence. List the criteria for an adequate oral orthosis.

10. In your own words, define three different etiologic factors that cause a CVA (*or stroke*).

11. What is a TIA?

12. What conditions increase an individual's risk for CVA?

13. What patient assessment technique, commonly used by dental hygienists, can provide information that may indicate your patient's increased risk for CVA.

14. Describe signs and symptoms commonly observed in a patient with a history of CVA.

15. What is aphasia?

16. If your patient has a history of CVA damage to the right-hand side of the brain, that patient would exhibit __________-side hemiplegia, have difficulty with action requiring ____________ and would likely behave in an ____________________ manner.

17. If your patient has a history of CVA damage to the left-hand side of the brain, that patient would exhibit ____________ -side hemiplegia, have difficulty with ____________ communication, and would likely behave in a ____________ manner.

18. Complete Infomaps 59-1 and 59-2 with just enough basic information to help you identify and differentiate among the listed developmental and acquired disabling conditions.

INFOMAP 59-1 DEVELOPMENTAL CONDITIONS (ONSET BEFORE AGE 18)

CONDITION	CAUSE/OCCURRENCE	BASIC CHARACTERISTICS	CONSIDERATIONS FOR DENTAL HYGIENE CARE
Cerebral palsy			
Muscular dystrophy, Duchenne			
Muscular dystrophy, facioscapulohumeral			
Myelomeningocele			

19. What percent of patients with cerebral palsy also have brain damage that causes intellectual or cognitive impairment?

20. What additional disabling conditions can sometimes accompany a diagnosis of cerebral palsy?

21. What oral characteristics are associated with cerebral palsy?

22. What symptoms of muscular dystrophy can directly affect your patient's oral health status?

INFOMAP 59-2 ACQUIRED IMPAIRMENT (ONSET AFTER AGE 18)

CONDITION	CAUSE, OCCURRENCE, PATHOLOGY	BASIC CHARACTERISTICS	CONSIDERATIONS FOR DENTAL HYGIENE CARE
Bell's palsy			
Multiple sclerosis			
ALS			
Myasthenia gravis			
Parkinson disease			
Scleroderma, progressive systemic sclerosis			
PPS			

23. Describe the categories used to identify types of multiple sclerosis.

24. ALS is also sometimes called ____________

25. Describe early/onset symptoms for each of the two types of ALS.

26. Myasthenia gravis and scleroderma are both disabling conditions that have special significance for dental professionals. Why?

27. Care is taken when raising the dental chair after treatment of your patient with Parkinson's disease who is being treated with dopamine replenishment medications, because of the possibility of

____

28. Osteoarthritis is a chronic degenerative joint disease common in individuals who are

____

29. Describe the location and progression of osteoarthritis symptoms.

30. Describe osteoarthritis symptoms that can occur in the temporomandibular joint.

31. What is rheumatoid arthritis?

32. In your own words, describe the symptoms of rheumatoid arthritis.

33. What is juvenile rheumatoid arthritis?

34. How does rheumatoid arthritis affect the temporomandibular joint?

35. What modifications to standard treatment techniques can you use to increase the comfort of your patient who has arthritic involvement of the temporomandibular joint while you are providing dental hygiene treatment?

36. What is the relationship between rheumatoid arthritis and periodontal disease?

37. Drugs used for treatment of arthritis include pain medications such as NSAIDs. What additional drugs are used to control rheumatoid arthritis?

COMPETENCY EXERCISES

Apply information from the chapter and use critical thinking skills to complete the competency exercises. Write responses on paper or create electronic documents to submit your answers.

Read the Chapter 59 patient assessment summary to help you answer questions #1 through #3.

1. Anitha Jones presents for an initial visit dental hygiene appointment. Laura, Anitha's new caregiver, introduces herself as she assists you in transferring Anitha to the dental chair. While you are helping transfer Anitha to the dental chair, you note that she cannot control the constant disorganized movements of her arms, legs, and head. When you mistakenly startle her by reaching quickly to move the dental light out of the way, this uncontrolled movement becomes intensified. Anitha's hand flings out and bumps into the instrument tray, scattering instruments all over the floor. Anitha's face muscles are in constant motion; she drools and breathes through her mouth. Describe steps you will take to determine modifications in your usual patient care procedures that will help to keep both you and Anitha safe and comfortable during dental hygiene treatment.

CHAPTER 59 – PATIENT ASSESSMENT SUMMARY			
Patient Name: *Ms. Anitha Jones*	Age: *30*	Gender: M F ☐	☑ Initial Therapy ☐ Maintenance
Provider Name: *D.H. Student*	Date: *Today*		☐ Re-evaluation
Chief Complaint: *Patient has recently moved into the area. She presents for routine 3-month maintenance and new patient examination.*			
Assessment Findings			
Health History • *Medical diagnosis of Cerebral Palsy* • *Spasticity, athetosis, facial movements* • *No intellectual or cognitive disability.* • *Takes anti-seizure medication once per day, but caregiver who accompanies her to the appointment is not sure what it is.* • *ASA Classification - III* • *ADL level - 3*	**At Risk For:**		
Social and Dental History • *Previous history of excellent professional dental care* • *Personal dental literacy is high* • *New caregiver with low dental knowledge*	**At Risk For:**		
Dental Examination • *Difficulty controlling jaw and face movements during examination* • *Bruxism; incisal attrition and history of anterior fractures* • *Evidence of past lip and cheek-biting trauma* • *Mouth breathing; slight anterior gingivitis* • *Increased gag reflex* • *Current posterior restorations in good repair* • *Healthy periodontal tissues; probing depths <3mm*	**At Risk For:**		

2. When she is trying to communicate, it takes Anitha a long time to say anything and you cannot understand her very well. What communication strategies will help you successfully determine answers to the questions you need to ask in order to complete your patient assessment?

3. As you complete assessment data, you realize that Anitha has enjoyed regular professional and personal dental care throughout her life. A caregiver has always provided daily oral biofilm removal. Laura admits to having very little dental knowledge, but she very much wants to learn how to keep Anitha's mouth as healthy as the previous caregiver has done. Use the assessment summary data for Anitha and a copy of the Dental Hygiene Care Plan template (Appendix B) or the care plan form used by your school clinic to complete a dental hygiene care plan for Anitha that includes appropriate education for Laura.

4. Mr. O'Brien, who has been recovering for about 9 months since experiencing a CVA, has been receiving physical and occupational therapy to help him learn how use his left hand to do what he used to do with his, now partially paralyzed, right hand and arm. He is very proud of his growing independence and slowly tells you about how he can now comb his own hair and brush his own teeth. While you are performing an oral examination, you note that his biofilm control is very poor and that there is a bolus of leftover food pocketed in his right cheek. The paralyzed muscles on that side of his face have affected his ability to self-clean and even to detect the food that is pouching there after he eats.
   - Explain how you can counsel Mr. O'Brien about his oral health needs and encourage him to let his wife help him clean his mouth, especially on the paralyzed side, while still respecting his desire to independently care for his own personal needs.

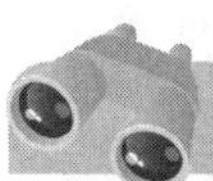

BOX 59-1 MeSH TERMS

Use a combination of MeSH terms and other key words to develop an effective and efficient PubMed literature search strategy.

- Dental care for disabled
- Neuromuscular diseases
- Parkinson disease
- Ischemia
- Ischemic attack, transient
- Paralysis
- Postpoliomyelitis syndrome
- Bell palsy
- Meningomyelocele
- Cerebral palsy (many specific types are also listed as MeSH terms)
- Muscular dystrophies
  - Muscular dystrophies, limb-girdle
  - Muscular dystrophy, Duchenne
  - Muscular dystrophy, Emery–Dreifuss
  - Muscular dystrophy, facioscapulohumeral
  - Muscular dystrophy, oculopharyngeal
- Arthritis
  - Arthritis, rheumatoid
  - Osteoarthritis

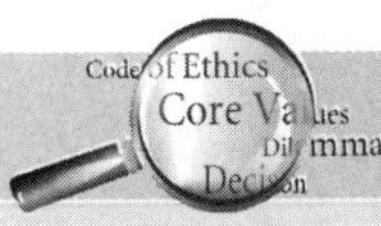

EVERYDAY ETHICS

Before completing the learning exercises below, reread and reflect on the Everyday Ethics Scenario and Questions for Consideration in this chapter of the textbook. It may also be useful to review the Dental Hygiene Ethics discussion in Chapter 1, the Ethical Applications in the introduction pages for each section in the textbook, as well as the Codes of Ethics in textbook Appendices I–IV.

Cooperative Learning Activity

Answer each of the questions for consideration at the end of the scenario in the textbook. Compare what you wrote with answers developed by another classmate and discuss differences/similarities.

Discovery Activity

Investigate the practice act in your state to determine the legal issues involved as the dental hygienist in this scenario contemplates what action to take.

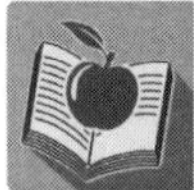

Factors To Teach The Patient

This scenario is related to the following factors listed in this chapter of the textbook:

- ▷ That daily, thorough biofilm removal is particularly necessary to reduce the occurrence of oral disease.
- ▷ That regular maintenance appointments are important to promote oral health.
- ▷ Why maintaining periodontal health has added value for teeth used as abutments for a mouth-held implement.
- ▷ How to clean and maintain the mouth-held implement.
- ▷ The need to maintain teeth in order to tolerate a mouth-held aid.

Once a month, your employer, Dr. Tom Buckner, and his entire dental team provide care in the little dental clinic inside a nearby assisted-living residence. Your next patient, Terry Biensfield, 25 years old, sustained a level C5 spinal-cord injury in a motorcycle accident several years ago. He has worked hard in his physical-therapy sessions to maximize his level of function in activities of daily living by using adaptive aids. You have taught him how to brush his own teeth using a modified, long-handled toothbrush attached to one hand, but he still needs some caregiver support and reminders that he must complete his daily oral care routine.

Last month, Dr. Buckner and the physical therapist devised a mouthstick appliance that allows Terry to use a computer. Terry has been practicing with the computer every day, when he participates in an online discussion for people with spinal-cord injuries. He now has lots of new ideas for ways he can use his mouthstick to be more independent and creative in his daily life.

Use a motivational interviewing approach (see Appendix D) to write a statement explaining to Terry how important it is for him to maintain an optimum level of oral health so his teeth can continue to support the use of the mouthstick.

60

The Patient with a Sensory Impairment

LEARNING OBJECTIVES

Upon successful completion of these exercises, you will be able to:

1. Identify and define key terms and concepts related to sensory impairment.
2. Describe the causes of sensory impairments.
3. Identify factors that affect interpersonal communication and patient education.
4. Plan and document adaptations that enhance dental hygiene care for a patient with a sensory impairment.

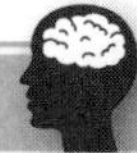

KNOWLEDGE EXERCISES

1. In what way does the ADA define the responsibility of the dental practitioner in meeting the needs of a patient with a hearing or vision impairment?

2. In your own words, define *visual impairment*.

3. Explain the term *legally blind*.

4. For each descriptive term for the two types of visual impairment often corrected by prescription eyeglasses, provide the medical term and characteristics associated with it.

   Farsighted

   Nearsighted

5. An astigmatism, also often corrected with prescription glasses, is caused by what?

____

____

6. An ____________ measures visual acuity and prescribes lenses for the correction of visual defects; an ____________ is the technician who prepares the adaptive lenses prescribed by the specialist.

7. An ____________ is a physician specializing in treatment of defects, injuries, and diseases of the eye.

8. ____________ during pregnancy is the cause of at least half of the blindness in children.

9. ____________ is an inflammation of the retina.

10. What is retinopathy?

____

____

11. Identify and describe the condition that causes blindness in infants who must be treated at birth with very high concentrations of oxygen.

____

____

____

____

12. In your own words, define *glaucoma*.

____

____

____

13. A patient with glaucoma has limited ____________.

14. What terms refers to a visual impairment that can be caused by a vitamin deficiency?

____

15. Briefly explain some actions the dental hygienist can take to assure understanding when providing oral hygiene instructions for the patient with a visual impairment.

____

____

____

16. Why do you always speak to patients who have a significant visual impairment each time before you enter or leave the room and each time before you touch them during dental hygiene treatment?

____

____

17. A person can hear when the ____________ vibrates and sound waves are transmitted to nerve endings by the ossicles of middle ear, to cochlea in the inner ear, and then to the brain.

18. What is tinnitus?

____

____

19. What is vertigo?

____

____

____

20. What is the abbreviation for decibel?

____

21. Your patient is considered deaf when his or her hearing impairment is at what level?

____

____

22. What descriptive phrase is sometimes used for a patient who cannot hear as well as someone with normal hearing?

____

____

23. List factors that may contribute to hearing loss.

____

____

____

____

____

____

24. What is an audiologist?

____

____

____

25. How does the audiologist determine an individual's degree and type of hearing ability?

26. An otologist would most likely be the healthcare worker involved with treating otitis media. What is otitis media?

27. Identify the four types of hearing loss and briefly identify the damaged body structure(s) associated with each type.

28. How does a hearing aid function?

29. Why should you remind your patient who uses a hearing aid to either turn it off or take it out during dental hygiene treatment?

30. Describe a cochlear implant.

31. In your own words, what is ASL?

32. What is speech reading?

33. If your patient is speech reading, what can you do to enhance his or her understanding during oral hygiene instructions?

34. The best way to teach skills, such as biofilm removal, to your patient with a hearing loss is by ___________ rather than by explanation.

COMPETENCY EXERCISES

Apply information from the chapter and use critical thinking skills to complete the competency exercises. Write responses on paper or create electronic documents to submit your answers.

1. You have completed Mr. Corkman's dental hygiene treatment for today, and you direct him down to Jenny, the appointment manager, so he can schedule his next visit while you clean and disinfect the treatment room for your next patient. When he gets to the end of the hallway, you hear him say, "Delighted to meet you, Benny!" in a very loud voice. You observe him at the front desk for a bit and then walk up to him and remind him that he turned his hearing aid off when you were using the ultrasonic scaler during his treatment. What did you observe to indicate Mr. Corkman had forgotten to turn it on again?

2. Ask one of your student colleagues to role-play the part of Anastasia Binghamton, 16 years old, your patient who is profoundly deaf. Her preferred method of communicating is using a combination of ASL and finger spelling. Use the pictures in Figures 60-2 and 60-3 in the textbook to help you practice asking her the following questions.
   - Are there any changes in your health history?
   - Is there any pain in the area where tooth 32 was extracted last month?
   - Can you please open wider so that I can polish the back teeth?
   - I will show you how to position your toothbrush in order to get all the bacteria off the gums.
   - The dentist will be right in to examine your mouth.
   - Please make your next appointment in 6 months.

3. Patty Ricalde, 25 years old, is one of your favorite patients. She usually arrives for her appointment clinging to the arm of her younger sister; both of them are out of breath, laughing uproariously, and looking as though they had just returned from some astonishing adventure. Sometimes they have, as you found out last year, when they came in with photographs of a desert hiking adventure in southern Utah! Sometimes, when you listen to the two of them, you forget that Patty is designated as legally blind. She also wears a hearing device that allows her to communicate with anyone who will take the time to talk slowly and clearly.

   You will be developing a new dental hygiene care plan for Patty, and you want to designate her ADL level to indicate her ability to manage daily oral care. (*Hint:* Refer to Table 24-3 in Chapter 24 of the textbook.)

   Discuss the ADL level you will assign to Patty.

4. What ASA classification will you assign to Patty? (*Hint:* Refer to Table 24-1 in Chapter 24 of the textbook.)

5. Your next patient, Damian, arrives with a huge golden retriever guide dog he calls Harrison. You are a bit flustered and you hold out your hand to greet Damian without first letting him know you have come into the room with him. He bumps into you as he turns to return your greeting and you realize Damian is almost totally blind. You aren't quite sure what to do next. You cover your distress by complimenting him on the beauty of his dog and bending down to hug the dog.

   You gently take Harrison by the collar and lead him down the hall to the door of your treatment room. Damian follows you and his dog into the room. You raise the chair up a bit higher, so the seat is just above the level of Damian's knees and you turn him around and gently ease him back until he is sitting against the edge of the dental chair. You tell him you will place the dog out in the hall where there is significantly more room. He seems uneasy about that, but you reassure him that no one will be going by to step on the dog, as your treatment room is the last one down the hall.

   As you return to the room, Damian pushes himself up and back into the chair, turns, and slides his feet up on the footrest. You wince as his head just misses the dental light, but he doesn't hit it and you breathe a sigh of relief. You notice the time is running out for your appointment, so you quickly update his health history (no significant findings), lower the chair, and then tell Damian to grab hold of the armrests before you tilt him back. You complete your oral assessment and begin scaling.

   Later, after polishing his teeth, you squirt lots of water so he can rinse her mouth. Damian raises himself from the chair, swallows twice, and then apologizes and asks for a cup to rinse. After you help him rinse with a cup, you are feeling that this appointment has been very stressful for both of you, and you would love to have a quiet minute to recover your calm. As Damian gets out of the dental chair, you walk out into the hallway to bring Harrison back in to him.

   What could you have done differently to manage Damian's care in a way that reduces both his stress and your own during this appointment?

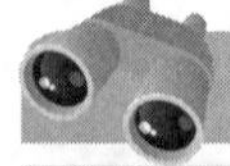

BOX 60-1 MeSH TERMS

Use a combination of MeSH terms and other key words to develop an effective and efficient PubMed literature search strategy.

Vision disorders	Hearing disorders
Vision, low	Hearing loss
Diabetic retinopathy	Tinnitus
Retinopathy of prematurity	Hearing aids
Glaucoma	Cochlear implants
Macular degeneration	Lipreading
Cataracts	Manual communication

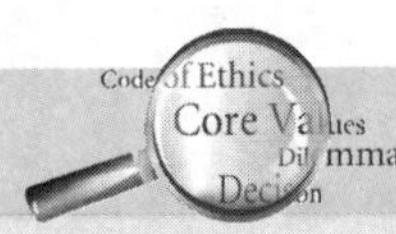

EVERYDAY ETHICS

Before completing the learning exercises below, reread and reflect on the Everyday Ethics Scenario and Questions for Consideration in this chapter of the textbook. It may also be useful to review the Dental Hygiene Ethics discussion in Chapter 1, the Ethical Applications in the introduction pages for each section in the textbook, as well as the Codes of Ethics in textbook Appendices I–IV.

Individual Learning Activity

Imagine the scenario from the patient's perspective. How might the patient's response to the questions following the scenario be different from those of the dental hygienist involved?

Collaborative Learning Activity

Work with another student colleague to role-play the scenario. The goal of this exercise is for you and your colleague to work though the alternative actions in order to come to consensus on a solution or response that is acceptable to both of you.

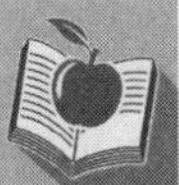

Factors To Teach The Patient

This scenario is related to the following factor:

▷ The importance of oral care for the guide dog.

When you have completed care for Damian (introduced in the Competency Exercises) for the day, he tells you laughingly that the vet told him Harrison's teeth need to be brushed regularly to keep him healthy. You reply that, of course, regular oral hygiene is as important for the dog as it is for Damian. You agree to teach him how. Damian states he already has a toothbrush and some special chicken-flavor toothpaste at home.

Keeping in mind that this patient is blind, use what you learned in this chapter and also the motivational interviewing principles summarized in Appendix D as a guide to prepare a conversation to teach Damian about maintaining his guide dog's oral health.

61

The Patient with a Neurodevelopmental Disorder

LEARNING OBJECTIVES

Upon successful completion of these exercises, you will be able to:

1. Identify and define key terms and concepts related to the patient with a neurodevelopmental disorder.
2. Identify the dimensions, intellectual functioning levels, risk factors, and etiologies associated with neurodevelopmental disorders.
3. Describe the specific characteristics of individuals with an intellectual disorder, Down syndrome, and autistic spectrum disorder.
4. Plan and document modifications necessary for dental hygiene care and effective oral hygiene instruction for persons with a neurodevelopmental disorder.

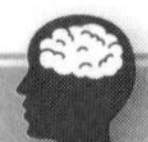

KNOWLEDGE EXERCISES

Write your answers for each question in the space provided.

1. List examples of neurodevelopmental disorders that are usually first diagnosed before or during adolescence.

2. List the five interrelated dimensions that contribute to testing the functioning level of an individual with an intellectual disorder.

3. In your own words, briefly summarize the characteristics for each classification of intellectual functioning that will impact the dental hygienist's approach to providing oral health education and oral hygiene instruction.

Mild

Moderate

Severe

Profound

4. Identify four categories of risk factors for intellectual disability.

5. What behavior-related factors during pregnancy may result in an infant with an intellectual disorder?

6. What can happen during the infant's birth that can lead to an intellectual disorder?

7. What two early childhood situations can lead to intellectual disorders?

8. Identify characteristic physical features or anomalies you might observe when performing an extraoral examination for your patient with an intellectual disorder.

9. List five intraoral findings common in individuals with intellectual disorders.

10. List five characteristics that can help you identify an individual with Down syndrome.

11. Most individuals with Down syndrome have pleasant personalities. Identify three personal characteristics that make these individuals likable and easy to be around.

12. Why do patients with Down syndrome often present for dental treatment with very cracked and dried lips?

13. Identify physical/medical health problems commonly found in individuals with Down syndrome that require special consideration or modifications during dental hygiene treatment.

14. Briefly describe the characteristics that distinguish each of the five variations of autism spectrum disorder.

15. In your own words, briefly summarize three main characteristics you are likely to observe during a dental hygiene appointment with your patient who has been diagnosed with an autism spectrum disorder.

16. Describe two types of treatment used to manage symptoms and increase the ability of the patient with autism to live a normal life.

17. Identify specific actions you can initiate during dental hygiene appointments to help your patient with an autistic spectrum disorder or any other neurodevelopmental disorder to learn how to cooperate.

COMPETENCY EXERCISES

Apply information from the chapter and use critical thinking skills to complete the competency exercises. Write responses on paper or create electronic documents to submit your answers.

1. Next week you will be starting a new part-time position as the dental hygienist for 50 resident patients in a small private residential facility. You will go once a week to work with Dr. Sally Roderick, the dentist who has been providing dental care at the residence for 25 years. The individuals living in the residence are classified as having severe or profound intellectual disorder. You are excited about the opportunity to work with Dr. Roderick and to learn about this population, which you have only read about in your textbook.
   To prepare for this new challenge, create a list of planning measures you can take and modifications you can make to your usual treatment procedures so you can increase your effectiveness when providing dental hygiene care for these patients.

2. On the first day at the residential center, you find that Dr. Roderick has done very well providing patients with restorative care, but not much attention has been paid to dental hygiene care and education. The patient in your clinic chair right now is Bonne. She is 22 years old and is classified as having a profound intellectual disability.
   One of the nurse's aides, who is her regular caregiver, helps you place Bonne in the papoose board and sits by the side of the dental chair to help when she can. You have some difficulty examining Bonne's mouth, but you can readily see that she has extensive biofilm

buildup and significant amounts of calculus in all areas of her mouth.

You know that it will take more than one appointment to assess Bonne's dental hygiene needs thoroughly and to make a full plan for care. However, Dr. Roderick asks you to write up a formal dental hygiene care plan for what you will accomplish in the next three or four appointments so the plan can be recorded in Bonne's medical record. You know that you must plan enough time for the complete assessment you need to accomplish before you can fully understand Bonne's oral condition. You must also plan to educate the aide for daily biofilm control.

Use the Dental Hygiene Care Plan Template in Appendix B to develop a formal, written care plan for clinical procedures and educational interventions you will provide during the four appointments you will schedule in the next few weeks for Bonne and her caregiver.

3. Today when you saw Bonne in the clinic, you reviewed her medical history, provided a limited intraoral assessment examination, and developed a written care plan. Use your institution's guidelines for writing in patient records to document these procedures.

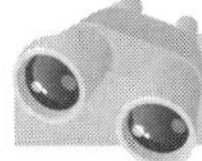

BOX 61-1 MeSH TERMS

Use a combination of MeSH terms and other key words to develop an effective and efficient PubMed literature search strategy.

Intellectual disability
Developmental disabilities
Dental care for disabled
Child development disorders, pervasive
Asperger syndrome
Autistic disorder
Down syndrome
Tic disorders
Language disorders

EVERYDAY ETHICS

Before completing the learning exercises below, reread and reflect on the Everyday Ethics Scenario and Questions for Consideration in this chapter of the textbook. It may also be useful to review the Dental Hygiene Ethics discussion in Chapter 1, the Ethical Applications in the introduction pages for each section in the textbook, as well as the Codes of Ethics in textbook Appendices I–IV.

Individual Learning Activity

Imagine that you have observed what happened in the scenario, but are not one of the main characters involved in the situation. Write a reflective journal entry that:

describes how you might have reacted (as an observer–not as a participant),

expresses your personal feelings about what happened,

or

identifies personal values that affect your reaction to the situation.

Collaborative Learning Activity

Answer each of the questions for consideration at the end of the scenario in the textbook. Compare what you wrote with answers developed by another classmate and discuss differences/similarities.

Factors To Teach The Patient

This scenario is related to the following factors listed in this chapter of the textbook:

For the patient

- ▷ How to perform oral self-care procedures.
- ▷ Why assistance from others is an important supplement to the patient's own efforts.
- ▷ How to use and show cooperation skills.

For the caregiver

- ▷ Why a total preventive program is important.
- ▷ How to incorporate behavior modification into oral care procedures.
- ▷ The importance of repeating "show–tell–do" instructions often.

Use information in Chapter 61 in the textbook and the motivational interviewing approach (see Appendix D) to develop a conversation you will use to provide oral hygiene instructions for a patient who is classified with a moderate intellectual disability. Include the patient's caregiver as you discuss strategies for daily oral care.

Use the conversation you create to role-play this situation with a fellow student. If you are the patient or the caregiver in the role-play, be sure to ask questions. If you are the dental hygienist, try to anticipate questions and answer them in your explanation. Modify your conversation based on what you learned.

Crossword Puzzle

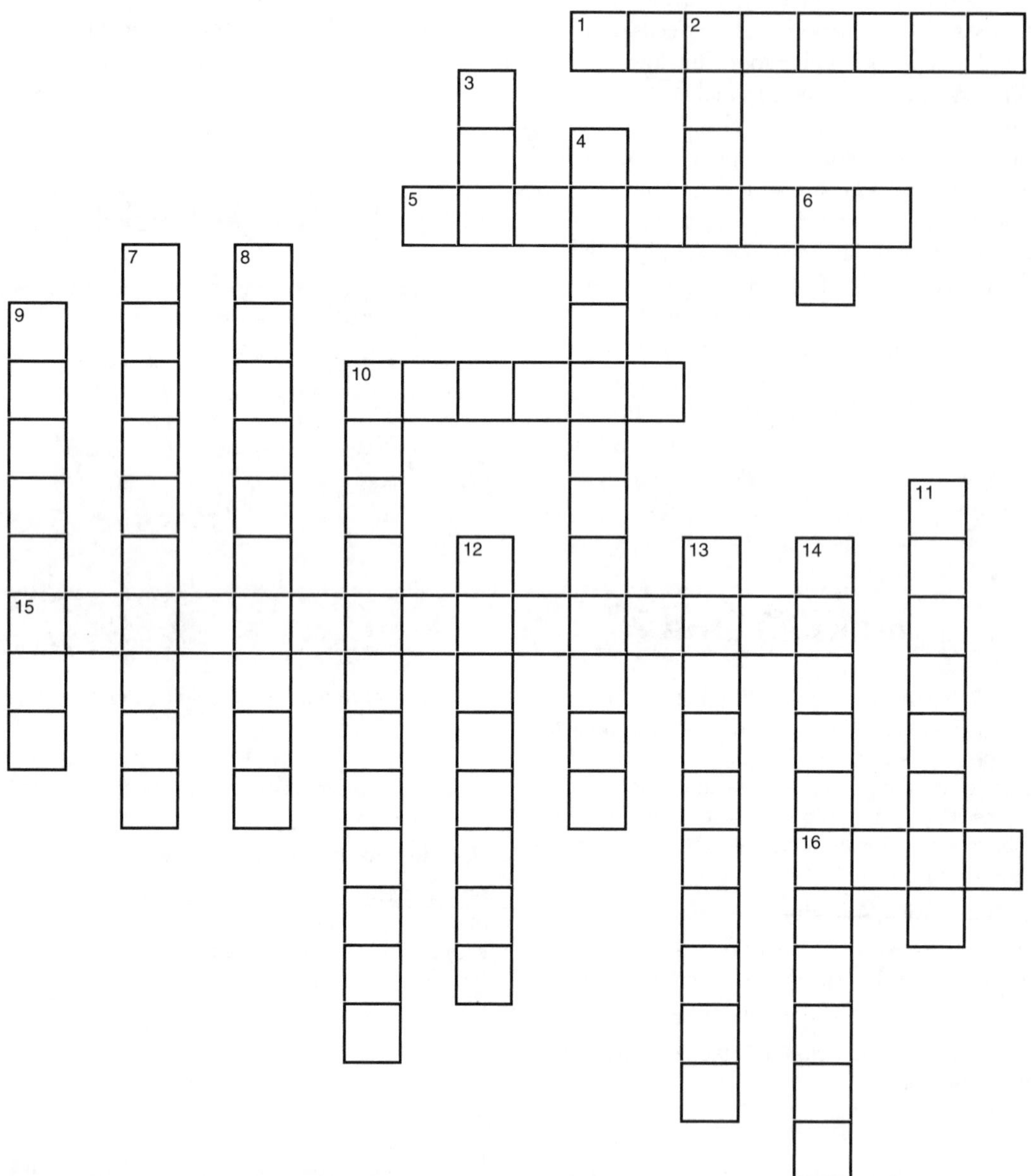

Puzzle Clues

Across

1. An autistic spectrum disorder characterized mainly by impairment in social interactions.
5. The involuntary repetition of a word or sentence just spoken by another person.
10. Inability or refusal to speak.
15. The reflection or transmission of ultrasonic waves in body tissues; can be used to examine a fetus to determine birth defects.
16. An autism spectrum disorder that occurs only in girls; characterized by repetitive hand movements.

Down

2. Persistent craving/eating of nonnutritive substances or unnatural articles of food.
3. Sudden nonrhythmic motor movement or vocal sound
4. Trisomy 21 syndrome (two words).
6. Numeric rating of the relationship of mental age to chronologic age.
7. Repeated regurgitation of food.
8. Involuntary utterance of vulgar words.
9. Classification of intellectual function for which the individual would most likely need to have all daily oral hygiene measures provided by a caregiver.
10. Very large tongue.
11. Category of intellectual function in which the individual could most likely attend to personal oral care with some reminders from a caregiver.
12. Refers to coexisting medical conditions.
13. A vertical fold of skin on either side of the nose; a normal characteristic of persons of some races that is also associated with Down syndrome.
14. Abnormality in morphologic development.

62

Family Abuse and Neglect

LEARNING OBJECTIVES

Upon successful completion of these exercises, you will be able to:

1. Identify and define key terms and concepts related to family abuse and neglect.
2. Describe various categories of family maltreatment.
3. Recognize and document signs and behavioral indicators of abuse.
4. Identify the dental hygienist's role in recognizing and reporting abuse and neglect.

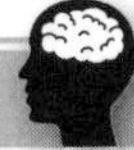

KNOWLEDGE EXERCISES

Write your answers for each question in the space provided.

1. Define *forensic dentistry*.

2. Identify three programs you can explore further to help you learn more about how to assess and respond to suspected abuse during a patient/provider interaction.

The factors involved in the recognition and management of suspected maltreatment of children, the elderly, people with disabilities, and women are similar. When answering the following questions, be sure to take all of these potential at-risk groups into consideration, unless the question specifics a particular group or groups.

3. List four major types of maltreatment that can occur in families.

4. Identify two types of maltreatment of elders that do not usually occur in cases involving children.

5. In your own words, define *dental neglect*.

6. When children state that there is no one at their house to help them brush their teeth, what additional appearance and behavioral indicators might lead you to suspect that your patient is neglected?

7. Identify the signs of lice infestation.

8. Identify personal appearance factors that might lead you to suspect that an individual is being physically abused.

9. In your own words, describe the raccoon sign.

10. What is an area of baldness that is caused by pulling out hair by the roots?

11. What is the medical term used to identify a bruise?

12. Describe what you might notice about site of an accidental injury versus the common sites you might notice if the injuries are inflicted or deliberate.

13. Identify intraoral signs of physical abuse.

14. Identify general signs of physical abuse and neglect in a child patient.

15. In what way do these general signs compare with what you might notice if an elderly patient is being mistreated?

16. Extremely aggressive behavior by a child when you try to examine his or her mouth can be a behavioral indicator for ____________________ as well as for physical abuse.

17. Identify intraoral signs of sexual abuse.

18. List nonabuse-related conditions that can mimic the physical signs of abuse.

19. One important role for the dental hygienist in cases of suspected abuse is to document the observable facts in the patient's record. What information is necessary to have available when you are reporting abuse to state authorities?

____

____

____

____

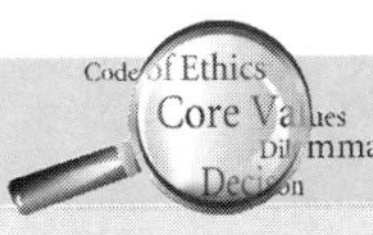

COMPETENCY EXERCISES

Apply information from the chapter and use critical thinking skills to complete the competency exercises. Write responses on paper or create electronic documents to submit your answers.

1. Read the information in the Everyday Ethics case study for this workbook chapter. Using your institution's guidelines for writing in patient records, document your findings regarding Sarah. Important note: write your progress note entry so that it includes only factual, objective information about the dental hygienist's observations and no subjective statements or personal opinions.

2. Outline the thought process you will use when making a decision to report suspected child abuse to state authorities. Discuss your outline with a small group of your student colleagues. Use the results of this discussion to write an office protocol for reporting suspected abuse.

DISCOVERY EXERCISES

1. Investigate the laws and the processes for reporting child, elder, or spouse abuse in your state.

2. Investigate the agencies in your area where abused elders or battered spouses can obtain help or emergency assistance.

3. Investigate the PANDA program, the AVDR Tutorial for Dentists, or project RADAR to learn more about recognizing and reporting family abuse and neglect.

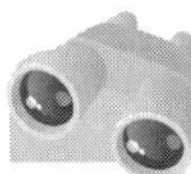

BOX 62-1 MeSH TERMS

Use a combination of MeSH terms and other key words to develop an effective and efficient PubMed literature search strategy.

Child abuse	Elder abuse
Child abuse, sexual	Mandibular injuries
Battered child syndrome	Maxillofacial injuries
Spouse abuse	Mandatory reporting

EVERYDAY ETHICS

Before completing the learning exercises below, reread and reflect on the Everyday Ethics Scenario and Questions for Consideration in this chapter of the textbook. It may also be useful to review the Dental Hygiene Ethics discussion in Chapter 1, the Ethical Applications in the introduction pages for each section in the textbook, as well as the Codes of Ethics in textbook Appendices I–IV.

Collaborative Learning Activities

Identify a situation in which you have resolved an ethical dilemma and share the story with a classmate. Discuss how that person might have acted differently to resolve the situation.

Work with a small group to develop a 2- to 5-minute role-play that introduces the everyday ethics scenario described in the chapter (a great idea is to video record your role-play activity). Then develop separate 2-minute role-play scenarios that provide at least two alternative approaches/solutions to resolving the situation. Ask classmates to view the solutions, ask questions, and discuss the ethical approach used in each. Ask for a vote on which solution classmates determine to be the "best."

Factors To Teach The Patient

This scenario is related to the following factors listed in this chapter of the textbook:

- ▷ The value of oral hygiene with age-appropriate materials.
- ▷ What the bacterial biofilm is on teeth, using a disclosing agent.
- ▷ How to use the new toothbrush the child just received.
- ▷ Why it is especially important to brush the teeth and tongue just before going to sleep.

Johnny is 8 years old. This is his first dental hygiene visit with you, and his dental history indicates that he has not seen a dentist since the HeadStart program required a dental examination when he was 3 years old. His parents scheduled this dental appointment as a result of a directive from state authorities after a report by his teacher.

Johnny is very shy, but after he gets to know you a bit during his appointment, he seems interested in what you are doing and asks all kinds of questions. You note during your intraoral examination that his teeth are completely covered with dental biofilm. Johnny states he doesn't really have a very good toothbrush. He obviously is not performing daily self-care, and you suspect that his parents are not helping or encouraging him in any way. Fortunately, there are no carious lesions, but his gingival tissue is red and bleeds easily when you touch it.

Use the principles of motivational interviewing (see Appendix D) as a guide, and use language appropriate for a child to explain to Johnny why he needs to brush his teeth every day.

63

The Patient with a Seizure Disorder

LEARNING OBJECTIVES

Upon successful completion of these exercises, you will be able to:

1. Identify and define key terms and concepts related to seizure disorders.
2. Identify cause, classifications, clinical manifestations, and emergency management of seizures.
3. Discuss oral considerations related to management of seizures.
4. Plan and document dental hygiene care for a patient with a history of seizure disorder.

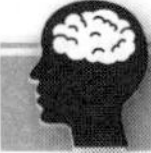

KNOWLEDGE EXERCISES

Write your answers for each question in the space provided.

1. In your own words, describe a seizure?

2. Although most seizure disorders tend to be stable, some individuals experience a random pattern of seizures that disrupt their lives. List some activities that may be compromised for an individual who experiences recurrent seizures.

3. If your patient has a history of seizure activity, when should you contact/consult with your patient's physician?

4. In what three ways are epileptic syndromes classified?

5. Briefly describe the physical manifestations of a tonic–clonic seizure.

6. In your own words, briefly describe the clinical manifestations of an absence seizure.

7. What is a partial seizure?

8. List some of the medical conditions that can cause seizures.

9. What kinds of stimuli, common in a dental practice, could potentially precipitate a seizure during patient care for a susceptible patient?

10. List other medical conditions you should consider if your patient is manifesting some clinical signs of a seizure, particularly if the patient's medical history does not indicate a seizure disorder. (*Hint*: Think "differential diagnosis.")

11. If your patient does have a seizure during dental hygiene treatment, what emergency measures will you take to protect your patient from injury?

12. What oral injuries are associated with tonic–clonic seizures?

13. What action should you take in the event that your patient's tonic–clonic seizure continues for longer than 5 minutes?

14. Describe status epilepticus.

15. List the types of surgical interventions used to medically treat patients with seizure disorders.

16. Your patient with a seizure disorder is likely to be taking an antiepileptic medication. In your own words, briefly describe the mechanism, incidence, appearance, and effects of phenytoin-induced gingival hyperplasia.

17. What medications, in addition to phenytoin, are associated with gingival overgrowth?

18. Identify dental hygiene treatment and education interventions that can prevent or inhibit the growth of gingival tissues in your patient who is taking phenytoin or another medication associated with gingival enlargement.

19. What surgical options are available for treating phenytoin-induced gingival hyperplasia?

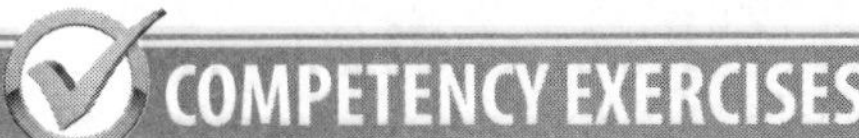

COMPETENCY EXERCISES

Apply information from the chapter and use critical thinking skills to complete the competency exercises. Write responses on paper or create electronic documents to submit your answers.

1. You can tell your new patient has a very business-like approach to his health care. Mr. Arakawa is a 45-year-old chief executive officer in a major corporation in town. As you lead him back to your treatment room, he stops briefly at the front desk to make sure of the procedure for submitting today's charges to his dental insurance. He mentions that he is on a tight schedule and wants to be sure about what time his appointment will end.

   He fills out the health history form you hand him with short, efficient strokes of his pen and hands it back to you. The only positive answers on the form are for seizure activity and medication, but he does not indicate what drug he is taking. You know that to completely understand Mr. Arakawa's condition, you must ask him more questions. Create a list of questions you will ask Mr. Arakawa as you clarify his health history information.

2. When you begin to ask Mr. Arakawa the questions you formulated, he briskly states that his history of seizures is not relevant to his dental treatment. He states that his previous dental provider never asked such questions, and, besides, he has not had a seizure for a long time. He tells you about the medication he is taking but is clearly not happy about answering the other questions you are asking.

   You know he needs to understand why it is important for you to learn about his history of seizures. What information will you include in your discussion with Mr. Arakawa as you convince him to comply with your request for information about his seizures?

3. Your education/counseling approach is successful and you find out Mr. Arakawa has been experiencing seizures for almost 30 years. The severity of the tonic–clonic-type seizures he experiences has decreased since his teenage years, and in fact, the seizures are now fairly well under control.

   The medication he is currently taking is an ethosuximide, but his previous prescription was a phenytoin (Dilantin), which he took for almost 20 years. About 10 years ago, he had gingival surgery to control gingival overgrowth he experienced from taking the phenytoin and fears that his gums are growing again.

Mr. Arakawa experienced some fairly serious dental trauma when he lost consciousness and fell during a seizure, and his maxillary anterior teeth have been replaced with a porcelain bridge. He has often bitten his lips and tongue when he is convulsing. One time when he was young, he experienced a seizure during routine dental treatment and that is why he was at first reluctant and embarrassed to share much information about his seizures with you. He describes the aura that he experiences before a seizure, which appears as flashes of light just outside the direct view of his left eye. He also mentions that sometimes changing patterns of light have caused a seizure to happen and asks you to be careful when positioning the dental light during his treatment. His last seizure was about 2 years ago.

Using your institution's guidelines for writing in patient records, document what you have learned about Mr. Arakawa's medical condition.

4. You know that many medications prescribed to control seizures have numerous side effects, other than gingival hyperplasia, that are a concern for dental professionals. Refer to the list of potential side effects in the "Treatment" section of Chapter 63 in the textbook and indicate which side effects have implications for patient education or treatment modifications during Mr. Arakawa's dental hygiene appointments.

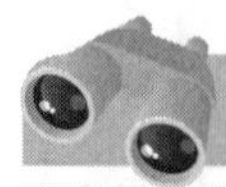

BOX 63-1 MeSH TERMS

Use a combination of MeSH terms and other key words to develop an effective and efficient PubMed literature search strategy.

Seizures
Epilepsy, generalized
Epilepsy, absence
Epilepsy, tonic–clonic
Epilepsy, complex partial
Status epilepticus
Anticonvulsants

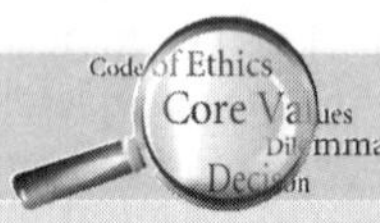

EVERYDAY ETHICS

Before completing the learning exercises below, reread and reflect on the Everyday Ethics Scenario and Questions for Consideration in this chapter of the textbook. It may also be useful to review the Dental Hygiene Ethics discussion in Chapter 1, the Ethical Applications in the introduction pages for each section in the textbook, as well as the Codes of Ethics in textbook Appendices I–IV.

Collaborative Learning Activity

Answer each of the questions for consideration at the end of the scenario in the textbook. Compare what you wrote with answers developed by another classmate and discuss differences/similarities.

Discovery Activity

Ask a dental hygienist who has been practicing for a year or more to read the scenario. Provide a copy of the Code of Ethics as well. Share the responses you have made to answer each question and ask that person to discuss the situation with you. What insights did you have or what did you learn during this discussion?

Factors to Teach the Patient

This scenario is related to the following factors listed in this chapter of the textbook:

- Relationship of systemic health to oral health.
- Importance of careful daily care of mouth.
- Antiepileptic medication side effects, including gingival enlargement and how to minimize its growth.
- Seek immediate care if any oral change or injury is suspected.

Use the information provided in Chapter 63 in the textbook as a guide to prepare a conversation that you could use to provide patient education for Mr. Arakawa (introduced in the Competency Exercises). As you prepare the conversation, remember that you have already observed Mr. Arakawa's business-like approach to health care. Use the motivational interviewing approach (see Appendix D) to be sure your education approach suits his personality and level of readiness for behavior change.

Use the conversation you create to role-play this situation with a fellow student. If you are the patient in the role-play, be sure to ask questions. If you are the dental hygienist, try to anticipate questions and answer them in your explanation.

Crossword Puzzle

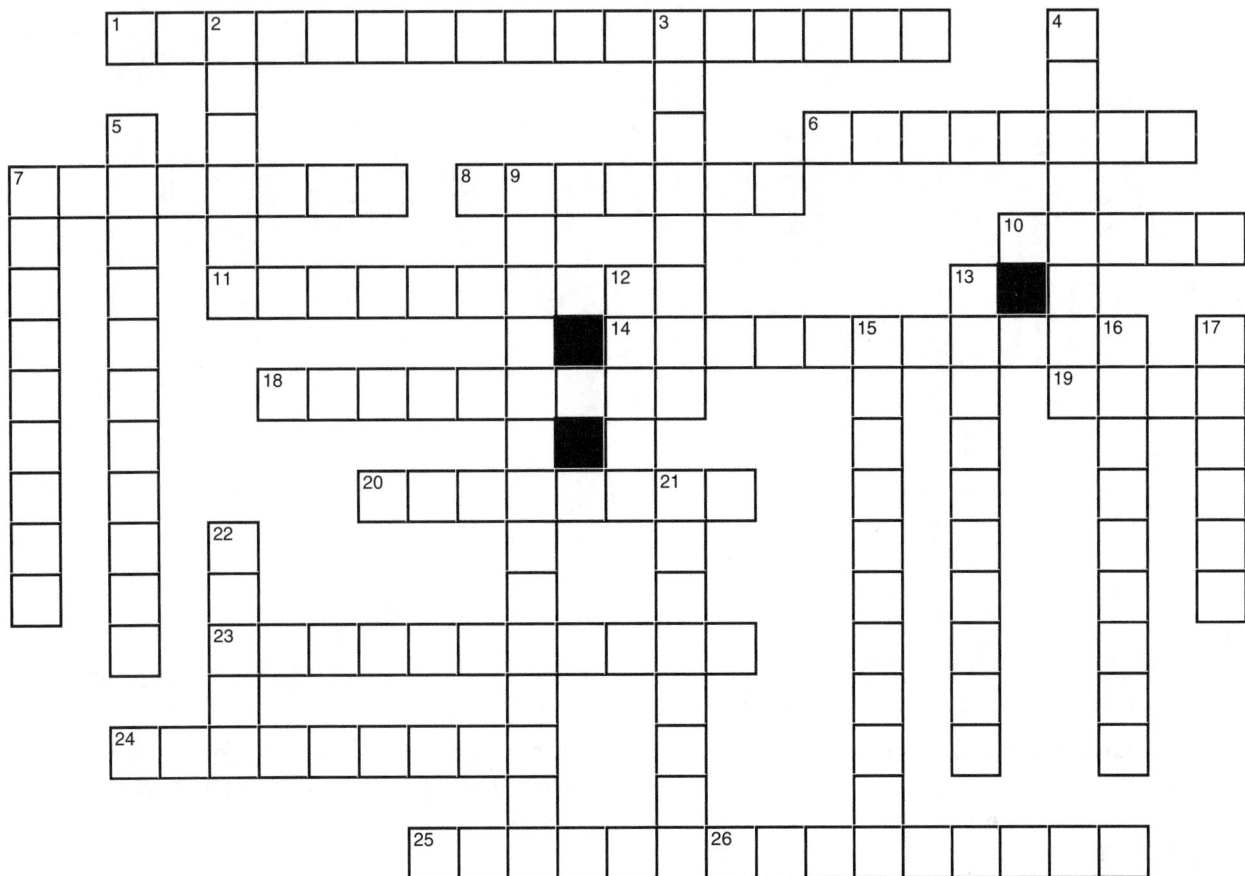

Puzzle Clues

Across

1. A life-threatening emergency related to seizure disorders (two words).
6. A group of functional disorders of the brain characterized by recurrent seizures.
7. The sudden recurrence or intensification of sharp spasms or convulsions.
8. A seizure that involves only part of the brain.
10. A state of continuous, unremitting muscular contractions.
11. Uncontrolled motor activity, such as repeated swallowing.
14. Abnormal burning, prickling, or tingling sensation.
18. The phase following a seizure when rest, reassurance, and palliative care for any oral trauma are administered.
19. A peculiar prodromal sensation experienced by some people immediately preceding a seizure.
20. Former term for a type of tonic–clonic epileptic seizure (two words).
23. A seizure that affects the entire brain at the same time.
24. Impaired digestive function.
25. Active, acute phase of an epileptic seizure.
26. Shock-like contractions of muscles or groups of muscles.

Down

2. Irregular muscle action.
3. Former term for absence seizure (two words).
4. Double vision.
5. A disorder for which the cause is hidden.
7. Class of anticonvulsant drugs highly correlated with gingival hyperplasia.
9. Drug that inhibits convulsions.
12. Sudden, involuntary contraction.
13. A seizure disorder that does not resolve following treatment with a basic, single drug therapy.
15. Type of seizure in which there is alternate contraction and relaxation of muscles (two words).
16. Term associated with symptoms such as pallor, flushing, sweating, pupillary dilation, cardiac arrhythmia, or incontinence.
17. Refers to expression or appearance of the face.
21. A type of seizure in which the person experiences a brief impairment of consciousness before a return to awareness with no recollection of the seizure.
22. Nerve that is stimulated by a pacemakerlike device implanted to reduce seizures.

64

The Patient with a Mental Health Disorder

LEARNING OBJECTIVES

Upon successful completion of these exercises, you will be able to:

1. Identify and define key terms and concepts related to psychiatric disorders.
2. Describe the symptoms, treatment, and oral implications of a variety of psychiatric and mood disorders.
3. Plan and document dental hygiene care and oral health education for a patient with a psychiatric disorder.

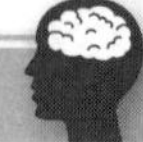

KNOWLEDGE EXERCISES

Write your answers for each question in the space provided.

1. Why is it more appropriate to refer to your patient as "an individual with bulimia" rather than as "a bulimic"?

2. List the four types of anxiety disorders described in the textbook.

3. Briefly describe each of the three types of treatment provided for a patient with anxiety disorder.

4. What oral problems are associated with anxiety disorders?

5. List ways to reduce anxiety and enhance the patient's feeling of being in control while you are providing dental hygiene care.

6. Briefly describe postpartum depression.

7. List common signs and symptoms that may indicate someone is experiencing an episode of depression.

8. In addition to those discussed for anxiety disorders, what additional treatment modality is sometimes provided for a patient with a depressive disorder?

9. List the types of antidepressant medications you may see on the medical history of a patient being treated for a depressive disorder.

10. What is the most common oral side effect of the antidepressant medications used by patients with depression?

11. Briefly describe why a patient with depression is at higher risk for dental caries.

12. Why might you consider offering tinted protective eyewear for a patient who is taking medications to treat depression?

13. List one specific behavior to avoid in your approach to oral health education for a patient with depression.

14. Define *euphoria*.

15. In what way is bipolar disorder different from a depressive disorder?

16. In your own words, briefly summarize the characteristics common to the manic phase of bipolar disorder.

17. List the categories of drugs used to treat bipolar disorder.

18. What drug used to treat bipolar disorder can impart a metallic taste in your patient's mouth?

19. Define dysguesia.

20. What is pica?

21. In your own words, briefly describe and compare the major eating disorders listed below.

Anorexia nervosa:

Bulimia nervosa:

Binge-eating disorder:

22. What medical complication related to the orofacial region can arise from excessive purging behaviors?

23. Discuss the effects of perimolysis as it relates to purging behaviors.

24. Briefly describe factors that increase risk for negative oral effects when a patient has an eating disorder.

Dental caries:

Mucosal lesions:

Periodontal disease:

Hypersensitive teeth:

Trauma:

25. What changes in saliva contribute to oral problems often identified in patients with an eating disorder?

26. In your own words, define *schizophrenia*.

27. List and briefly describe each of the three categories of symptoms you might observe in a patient with schizophrenia.

____

____

____

____

____

28. Identify the concept or term defined by each of the following statements.

A false sensory perception in the absence of an actual external stimulus:

____

A mental impression derived from misinterpretation of an actual sensory stimulus; a false perception:

____

A false belief firmly held although contradicted by social reality:

____

A psychiatric disorder characterized by delusions of persecution, illusions of grandeur, or a combination of both:

____

29. Unfortunately, many people diagnosed with schizophrenia also have high rates of _______________.

30. List the major categories of psychotropic medications.

____

____

____

____

31. List the potential oral effects of antipsychotic medications.

____

____

____

____

____

32. List potential physical side-effects of antipsychotic medication that may require modifications during dental hygiene care.

____

____

____

____

____

____

____

____

33. In your own words define *dysarthria*?

____

____

34. What is tardive dyskinesia?

____

____

35. During a scaling and root planing procedure, how can you facilitate safety and comfort of your patient with tardive dyskinesia?

____

36. In your own words, describe measures you can take to prevent or prepare for a psychiatric emergency.

____

____

____

____

37. If your patient has a panic attack while you are providing dental hygiene care, what will you do?

____

____

____

____

____

____

COMPETENCY EXERCISES

Apply information from the chapter and use critical thinking skills to complete the competency exercises. Write responses on paper or create electronic documents to submit your answers.

1. Study the list of potential effects of antipsychotic medications in Table 64-1 in the textbook. Identify at least three modifications you can make beyond your usual clinical routines to ensure the comfort and safety of your patient who is taking an antipsychotic medication.

2. When you check his health history before calling Jack into your treatment room at the VA hospital, you notice he has been diagnosed with posttraumatic stress disorder. You greet him cheerfully, talk to him brightly all the way down the hall to your room about how beautifully the sun is shining today. You ask him, with a smile, if there have been any changes in his medications since he was last seen in the dental clinic.

   But you notice that his only response is to stand beside you trembling and shaking. You immediately suspect that he is displaying symptoms of a panic attack. Describe what additional assessment measures are appropriate to help determine if your suspicion is correct. Describe how you will you react to Jack's obvious distress?

3. After he has calmed down, you and Jack decide together to reschedule his dental hygiene appointment for another day. Use the SOAP note format or your clinic's form for recording a patient visit to develop a progress note to document what happened at today's appointment.

4. Shaun Kennedy, a newspaper reporter, has been your patient for several years. You always enjoy the stories he tells about working for the newspaper. His oral hygiene has never been particularly good, and you have been really working with him each time he comes in to make sure he understands how his risk for oral disease increases when he doesn't thoroughly remove the dental biofilm from his teeth every day. You know that he is receiving treatment for bipolar disorder, but, so far, you have not noticed that he ever displays any symptoms of either the manic phase or the depressive phase of his disease.

   Today Shaun is talking a mile a minute about a new novel he has started writing. As he gets more excited about telling you the plot of the novel, he actually pushes your hands aside, leaps up from the chair, and walks back and forth in your small treatment space! You would really like to convince him to get back in the dental chair so you can complete your oral hygiene instructions in a timely manner. What can happen if you pressure him to comply? Given Shaun's behavior today, how can you sensitively and realistically approach this situation?

5. Isabella Stamos, 13 years old, is a beautiful girl with long curly blond hair, huge green eyes, and an already successful modeling career. You still have not started your intraoral examination, but after talking with her and observing her for several minutes, you suspect that she has an eating disorder. What clinical clues or signs can you look for to help confirm your impressions? What questions will you ask Isabella to help you determine if your suspicions are correct?

6. After you have questioned Isabella and completed an intraoral examination, it becomes clear that she is battling with bulimia nervosa. What ethical factors will you take into consideration when you discuss your assessment findings and Isabella's oral health needs with her mother at the end of the appointment?

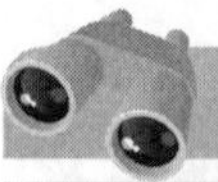

BOX 64-1 MeSH TERMS

Use a combination of MeSH terms and other key words to develop an effective and efficient PubMed literature search strategy.

Anxiety disorders	Depression, postpartum
Obsessive-compulsive disorder	Bipolar disorder
Panic disorder	Schizophrenia pica
Stress disorders, traumatic	Anorexia nervosa
Depression	Bulimia nervosa
Depressive disorder	Binge-eating disorder

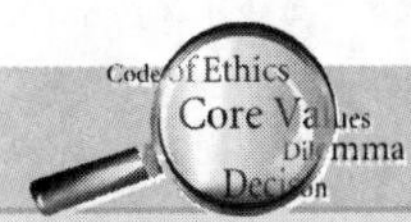

EVERYDAY ETHICS

Before completing the learning exercises below, reread and reflect on the Everyday Ethics Scenario and Questions for Consideration in this chapter of the textbook. It may also be useful to review the Dental Hygiene Ethics discussion in Chapter 1, the Ethical Applications in the introduction pages for each section in the textbook, as well as the Codes of Ethics in textbook Appendices I–IV.

Individual Learning Activity

Imagine that you are the dental hygienist in this scenario. Answer each of the questions for consideration at the end of the scenario.

Discovery Activity

Ask a dental hygienist who has been practicing for a year or more to read the scenario. Provide them with a copy of the Code of Ethics as well. Share the responses you have made to answer each question and ask that person to discuss the situation with you. What insights did you have or what did you learn during this discussion?

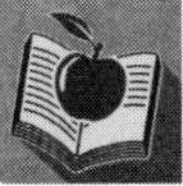

Factors To Teach The Patient

This scenario is related to the following factors listed in this chapter of the textbook:

- ▷ The causes and effects of enamel erosion; the high acidity of the vomitus from the stomach.
- ▷ How to rinse after vomiting but not brush immediately; demineralization begins promptly after the acid from the stomach reaches the teeth, and brushing can cause abrasion of the demineralizing enamel.
- ▷ The need for multiple fluoride applications through use of home dentifrice, rinse, and brush-on gel, as well as professional application of varnish or gel-tray at regular dental hygiene appointments.

You have talked with Isabella (introduced in the Competency Exercises in this chapter) about some ways she can receive help with her eating disorder, but as a dental hygienist, you know that the most important thing you can do is educate her about the risks to her oral health.

Use the principles of motivational interviewing (Appendix D) as a guide, and taking into account the personal factors that often accompany this disorder, educate Isabella about the negative oral findings common in a patient with bulimia. Discuss strategies for protecting her teeth and gums until she gets her eating behaviors under control.

65

The Patient with a Substance-Related Disorder

LEARNING OBJECTIVES

Upon successful completion of these exercises, you will be able to:

1. Identify and define key terms and concepts related to alcohol and drug use.
2. Identify physical and behavioral factors associated with alcohol and drug use.
3. Describe health-related effects of alcohol and drug use, abuse, and withdrawal.
4. Plan dental hygiene care and oral hygiene instructions for the patient with a substance-related disorder.

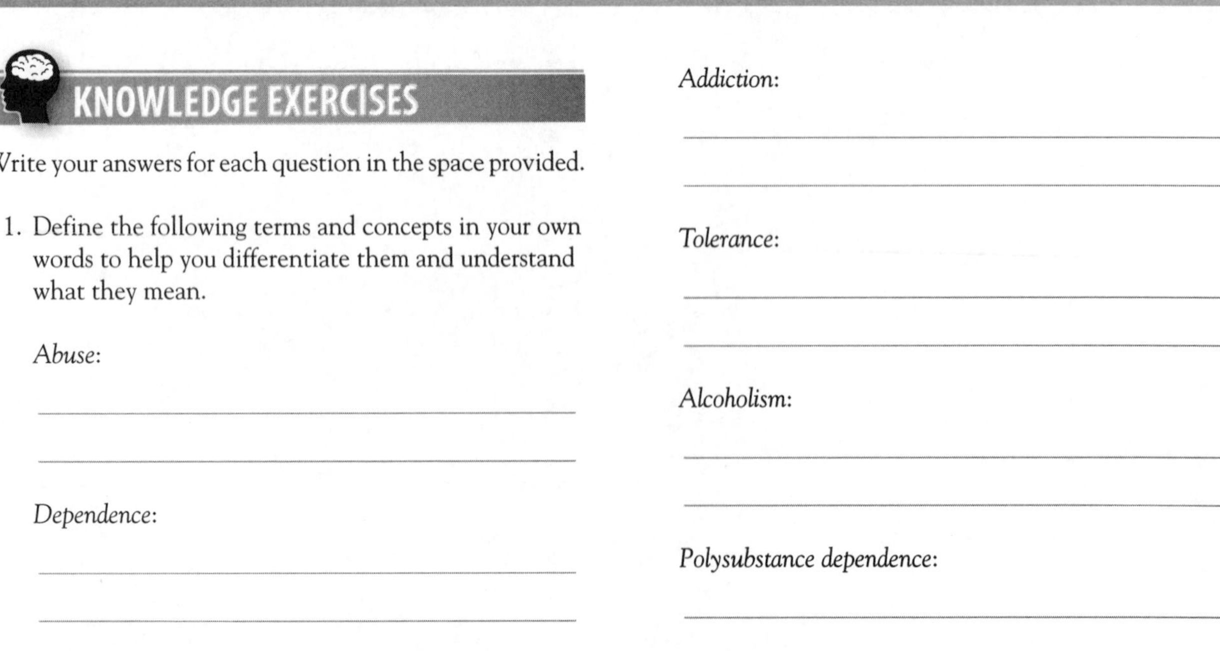

KNOWLEDGE EXERCISES

Write your answers for each question in the space provided.

1. Define the following terms and concepts in your own words to help you differentiate them and understand what they mean.

   Abuse:

   Dependence:

   Addiction:

   Tolerance:

   Alcoholism:

   Polysubstance dependence:

2. What is the difference between chemical, physical, and psychological dependence?

3. Identify the levels in the spectrum of alcohol use.

4. Identify the signs of alcoholism.

5. What is *acne rosacea?*

6. What factors contribute to the etiology of alcoholism?

7. How is the concentration of alcohol in the blood measured?

8. What behavioral characteristics, if you observe them in an otherwise healthy patient, might indicate that your patient is intoxicated?

9. Define *nystagmus*.

10. The liver is the organ most severely affected by chronic alcohol abuse. Briefly describe the adverse effects of excessive or prolonged alcohol use on each of the following body systems.

Immune system:

Digestive system:

Cardiovascular system:

Nervous system:

Reproductive system:

11. In what ways does excessive alcohol consumption affect nutritional intake?

____

____

____

____

12. Describe the two types of complications that can occur if an individual abruptly withdraws from alcohol use.

Alcohol hallucinosis:

____

____

____

Alcohol withdrawal delirium (DTs):

____

____

____

____

____

13. Identify factors that can increase the severity of the symptoms that a person with alcoholism may experience if he or she abruptly ceases drinking.

____

____

____

____

14. What is the overall objective of treatment provided to support an individual who is recovering from alcoholism?

____

____

15. List the four components of an alcohol treatment program.

____

____

____

____

16. Your patient who is participating in an alcohol recovery program may be taking an alcohol-sensitizing agent because these drugs act as a deterrent to consuming alcohol. If alcohol is taken, this drug interferes with the conversion of __________ to __________ in the liver and makes the patient very ill.

17. Identify the drug prescribed for the recovering alcoholic to help inhibit or decrease the desire to consume alcohol.

____

18. Use of alcohol during pregnancy can seriously threaten the health of the baby because __________.

19. The mother's general health and nutritional status, __________ use, and abuse of __________ are additional factors linked with alcohol intake that may influence the baby's health.

20. Describe the physical features that can be observed in an infant with a FASD.

____

____

____

____

21. Identify behavioral, cognitive, and psychomotor factors associated with FASD.

____

____

____

____

____

22. List the categories of drugs that are most commonly abused.

____

____

____

____

____

23. Describe the characteristics of a drug classified as a US Drug Enforcement Administration Schedule II drug.

24. Identify oral manifestations associated with the use of each of the following drugs.

Methamphetamine:

Speed, Ecstasy, and other amphetamine-based drugs:

Cocaine:

Cannabis:

25. Which body systems can be adversely affected by excessive use of drugs?

26. Identify medications commonly used to assist in lessening withdrawal symptoms during treatment for drug abuse.

27. In your own words, summarize the responsibility of dental team members in managing the risk for prescription drug abuse.

28. List actions that healthcare providers can take to avoid prescription pad theft.

COMPETENCY EXERCISES

Apply information from the chapter and use critical thinking skills to complete the competency exercises. Write responses on paper or create electronic documents to submit your answers.

1. Explain why it is especially important to inspect intraoral tissues each time you assess a patient who has a past or current history of excessive alcohol consumption or drug use.

2. The CAGE questionnaire (Box 65-8) provides a reliable score for determining potential alcohol dependence and is beneficial for use as a screening tool in clinical settings. Asking additional questions can obtain additional information to assist in providing appropriate patient care. Discuss the kind of communication approach that would be most successful in eliciting honest answers from patients.

3. Your afternoon patient is 20 minutes late for her appointment; she is a well-dressed woman in a businesses suit and is new patient to the office. As you review her medical history you notice her breath smells of alcohol and she answered "yes" to the question concerning having 1 or more drinks a day. You explain the office policy that a "yes" answer to that question requires you to give her an additional questionnaire; you ask if she is willing to answer additional questions and she complies. The patient answers "yes" for all four questions in the CAGE questionnaire; she immediately engages you in a discussion concerning her answers. The patient admits that she has been trying to stop drinking because she has noticed red areas in her mouth; she states that no matter how much she brushes her gums bleed, and they are red and swollen all the time. The patient lives alone and feels very guilty about her habit; lately she needs a drink in the morning before going to work and at night before going to sleep. She has no family.

   As you question her further, you determine that her colleagues make annoying comments about her breath and criticize her for drinking. The patient has also answered "yes" to increasing pains in her stomach.

   According to the CAGE questionnaire, explain what degree of suspicion of alcohol consumption you would assign to this patient and why.

   What medical referral would this patient require and why?

   Is this patient at increased risk for drug abuse and why?

4. Your next patient is Justin Townsley, age 21. He has just returned home from his first year away at college. His mother has made a dental hygiene appointment for him because he has not had his teeth examined in at least three years. She also wants him to have his wisdom teeth extracted before he is no longer covered under her dental insurance plan. When you go to greet Justin in the reception area, you overhear the end of a cell phone conversation in which he is planning to meet his buddies later on this evening to go out partying. "And, we'll stay out all night so we can have even more fun *this* time than we did *last* time," he says just before he hangs up the telephone to greet you. He stumbles just a bit as he rises from the chair but recovers quickly to follow you to the treatment room. As he walks past you into the chair, you distinctly catch the odor of alcohol on his breath.

   Justin's health history is unremarkable except for having an arm broken in an automobile accident last year. He states that he does not take any regular medications. When you take his pulse and blood pressure today, both are slightly elevated.

   Your intraoral findings include generalized poor oral hygiene, significant calculus deposits, coated tongue, dry oral mucosa, red and swollen gingiva, generalized 4- to 6-mm probing depths, and generalized bleeding on probing. Justin states that "the left side of my jaw has been aching a lot lately, probably from grinding my teeth." A front tooth and the cusp of an upper premolar are both slightly chipped, findings that were not previously noted. As you are working to complete your oral assessment, Justin keeps up a constant conversation about how much fun he has had this year while he was away at college. He sheepishly admits that his daily oral care has suffered, saying, "I stay up all night sometimes—to study for all those mid-term and final exams, you know. Sometimes I just forget to brush."

   You decide that you need to ask Justin about his drinking and the possible use of stimulant drugs. Identify the assessment findings that lead you to this decision.

   What oral signs and symptoms will you look for as you continue your assessment?

   What additional follow-up questions will you ask Justin to help you determine his patterns of alcohol and/or drug use?

5. Your careful and sensitive questioning leads you to believe that Justin's level of alcohol consumption and possible use of street drugs is probably having some detrimental impact on his health status. You

are concerned enough that you discuss the matter with him and you give him a brochure about the oral effects of alcohol. You plan to bring your concerns for his health up again at his subsequent appointments. When you write a dental hygiene care plan for Justin, you will plan two additional visits for scaling and root planing his entire mouth. What education/counseling and oral hygiene instructions/home care interventions will you plan to help Justin maximize healing and tissue response during and after oral debridement? (*Hint*: If you write dental hygiene diagnosis statements for Justin it may help you decide on your planned interventions.)

6. Using your institution's guidelines for writing in patient records, document progress notes for your first appointment with Justin.

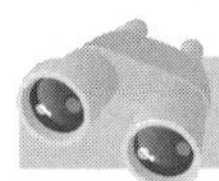

BOX 65-1 MeSH TERMS

Use a combination of MeSH terms and other key words to develop an effective and efficient PubMed literature search strategy.

Substance-related disorders	Amphetamine-related disorders
Substance abuse detection	Alcoholics
Street drugs	Alcoholism
Methamphetamine	Alcohol drinking
Abnormalities, drug-induced	Alcoholic intoxication
Cocaine-related disorders	Alcohol induced disorders
Crack cocaine	Fetal alcohol syndrome
Marijuana abuse	

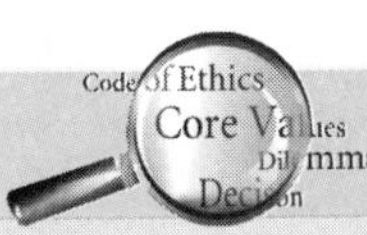

EVERYDAY ETHICS

Before completing the learning exercises below, reread and reflect on the Everyday Ethics Scenario and Questions for Consideration in this chapter of the textbook. It may also be useful to review the Dental Hygiene Ethics discussion in Chapter 1, the Ethical Applications in the introduction pages for each section in the textbook, as well as the Codes of Ethics in textbook Appendices I–IV.

Individual Learning Activity

Imagine that you have observed what happened in the scenario, but are not one of the main characters involved in the situation. Write a reflective journal entry that:

describes how you might have reacted (as an observer—not as a participant),

expresses your personal feelings about what happened,

or

identifies personal values that affect your reaction to the situation.

Discovery Activity

Summarize this scenario for faculty member at your school and ask them to consider the questions that are included. Is their perspective different than yours or similar? Explain.

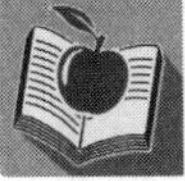

Factors To Teach The Patient

This scenario is related to the following factors listed in this chapter of the textbook:

- ▷ Drug abuse is a great risk to overall health.
- ▷ The risk of oral cancer is increased by the use of alcohol.
- ▷ Routine oral screening is needed at least twice a year to check for signs of early cancer.
- ▷ Drinking alcohol and using other drugs (prescription or over the counter) can lead to medical emergencies. Always check each drug and its action before using it in combination with alcohol or in combination with another drug.

Discussing your concerns about potential substance abuse with a patient like Justin Townsley (introduced in Competency Exercises question #4) requires building trust. You will be more successful in educating Justin and changing his health behaviors if you approach him without disapproval or judgment, but instead provide important information that motivates him to make changes in his own behaviors.

Use information in Chapter 65 of the textbook and the principles of motivational interviewing (see Appendix D) as guides to develop a conversation you will use to discuss the negative effects that alcohol and other drugs can have on Justin's health status.

Use the conversation you create to role-play this situation with a friend or fellow student. If you are the patient in the role-play, be sure to ask questions. If you are the dental hygienist, try to anticipate questions and answer them in your explanation. Modify your conversation based on what you learned.

66

The Patient with a Respiratory Disease

LEARNING OBJECTIVES

Upon successful completion of these exercises, you will be able to:

1. Identify and define key terms and concepts related to respiratory diseases.
2. Differentiate between upper and lower respiratory tract diseases.
3. Describe a variety of respiratory diseases.
4. Plan and document dental hygiene care and oral hygiene instructions for patients with compromised respiratory function.

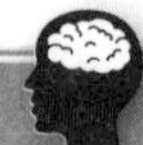

KNOWLEDGE EXERCISES

Write your answers for each question in the space provided.

1. Describe four additional infection control practices that can be implemented to help prevent transmission of respiratory infections.

2. What vital signs, related to respiratory function, are assessed at each patient visit?

3. Define *dyspnea.*

4. What medical test measures various aspects of breathing and lung function?

5. When performing a pulse oximetry test, what level of blood oxygen saturation signifies poor oxygen exchange?

6. What should you do if you recognize your patient is experiencing symptoms of respiratory distress during dental hygiene treatment?

7. A patient in respiratory distress may experience hypoxia. What patient signs and symptoms characterize hypoxia?

8. ____________ is defined as a breathing rate of greater than 20 breaths per minute. A patient who is breathing very rapidly can experience ____________, which may lead to dizziness and possible syncope.

9. What body structures are considered to be in the upper respiratory system?

10. What body structures comprise the lower respiratory system?

11. What are the pleura?

12. Identify two functions of the mucus secreted from goblet cells in respiratory mucosa?

13. What happens when an inflammatory disease causes an overproduction of mucus?

14. Identify three upper respiratory diseases more likely to be viral rather than bacterial infections.

15. What medication is used primarily to treat bacterial respiratory infections but is not prescribed for infections caused by a virus or fungus?

16. How are upper respiratory infections transmitted?

17. How can you best prevent transmission of pathogens while you are providing dental hygiene treatment?

18. What type of upper respiratory infection can cause tooth pain?

19. Identify two oral side effects of medications commonly used to treat upper respiratory infections.

20. What oral lesions can accompany the infectious stage of an upper respiratory infection?

21. List the lower respiratory tract diseases described in this chapter.

22. Identify three types of organisms that can cause pneumonia.

23. What medical treatment is provided for each type of pneumonia identified in question 22?

24. What pathogen causes a type of pneumonia most often associated with immune-impaired individuals?

25. Pneumonia infection that occurs from person-to-person transmission (not in a healthcare facility) is called:

26. What is one potential cause for HCAP or NCAP pneumonia?

27. What signs and symptoms are associated with tuberculosis?

28. How is tuberculosis transmitted?

29. How is clinically active tuberculosis diagnosed?

30. What two diagnostic tests are used to determine a latent tuberculosis infection?

31. What medication regimen is used to treat the clinically active stage of tuberculosis?

32. What oral condition is associated with the causative agent of tuberculosis?

33. List five types of asthma based on pathophysiology.

34. List the four National Asthma Education and Prevention Program classifications of asthma.

35. What are the signs and symptoms of an asthma attack?

36. True or False? Corticosteroids and mast call stabilizers are examples of *short-term control* medications for asthma.

37. List the types of drugs an individual with asthma needs to avoid and briefly describe the reason for each.

38. What ingredient in local anesthetic solutions can be a risk factor for asthma attack?

39. What oral condition(s) may occur in patients being treated for asthma?

40. What is the primary cause of COPD?

41. Patients with COPD who are chronic smokers have an increased risk for which oral conditions?

42. The term *blue bloater* is related to ______________.

43. Describe the cough of an individual with chronic bronchitis?

44. What are the symptoms of emphysema?

45. Cystic fibrosis is an autosomal recessive gene disorder that affects the ______________ tract, the ______________ tract, and the ______________.

46. What oral changes are likely to occur as cystic fibrosis progresses?

47. In your own words, briefly describe sleep apnea and summarize dental hygiene care protocols for the patient who uses a CPAP machine.

48. Complete Infomap 66-1 to compare three types of hypersensitivity reactions.

INFOMAP 66-1

CONDITION	PATHOGENESIS	SIGNS/SYMPTOMS
Allergic rhinitis (hay fever)		
Atopic asthma		
Anaphylaxis		

COMPETENCY EXERCISES

Apply information from the chapter and use critical thinking skills to complete the competency exercises. Write responses on paper or create electronic documents to submit your answers.

1. Charles Marcin, a handsome blond gentleman who is 67 years old, has been a patient in the practice for many years; however, this is the first time you have met him. His health history confirms your first impression of Mr. Marcin as a patient with COPD, and you remember the term *pink puffer* from your textbook. You observe Mr. Marcin carefully as he walks the short distance from the reception room to your treatment room. He rests with his head bent and his hands on the back of the dental chair to catch his breath before he sits down.

   Describe what you observe as you watch Mr. Marcin's breathing pattern and explain how it is different from the breathing pattern of an individual with other respiratory diseases.

2. When he can talk again, Mr. Marcin reminds you to call him Charlie. He says he has recently had a bit of a cold but is feeling somewhat better now. He tells you that his cough has pretty much gone away, and he isn't blowing his nose every 5 minutes any more. He complains that this is already his second cold this year, and once he was treated for a sinus infection. He mentions his teeth are stained because he has been drinking so much hot tea lately, and he is excited about being in your office today so that he can have an especially bright smile for his daughter's wedding this coming weekend. You think back to everything you learned about respiratory diseases as you plan Mr. Marcin's appointment for today. What safety and comfort factors will you need to assess and consider as you provide care during Mr. Marcin's dental hygiene appointment today?

3. Mr. Mitch Angelo is currently taking several medications to treat his asthma. When you are examining his mouth, you notice enamel erosion on the lingual areas of the anterior teeth. Explain what is happening that may be contributing to this oral condition.

4. When you have completed the first quadrant of scaling and root planing, you mention to Mr. Angelo that the gingival tissue in that area might be a bit sensitive later on today. He asks you what he should do if he feels pain. Which analgesics does a patient with asthma need to avoid?

5. When you update his medical history, Mr. Ben Samuelson, a 45-year-old businessman, tells you that he has been taking a new medication called isoniazid. When you question him further, he states that he does not know why he is taking it. What follow-up questions will you ask Mr. Samuelson?

6. What additional steps will you take prior to beginning your assessment of Mr. Samuelson's oral condition?

7. Explain the role of oral bacteria as a potential pathogenic agent in pneumonia, particularly if the patient is debilitated or chronically ill.

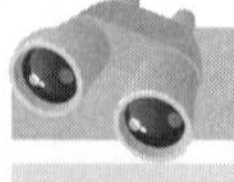

BOX 66-1 MeSH TERMS

Use a combination of MeSH terms and other key words to develop an effective and efficient PubMed literature search strategy.

Respiratory system	Asthma
Respiratory tract diseases	Pulmonary emphysema
Respiratory tract infections	Bronchitis
Lung diseases	Bronchitis, chronic
Pulmonary disease, chronic obstructive	

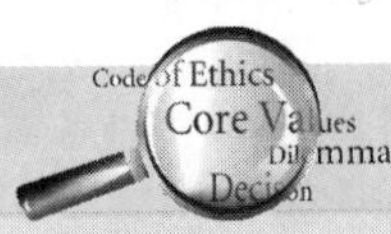

EVERYDAY ETHICS

Before completing the learning exercises below, reread and reflect on the Everyday Ethics Scenario and Questions for Consideration in this chapter of the textbook. It may also be useful to review the Dental Hygiene Ethics discussion in Chapter 1, the Ethical Applications in the introduction pages for each section in the textbook, as well as the Codes of Ethics in textbook Appendices I–IV.

Collaborative Learning Activity

Answer each of the questions for consideration at the end of the scenario in the textbook. Compare what you wrote with answers developed by another classmate and discuss differences/similarities.

Discovery Activity

Summarize this scenario for faculty member at your school and ask them to consider the questions that are included. Is their perspective different than yours or similar? Explain.

Factors To Teach The Patient

This scenario is related to the following factors listed in this chapter of the textbook:

- ▷ The need for frequent handwashing to help prevent transmission of respiratory disease.
- ▷ The need for thorough daily cleaning of toothbrushes to help prevent spread of infections.
- ▷ How using a new toothbrush and cleaning dentures/orthodontic appliances after bacterial infections can decrease the possibility of reinfection.
- ▷ Why elderly patients and those with chronic cardiovascular disease, diabetes, and other immunosuppressed conditions should receive a pneumonia vaccine and annual influenza immunizations.

Because of Mr. Marcin's chronic emphysema (patient introduced in Competency Exercises for this chapter), you are concerned about his recurring upper respiratory infections. Use the information in Chapter 66 in the textbook and the principles of motivational interviewing (see Appendix D) as guides to write a statement explaining ways that Mr. Marcin can reduce his risk for more serious acute respiratory diseases.

67

The Patient with a Cardiovascular Disease

LEARNING OBJECTIVES

Upon successful completion of these exercises, you will be able to:

1. Identify and define key terms and concepts related to cardiovascular disease.
2. Describe the cause, symptoms, prevention, and treatment of major cardiovascular diseases.
3. Identify clinical considerations and oral health factors related to cardiovascular conditions.
4. Plan and document dental hygiene care for a patient with cardiovascular disease.

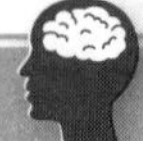

KNOWLEDGE EXERCISES

Write your answers for each question in the space provided.

1. Explain the two classifications of heart diseases.

2. Identify the various tissues in the heart that can be affected by cardiovascular disease.

3. In your own words, describe the progression and diagnosis of infective endocarditis.

4. List steps you can take to prevent infection during oral assessment and dental hygiene treatment if

you suspect your patient is at risk for infective endocarditis.

5. Refer to Figure 67-1 in the textbook to help you visualize the veins, arteries, and chambers of a healthy heart. Describe the sequence of the normal flow of blood.

6. Congenital heart disease is the result of anatomic anomalies that occur during the first ____________ weeks of fetal development. The exact cause is often unknown but is either ____________, ____________, or a combination of the two.

7. Refer to Figures 67-2 and 67-3 from the textbook to help you describe how the normal path of blood flow is compromised in each of the two types of congenital heart disease.

Ventricular septal defect:

Patent ductus arteriosus:

8. What symptoms of congenital heart disease may affect the delivery of dental hygiene care?

9. What is the etiology of rheumatic heart disease?

10. Describe how the flow of blood through the heart is altered when there is a mitral valve prolapse.

11. Recording blood pressure is an essential step in patient assessment before dental hygiene care. Blood pressure is recorded as a fraction; systolic/diastolic pressure in millimeters of mercury. In your own words, define systolic and diastolic blood pressure.

Systolic:

Diastolic:

12. Patient screening and early detection of hypertension are important components of dental hygiene care because, in early stages, this condition is often unrecognized owing to ____________.

13. Identify the sequelae of long-standing hypertension.

14. From memory (don't look in the book), list the systolic and diastolic values that determine normal adult blood pressure, prehypertension, and stage 1 and stage 2 hypertension.

15. What is malignant hypertension?

16. What blood pressure level triggers concern for your child patient? (*Hint:* You can also look at Table 11-1 in Chapter 11 for specific systolic and diastolic values.)

17. Identify modifiable patient lifestyle risk factors associated with essential hypertension.

18. List the causes of secondary hypertension.

19. Ischemic heart disease arises from ____________ to the heart muscle.

20. What is the principle cause of ischemic heart disease?

21. What are the modifiable (lifestyle) risk factors for ischemic heart disease?

22. What are the signs and symptoms of angina pectoris?

23. What is the difference between stable and unstable angina?

24. If your patient's medical history indicates medication for angina pectoris, where should the container with nitroglycerin be kept during a dental hygiene appointment?

25. The vasodilator (nitroglycerin) tablet is placed under the patient's tongue. What can you do to help the tablet to dissolve more quickly?

26. If your patient experiences an angina attack during dental hygiene treatment, what will you do? The steps are described below. Number the list in the correct order (1 = first step; 9 = last step).

Step Number	Description
_____	*Administer vasodilator (nitroglycerin)*
_____	*Administer oxygen*
_____	*Readminister vasodilator (if indicated)*
_____	*Call for staff/colleague assistance*
_____	*Call for medical assistance*
_____	*Position patient in upright, comfortable position*
_____	*Check patient response*
_____	*Check purchase date/potency of nitroglycerin*
_____	*Terminate dental hygiene treatment*

27. When do you record vital signs after an angina attack has been resolved by administering the patient's nitroglycerin?

28. What is the cause of myocardial infarction?

29. What is the most common artery associated with myocardial infarction?

30. The symptoms of myocardial infarction are similar to the symptoms of angina pectoris. What circumstances indicate that you should summon immediate medical assistance for your patient and be ready to administer basic life support?

31. If your patient who is experiencing symptoms of angina suddenly becomes unconscious, what should you do?

32. What symptoms may indicate the onset of a myocardial infarction?

33. After a myocardial infarction, your patient's elective dental and dental hygiene treatment is postponed until ____________.

34. What is congestive heart failure?

35. Identify the underlying causes and precipitating factors associated with congestive heart failure.

36. If your patient's medical history indicates chronic congestive heart failure, what symptoms can you observe that will indicate whether the right-hand or the left-hand side of the heart is affected?

Left-hand side of heart:

Right-hand side of heart:

What lifestyle changes are commonly recommended for patients with cardiovascular disease?

37. What surgical interventions can be used to treat heart disease?

38. A coronary stent is put in place to ___________ the blood vessel and prevent renarrowing of the lumen.

39. What is the purpose of a cardiac pacemaker or implantable defibrillator?

40. How will the dental hygiene clinician determine the need for antibiotic premedication when the patient has an implanted defibrillator?

41. Identify clinical procedures that will protect your patient who is receiving anticoagulant therapy for a cardiovascular condition.

COMPETENCY EXERCISES

Apply information from the chapter and use critical thinking skills to complete the competency exercises. Write responses on paper or create electronic documents to submit your answers.

1. Review your school's dental clinic policy and guidelines for screening and treating patients with hypertension and answer the following questions.

   At what intervals are patients' blood pressure readings recorded in the patient record?

   At what level are patients referred for a physician consult?

   At what level is administration of local anesthetic compromised?

   At what blood pressure classification or level will you suspend planned dental hygiene treatment and reschedule your patient after medical intervention?

2. What is the goal of providing dental hygiene treatment before and after cardiac surgery?

3. When you update her health history at her 3-month dental hygiene visit, Mrs. LaShawn Peal tells you her physician has recently prescribed anticoagulant therapy to treat a cardiac condition. She states she doesn't really understand what the medication is for, exactly, and that the Prothrombin Time test you ask her about was not recommended by her physician. She minimizes the issue and tells you if her doctor isn't worried about this kind of thing, then neither is she. She protests vehemently when you mention you need to contact her physician for a consultation before you begin her dental hygiene treatment. Using patient-appropriate language, explain why you will require a physician consult before you begin dental hygiene treatment for Mrs. Peal.

4. When you contact Mrs. Peal's physician, he tells you that he will order the test. Mrs. Peal can stop by any time to have it done. You return to the treatment room to explain the situation to Mrs. Peal. Using your institution's guidelines for writing in patient records, document why Mrs. Peal was dismissed today and her dental hygiene appointment rescheduled.

DISCOVERY EXERCISE

Visit the American Heart Association website at http://www.heart.org and use the website search box to learn more about conditions that put your patient at risk for infective endocarditis and access the latest guidelines for premedication.

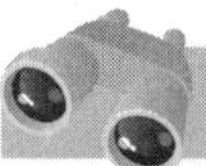

BOX 67-1 MeSH TERMS

Use a combination of MeSH terms and other key words to develop an effective and efficient PubMed literature search strategy.

Cardiovascular diseases	Hypertension
Coronary artery disease	Hypertension, malignant
Myocardial infarction	Prehypertension
Cardiovascular infections	Angina pectoris
Endocarditis, bacterial	Mitral valve prolapse
Atherosclerosis	Pacemaker, artificial
Arteriosclerosis	Rheumatic heart disease

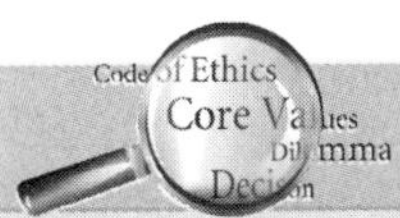

EVERYDAY ETHICS

Before completing the learning exercises below, reread and reflect on the Everyday Ethics Scenario and Questions for Consideration in this chapter of the textbook. It may also be useful to review the Dental Hygiene Ethics discussion in Chapter 1, the Ethical Applications in the introduction pages for each section in the textbook, as well as the Codes of Ethics in textbook Appendices I–IV.

Individual Learning Activity

Imagine that you have observed what happened in the scenario, but are not one of the main characters involved in the situation. Write a reflective journal entry that:

describes how you might have reacted (as an observer—not as a participant),
expresses your personal feelings about what happened,
or
identifies personal values that affect your reaction to the situation.

Collaborative Learning Activity

Work with a small group to develop a 2- to 5-minute role-play that introduces the Everyday Ethics scenario described in the chapter (a great idea is to video record your role-play activity). Then develop separate 2-minute role-play scenarios that provide at least two alternative approaches/solutions to resolving the situation. Ask classmates to view the solutions, ask questions, and discuss the ethical approach used in each. Ask for a vote on which solution classmates determine to be the "best."

Factors To Teach The Patient

This scenario is related to the *Stress Reduction Procedures* listed in the Factors to Teach the Patient section of this chapter in the textbook.

When you read the patient record before seating Mr. Pedro Valdez (age 58) for his dental hygiene continuing care appointment, you note that he has a very complex history of cardiovascular disease, including myocardial infarction 6 years ago. When you call his name in the reception area, he looks up at you while coughing into a tissue. He comments that you are not the dental hygienist he usually sees for his appointment. He rises wearily from the chair, complains briefly he has been waiting quite a long time, and walks with you to your treatment room.

As you stroll slowly beside him, you notice he is pale, and the back of his neck is sweating. When he reaches the dental chair, he collapses into it breathing heavily. While you take his blood pressure, you note that his skin feels quite cold, his fingernail beds look bluish, and his wrists and ankles appear quite swollen. You record a blood pressure of 135/95 mmHg on his right arm and a resting pulse of 83 beats per minute. When you begin to lower the dental chair for your intraoral examination, he becomes agitated, leans forward in the chair, and tells you that he has to sit up straight to be comfortable.

Use the information in Chapter 67 in the textbook and the motivational interviewing principles in Appendix D as guides to prepare an outline for a conversation that you might use to discuss the ways you will help Mr. Valdez to be comfortable and safe during his dental hygiene treatment.

Crossword Puzzle

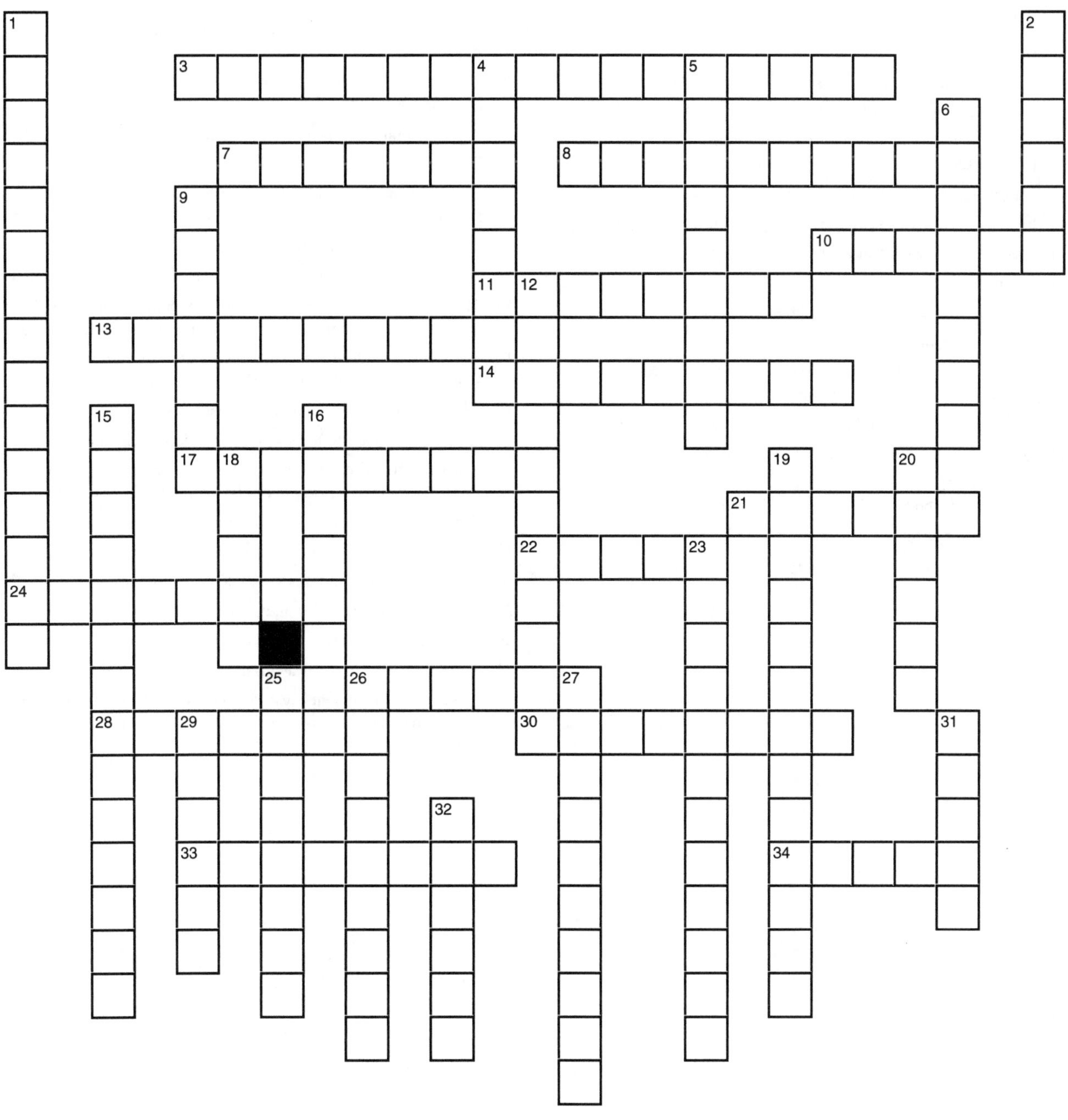

Puzzle Clues

Across

3. The record produced by recording electric currents generated by the heart; EKG.
7. Diminished availability of oxygen to blood tissues.
8. The middle layer of the heart wall.
10. The nonoxygenated blood that returns from body tissues to the heart and is pumped from the heart to the lungs.
11. Narrowing or constriction (of an artery).
13. Slowing of pulse to less than 60 beats per minute.
14. Characterized by hardening, thickening, and loss of elasticity.
17. Group or series of four.
21. A disease that causes acute, spasmodic pain attack.
22. Temporary cessation of breathing.
24. Deficiency of blood to supply oxygen (to the heart); result of constriction or obstruction of a blood vessel.
25. Deficiency of oxygen and increase of carbon dioxide in the blood.
28. Labored or difficult breathing that may be a symptom of cardiovascular disease.
30. Oxygenated blood that flows from the heart to nourish body tissues.
33. A blood clot attached to the interior of a blood vessel.
34. The channel inside a blood vessel.

Down

1. Narrowing of the lining of a blood vessel by fatty deposits containing cholesterol.
2. The surgical procedure that redirects blood flow around a narrowed heart artery.
4. Bluish coloration caused by reduced hemoglobin in the blood.
5. Blockage or closing (of a blood vessel).
6. Caused by an object (blood clot, air bubble, or clump of bacteria) that suddenly blocks an artery.
9. Localized area of ischemic necrosis in the heart.
12. Abnormally rapid heart rate; usually more than 100 beats per minute.
15. The record that is produced when a beam of ultrasonic waves is directed to record the position and motion of structures in the heart.
16. The downward displacement of the mitral valve between the left atrium and the left ventricle of the heart.
18. Abnormal accumulation of fluid in body tissues.
19. A substance that interferes with coagulation of the blood.
20. Related to the absence of oxygen in tissues; symptoms include deep respirations, cyanosis, increased pulse rate, and reduced coordination.
23. Lipid plaque that deposits on the lining of an artery.
25. Localized dilation of the wall of a blood vessel.
26. Mechanism that maintains a reliable heart rhythm.
27. Variation (of the heart) from its normal rhythm.
29. Dividing wall between left and right ventricles in the heart.
31. A term meaning passageway (as in patent ductus arteriosus).
32. Irregularity of heartbeat caused by turbulent flow of blood through a valve that has failed to close.

68

The Patient with a Blood Disorder

LEARNING OBJECTIVES

Upon successful completion of these exercises, you will be able to:

1. Identify and define key terms and concepts related to hematologic conditions.
2. Recognize blood components and normal reference values.
3. Describe the causes, symptoms, and oral effects of red and white blood cell disorders, bleeding disorders, and clotting deficiencies.
4. Plan and document dental hygiene education and treatment for patients with a blood disorder.

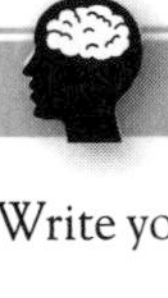

KNOWLEDGE EXERCISES

Write your answers for each question in the space provided.

1. List seven elements that make up blood.

2. What is the composition of plasma?

3. Identify the function of each of the plasma proteins.

4. Why are red blood cells termed *corpuscles*?

5. What is the purpose of red blood cells?

6. What is a normal hemoglobin value?

7. When the diagnosis is anemia, what has happened to the hemoglobin value?

8. Identify five basic causes of anemia.

9. Iron-deficiency anemia is more often seen in younger people than in older people; more often in ___________ than in ___________.

10. What can cause iron-deficiency anemia?

11. Identify two main types of anemia disorders in which red blood cells are destroyed.

12. Identify two causes of diminished production of red blood cells.

13. What genetic disorders are characterized by absent or decreased production of normal hemoglobin?

14. Which megaloblastic anemia is caused by a vitamin B_{12} deficiency?

15. What oral findings are related to anemia?

16. Which foods can you suggest to your patients as good sources of vitamin B_{12}?

17. Dietary factors are important in the treatment of folate-deficiency anemia, but this type of megaloblastic anemia may be more frequently related to ___________ than to inadequate intake.

18. What severe condition affecting newborns is also a result of folic acid deficiency?

19. Sickle cell disease is a form of ___________ anemia.

20. Individuals from which two ethnic populations are most at risk for sickle cell disease?

21. In your own words, briefly describe the clinical course of the chronic and acute phases of sickle cell disease.

Chronic anemia:

Acute vaso-occlusion or crisis:

22. Briefly describe preventive and disease state treatments for sickle cell disease.

Preventive:

____

During a crisis:

____

23. List oral manifestations associated with sickle cell disease that can be identified by the dental hygienist.

____

24. A red blood cell count ____________ normal levels is characteristic of polycythemia.

25. List symptoms of polycythemia that may be noted by the dental hygienist during an oral examination.

____

26. Identify two main types of white blood cells.

____

27. What is the main function of leukocytes?

____

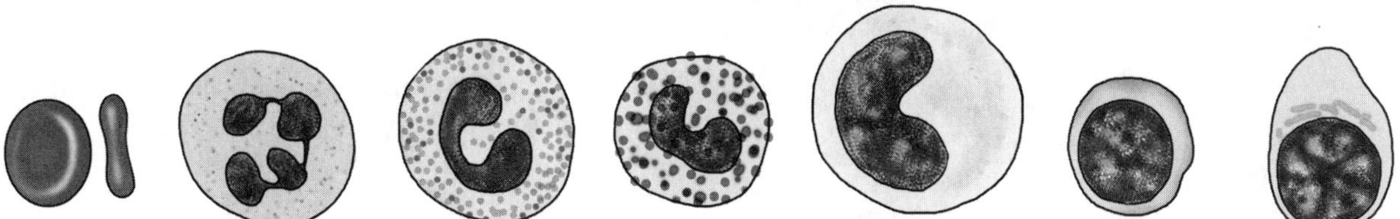

Erythrocytes | Neutrophil | Eosinophil | Basophil | Monocyte | Lymphocyte | Plasma cell

28. Match the name of the correct cell in the drawing above to the description of each white blood cell in the list below.

Functions to increase vascular permeability so that phagocytic cells can pass into inflamed areas.

____

Stains bright pink under the microscope; increases markedly during allergic conditions.

____

Multiplies when needed and moves back and forth between vessels and extravascular tissue.

____

Actively phagocytic; changes into macrophage in connective tissue.

____

Also called PMN; first in line to phagocytosis when the body is invaded by bacteria.

____

29. What is the normal reference value of leukocytes in the blood?

____

30. White blood cell counts can be used to detect and monitor disease because each cell type either ____________ or ____________ in association with certain conditions.

31. Identify the specific type of white blood cell associated with these approximate percentages of the total WBC count.

    60%–70%:

    ____

    20%–35%:

    ____

    2%–6%:

    ____

    1%–3%:

    ____

    1%:

    ____

32. Match each descriptive statement with the correct white blood cell disorder.

Disorder	Descriptive Statement
A. Neutropenia	____Caused by defects in myeloid cells.
B. Lymphocytopenia	____Abnormally low number of lymphocytes.
C. Leukocytosis	____Increase in circulating white blood cells.
	____Oral stomatitis and lymph mode enlargement are symptoms.
	____Symptoms include petechiae and mouth ulcers.
	____Can happen for many reasons including infection and excess exertion.
	____Symptoms include bruising and gingival bleeding.
	____Can be caused by protein-energy malnutrition or infection.
	____Decrease in numbers of neutrophils.
	____Can be associated with malignant neoplasms of immature white blood cells.
	____Can be caused by chemotherapy or radiation therapy.

33. List and briefly describe two platelet disorders.

    ____

    ____

    ____

    ____

34. List and briefly describe the cause of two types of coagulation disorders.

    ____

    ____

    ____

    ____

35. In your own words, describe the effects of hemophilia.

    ____

    ____

    ____

36. List at least five common herbs associated with increased bleeding if taken as a nutritional supplement.

    ____

    ____

    ____

    ____

    ____

    ____

    ____

    ____

37. What common pain medication alters the ability of platelets to stick together and form a clot?

    ____

38. Cancer treatments with chemotherapeutic agents put your patient at risk for which two blood disorders?

    ____

    ____

39. Consultation with the patient's primary care provider or ____________ may be a necessary component of a complete pretreatment assessment if the patient has a blood disorder.

40. What common dental hygiene interventions or actions can inadvertently cause increased risk for bleeding when the patient has a blood disorder?

    ____

    ____

    ____

    ____

COMPETENCY EXERCISES

Apply information from the chapter and use critical thinking skills to complete the competency exercises. Write responses on paper or create electronic documents to submit your answers.

1. When you update his health history, Jeremiah Bell tells you that his gums, which have always been healthy, have been bleeding profusely when he flosses. Once he woke up in the morning with blood in his mouth and on his pillow. What questions will you ask him?
2. Mr. Bell replies that he has seen his physician to be tested for a blood disorder and hands you a sheet of paper reporting the results of four tests. Which tests would you expect to see included in the report that evaluate bleeding time? (*Hint:* Table 68-1 will help you to answer this question).
3. If the report handed to you by Mr. Bell indicates a diagnosis of leukemia, what results would you expect to see for the blood tests?
4. You and the attending dentist decide together to postpone clinical dental hygiene treatment for Mr. Bell until you can arrange a telephone consultation with his physician. You provide oral hygiene instruction for Mr. Bell with an emphasis on what he can do on a daily basis to minimize oral effects of his blood disorder. Using your institution's guidelines for writing in patient records, document this appointment.
5. Mr. Weber presents for his continuing care appointment. He states that since his myocardial infarction 8 months ago, he is taking Warfarin daily. He is not sure of the amount nor his last anticoagulation test. What laboratory test(s) would you need to know before proceeding? What levels would be recommended for you to proceed today with treatment? What questions will you ask when you consult with his physician?

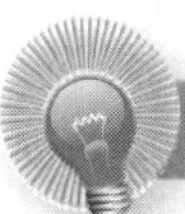

DISCOVERY EXERCISE

Explore the American Dental Association website or do a PubMed literature search to find information about the latest guidelines for management of dental patients who are taking anticoagulant or antiplatelet medications.

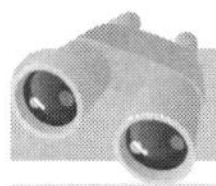

BOX 68-1 MeSH TERMS

Use a combination of MeSH terms and other key words to develop an effective and efficient PubMed literature search strategy.

Blood cells	Neutropenia
Blood platelets	Thrombocytopenia
Erythrocytes	Thrombocytosis
Neutrophils	Hemoglobins
Hemocytes	Anemia
Leukocytes	Hemorrhagic disorders
Hematologic diseases	Blood platelet disorders
Leukocyte disorders	

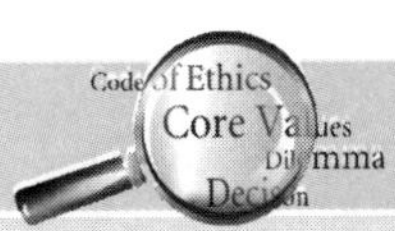

EVERYDAY ETHICS

Before completing the learning exercises below, reread and reflect on the Everyday Ethics Scenario and Questions for Consideration in this chapter of the textbook. It may also be useful to review the Dental Hygiene Ethics discussion in Chapter 1, the Ethical Applications in the introduction pages for each section in the textbook, as well as the Codes of Ethics in textbook Appendices I–IV.

Individual Learning Activity

Imagine that you are the dental hygienist in this scenario. Answer each of the questions for consideration at the end of the scenario.

Collaborative Learning Activity

Work with another student colleague to role-play the scenario. The goal of this exercise is for you and your colleague to work though the alternative actions in order to come to consensus on a solution or response that is acceptable to both of you.

Factors To Teach The Patient

This scenario is related to the following factors listed in this chapter of the textbook:

- ▷ Meticulous hygiene techniques to practice daily: toothbrushing, flossing, and other interdental cleaning devices.
- ▷ How to self-evaluate the oral cavity for deviations from normal; any changes should be reported to the dentist and dental hygienist.

When Mr. Bell (introduced in Competency Exercises in this chapter) returns in a few weeks for his follow-up appointment, he tells you that he has just started treatment for leukemia. He has been advised that it is very difficult to control all of the symptoms of his condition. He is very concerned about his oral health.

Use the information in Chapter 68 in the textbook the motivational interviewing principles in Appendix D to outline your education plan for Mr. Bell.

Use the outline you created to role-play this situation with a fellow student. If you are the patient in the role-play, be sure to ask questions. If you are the dental hygienist, try to anticipate questions and answer them in your explanation.

Crossword Puzzle

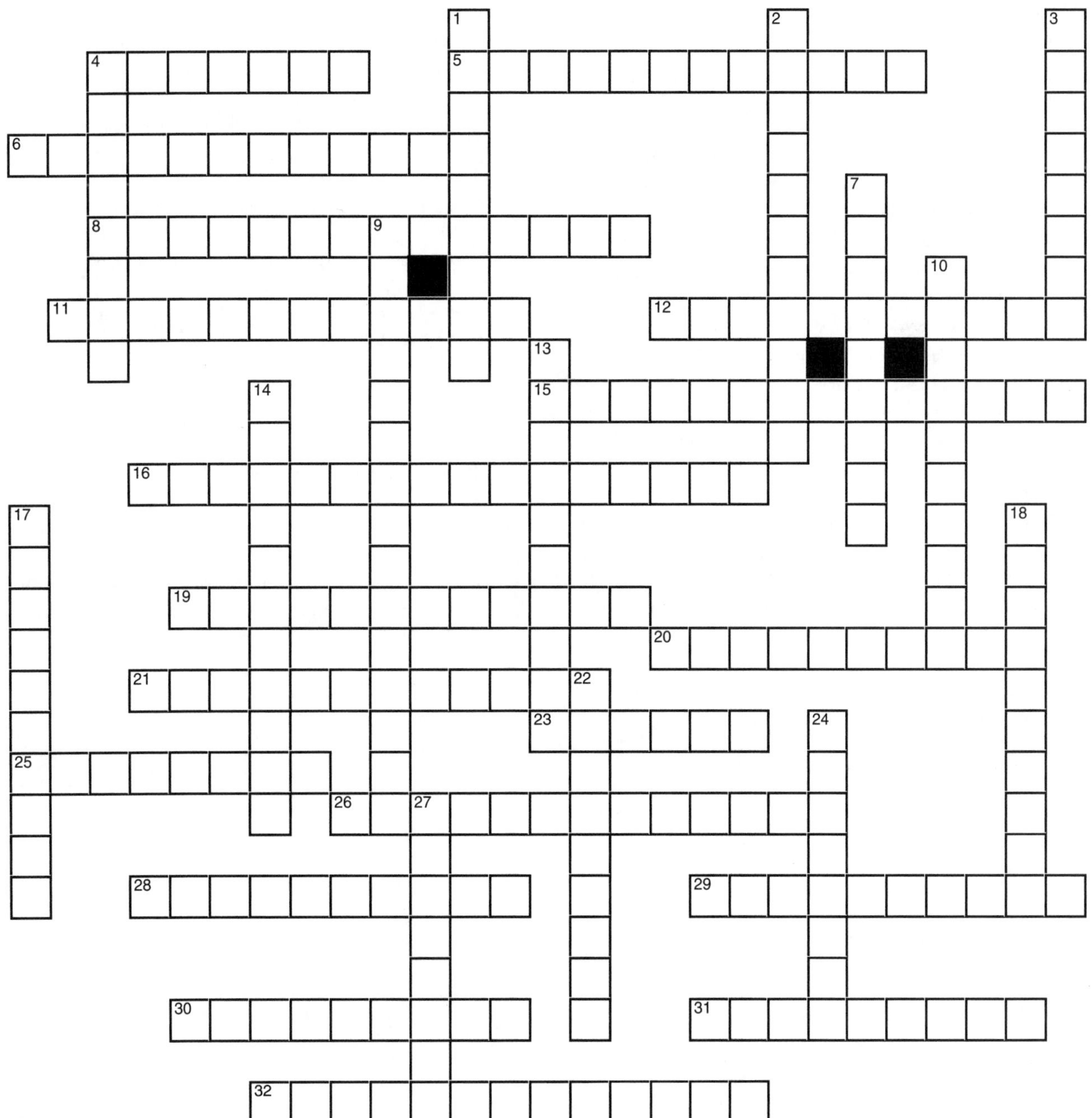

Puzzle Clues

Across

4. Hemorrhage into tissues.
5. Increase in total number of leukocytes.
6. Engulfing of microorganisms by phagocytes.
8. Formation of red blood cells.
11. Condition that can be caused by a variety of factors; characterized by an increase in the number of circulating white blood cells.
12. Diminished number of neutrophils.
15. Increase in the numbers of red blood cells.
16. A lowered number of platelets caused by decreased production in the bone marrow.
19. Test used for blood evaluation; normal range 4–8 minutes (two words).
20. Reduction in leukocytes in blood to less than 500 per mL.
21. Condition characterized by an increase in number and concentration of red blood cells; hemoglobin and hematocrit values are raised.
23. Some general signs and symptoms of this condition are paleness, weakness, headache, vertigo, and brittle nails.
25. Pinpoint-size hemorrhage.
26. Formation/development of blood cells, usually in the bone marrow.
28. A condition in which cell production cannot keep pace with turnover rate, resulting in a decreased total number of white blood cells.
29. Small, round agranulocyte with a large nucleus that nearly fills the cell; can multiply as immunologic need arises.
30. White blood cell.
31. Young cell found circulating in the blood in certain diseases.
32. Bright red blood; 97% saturated with oxygen.

Down

1. Inflammation of the tongue.
2. Factor in blood plasma that is essential to normal blood clotting.
3. The most extreme abnormal cause of leukocytosis.
4. Small element without a nucleus, about one-fourth the size of a red blood cell, that has a role both in clotting and clot dissolution after healing.
7. Rupture of erythrocytes with release of hemoglobin into plasma.
9. Test used for blood evaluation; normal range 11–15 seconds (two words).
10. Transmits molecular oxygen to body cells; normal range is 12–18 g per 100 mL.
13. A group of congenital disorders of the blood-clotting mechanism; related directly to the level of clotting factor in the circulating blood.
14. Pain in the tongue.
17. Most numerous of all white blood cells; first line of defense of the body.
18. Measure of red blood cells in whole blood; normal range is 37%–54%.
22. Loss of structural differentiation with revision to a more primitive type of cell.
24. Functions to increase vascular permeability during inflammation.
27. Large agranulocyte with indented nucleus that is actively phagocytic.

69

The Patient with Diabetes Mellitus

LEARNING OBJECTIVES

Upon successful completion of these exercises, you will be able to:

1. Identify and define key terms and concepts related to diabetes.
2. Explain the function and effects of insulin.
3. Identify risk factors for diabetes.
4. Describe etiologic classifications, signs and symptoms, diagnostic procedures, complications, and common medical treatment for diabetes.
5. React appropriately in a diabetic emergency.
6. Explain the relationship between diabetes and oral health.
7. Plan and document dental hygiene care and oral hygiene instructions for patients with diabetes.

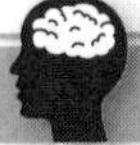

KNOWLEDGE EXERCISES

Write your answers for each question in the space provided.

1. What type of diabetes is related to genetics, obesity, and hormones during pregnancy?

2. Identify the health-related factors besides pregnancy that can result in diabetes.

3. What genetic syndromes are sometimes associated with diabetes?

4. Complete Infomap 69-1 by listing characteristics that will help you learn to differentiate between type 1 and type 2 diabetes.

INFOMAP 69-1 COMPARISON OF TYPE 1 AND TYPE 2 DIABETES

TYPE 1 CHARACTERISTICS	TYPE 2 CHARACTERISTICS

5. Diabetes is characterized by hyperglycemia. In your own words, define the range of measurements for *normal glucose blood level* and *hyperglycemia*.

6. Define the following symptoms of hyperglycemia.

   Polyuria:

   ____

   Polydipsia:

   ____

   Polyphagia:

   ____

7. List the common physical complications associated with uncontrolled diabetes.

   ____
   ____
   ____
   ____
   ____
   ____
   ____

8. What criteria are used to diagnose diabetes?

   ____
   ____
   ____

9. What self-administered tests are used for monitoring blood glucose levels during treatment of diabetes?

   ____
   ____
   ____
   ____
   ____
   ____

10. If your patient tells you the result of his fasting plasma glucose test this morning was less than______________, you know that his diabetes is well controlled and it is safe to provide dental hygiene treatment today.

11. If your patient tells you that her postprandial glucose level this morning was >200 mg per dL, you know that her diabetes is ______________________________.

12. What is the role of insulin in the human body?

   ____
   ____
   ____
   ____

13. Where is insulin produced in the human body?

   ____
   ____

14. What is exogenous insulin?

   ____

15. How is exogenous insulin administered?

   ____
   ____
   ____

16. What factors determine the dose of insulin administered for each patient?

   ____
   ____
   ____

17. Identify the duration of peak action for each of the classes of insulin.

   ____
   ____
   ____
   ____
   ____

18. What is the relationship of hypoglycemia from an inadequate nutritional intake to the level of insulin in the blood?

   ____
   ____
   ____
   ____

19. Describe the consequence when too little insulin is administered to control hyperglycemia.

   ____
   ____

20. Oral hypoglycemic agents act differently from insulin to control blood glucose levels. What is the mechanism of action of biguanides and thiazolidinediones?

21. If your patient is taking sulfonylureas or meglitinides to control type 2 diabetes, what side effect is important for you to watch for during dental hygiene treatment?

22. Your patient with uncontrolled diabetes is at risk for many long-term health complications. Identify the body systems or organs (other than the mouth) that can be affected.

23. Diabetes can be controlled, but to date, there is no known cure. List five factors important for maintaining the overall good health and well-being of an individual with diabetes or at risk for diabetes.

24. In one sentence, describe the relationship between poorly controlled diabetes and periodontal disease.

25. Uncontrolled glucose levels place your patient at risk for ____________________, an opportunistic oral infection.

26. What is the role of the dental hygienist in planning care for patients who are at risk for diabetes or who are exhibiting signs and symptoms of diabetes?

27. Why is stress prevention an important component of a dental hygiene care plan for a patient with diabetes?

28. Identify ways that the dental hygienist can reduce stress and prevent an emergency situation during an appointment with the patient with diabetes.

29. Why should you be very careful to avoid undue tissue trauma when providing dental hygiene care for your patient with diabetes?

COMPETENCY EXERCISES

Apply information from the chapter and use critical thinking skills to complete the competency exercises. Write responses on paper or create electronic documents to submit your answers.

1. In your own words, explain what can happen at the cellular level when glucose needed to supply energy cannot be accessed owing to either decreased supply or action of insulin.

Read the Section I Patient Assessment Summary to help you answer the following questions.

CHAPTER 69 – PATIENT ASSESSMENT SUMMARY

Patient Name: *Nicolas James Diamond*	Age: *57*	Gender: [M] F	☑ Initial Therapy ☐ Maintenance
Provider Name: *D.H. Student*	Date: *Today*		☐ Re-evaluation

Chief Complaint:
Patient presents for new patient examination. "I just want my teeth cleaned."

Assessment Findings

Health History • *Diagnosed several years ago with Type 2 Diabetes—Only monitors blood sugar levels when he isn't feeling well, tries to control the condition through diet and exercise.* • *No medical visits for two years—no current medications* • *Blood Pressure 145/95, Pulse 86 beats per minute.* • *Tobacco use: 1–2 packs per day for 35 years* • *Alcohol use: 1–2 drinks daily (usually beer)* • *ASA Classification—III* • *ADL level—0*	**At Risk For:**
Social and Dental History • *35 years in previous dental practice—dentist was a college roommate of his who recently retired.* • *No previous periodontal therapy—only received "dental cleanings" every 6 months.* • *Limited dental knowledge*	**At Risk For:**

Dental Examination
• *Generalized 6–8 mm probing depths*
• *Generalized recession on mandibular anterior and lingual of maxillary molars—sensitivity in molars*
• *Generalized slight mobility*
• *Generalized poor biofilm control*
• *Calculus lower anteriors*
• *Generalized bleeding on probing*
• *Generalized erythematous tissue*
• *Radiographic findings:*
  ◦ *Areas of horizontal and vertical bone loss*
  ◦ *Furcation involvement in mandibular molars*
  ◦ *Several large amalgam fillings with proximal overhangs*
  ◦ *Generalized subgingival and interproximal calculus visible on radiographs*
	At Risk For:

2. While you are waiting for Mr. Diamond, your first patient of the day, you look over the health history form he sent to the office a week earlier and note that he has been diagnosed with type 2 diabetes. Mr. Diamond finally arrives 15 minutes late for the appointment. He is extremely anxious, and states he is late because of the traffic. His morning, it seems, has not gone well, and everything is off schedule. As you bring him back to your treatment room, you notice that he is pale and trembling. He is perspiring profusely and seems agitated as he sits in the chair. What questions will you ask Mr. Diamond to add to the information you already know about his medical history?

3. Mr. Diamond responds irritably to your questions and gives vague answers. He says. "I have been having my teeth cleaned regularly for years and no one has ever asked these kinds of questions." When you take his vital signs, you note that his pulse is rapid and his blood pressure is a bit elevated. You are really conscious of your appointment time slipping away,

so you tilt the dental chair back to do an intraoral examination and begin your oral assessment. After 10 minutes, Mr. Diamond stops you and says "Please sit me upright." You note that his breath is coming in rapid gasps.

What is most likely to be happening and what will your response be?

4. Using your institution's guidelines for writing in patient records, document Mr. Diamond's appointment.

5. During a follow-up appointment several weeks later, when Mr. Diamond's medical situation has been stabilized, you are able to collect the rest of the assessment data. Use the information in Mr. Diamond's Patient Assessment Summary and a copy of the Patient-Specific Care Plan template in Appendix B to develop dental hygiene diagnosis statements and complete a dental hygiene care plan for providing initial therapy dental hygiene interventions for Mr. Diamond.

6. Discuss options for continuing care if Mr. Diamond's initial therapy outcomes are not optimal?

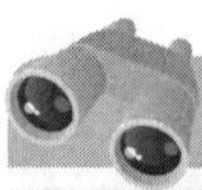

BOX 69-1 MeSH TERMS

Use a combination of MeSH terms and other key words to develop an effective and efficient PubMed literature search strategy.

- Diabetes mellitus, type 1
- Diabetes mellitus, type 2
- Diabetes, gestational
- Hyperglycemia
- Hypoglycemia
- Insulin
- Diabetes complications

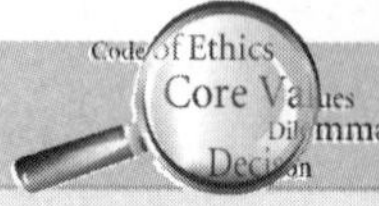

EVERYDAY ETHICS

Before completing the learning exercises below, reread and reflect on the Everyday Ethics Scenario and Questions for Consideration in this chapter of the textbook. It may also be useful to review the Dental Hygiene Ethics discussion in Chapter 1, the Ethical Applications in the introduction pages for each section in the textbook, as well as the Codes of Ethics in textbook Appendices I–IV.

Collaborative Learning Activity

Work with another student colleague to role-play the scenario. The goal of this exercise is for you and your colleague to work though the alternative actions in order to come to consensus on a solution or response that is acceptable to both of you.

Discovery Activity

Ask a friend or relative who is not involved in health care to read the scenario and discuss it with you from the perspective of a "patient" who receives services within the healthcare system. Discuss what you learned from the concerns, insights, or difference in perspective that person expressed.

Factors To Teach The Patient

This scenario is related to the following factors listed in this chapter of the textbook:

- ▷ Recognizing early warning signs of diabetes and seeking medical treatment.
- ▷ Reviewing practice of meticulous oral hygiene to prevent dental and periodontal disease.

Use the information from Chapter 69 in the textbook and the principles of motivational interviewing in Appendix D as guides to prepare a conversation that you might use to educate Ed (introduced in the textbook Everyday Ethics scenario) about the need to consult his physician related to signs and symptoms of diabetes, how diabetes can affect his oral health, and what he can do to prevent further health complications.

Use the conversation you create to role-play this situation with a fellow student. If you are the patient in the role-play, be sure to ask questions. If you are the dental hygienist, try to anticipate questions and answer them in your explanation.

SECTION IX Summary Exercises

Patients with Special Health Needs

Chapters 49-69

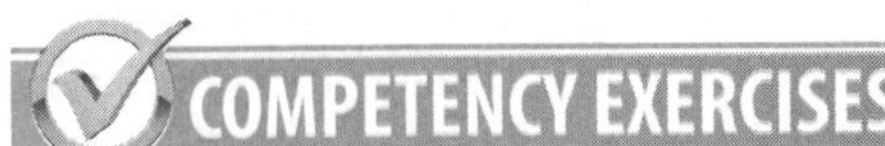

Apply information from the chapter and use critical thinking skills to complete the competency exercises. Write responses on paper or create electronic documents to submit your answers.

SECTION IX – PATIENT ASSESSMENT SUMMARY

Patient Name: *Nicolas James Diamond*	Age: *57*	Gender: [M] F	☑ Initial Therapy ☐ Maintenance
Provider Name: *D.H. Student*	Date: *Today*		☐ Re-evaluation

Chief Complaint:
Patient presents for new patient examination. "I just want my teeth cleaned."

Assessment Findings

Health History	**At Risk For:**
• *Diagnosed several years ago with Type 2 Diabetes—Only monitors blood sugar levels when he isn't feeling well, tries to control the condition through diet and exercise.* • *No medical visits for two years—no current medications* • *Blood Pressure 145/95, Pulse 86 beats per minute.* • *Tobacco use: 1–2 packs per day for 35 years* • *Alcohol use: 1–2 drinks daily (usually beer)* • *ASA Classification—III* • *ADL level—0*	
Social and Dental History	**At Risk For:**
• *35 years in previous dental practice—dentist was a college roommate of his who recently retired.* • *No previous periodontal therapy—only received "dental cleanings" every 6 months.* • *Limited dental knowledge*	

Dental Examination

- *Generalized 6–8 mm probing depths*
- *Generalized recession on mandibular anterior and lingual of maxillary molars—sensitivity in molars*
- *Generalized slight mobility*
- *Generalized poor biofilm control*
- *Calculus lower anteriors*
- *Generalized bleeding on probing*
- *Generalized erythematous tissue*
- *Radiographic findings:*
  - *Areas of horizontal and vertical bone loss*
  - *Furcation involvement in mandibular molars*
  - *Several large amalgam fillings with proximal overhangs*
  - *Generalized subgingival and interproximal calculus visible on radiographs*

At Risk For:

1. Use the information in the Chapter 69 Patient Assessment Summary for Mr. Nicholas Diamond and a copy of the Patient-Specific Care Plan template in Appendix B (or the form your clinic uses for a patient care plan) to develop a care plan for a series of initial dental hygiene therapy appointments.

2. The best way to become competent in planning and providing dental hygiene care for patients with special needs is, of course, to practice planning and providing care. The learning that comes from practicing your skills is always enhanced by taking time to record the process in some sort of written format so that you can later reflect on what you have done, how you did it, and why things did or did not work out as you had planned.

   Select one or more patients for whom you provide care in your school clinic who have one (or more) of the special needs identified in the textbook. To complete this exercise, gather the assessment data from each patient's record, a copy of the patient-specific dental hygiene care plan template in Appendix B (or from your clinic), the information from the appropriate chapters in the textbook, and any other source of information you think might be important (such as a drug reference book).

   Use the patient-specific care plan template to develop a comprehensive written dental hygiene care plan for each patient you select.

DISCOVERY EXERCISES

1. Gather as much information as you can about a specific special-need condition that interests you. Use PubMed (and the appropriate MeSH terms from the chapters in the textbook) to help you search the professional literature and/or look for online sources of information about the condition. The information in the scientific literature will probably be the most valid and reliable about the condition you select. Online sources can be variable, and it is important to determine that the host of the website is a reliable source of data and provides information about the condition that is supported by scientific principles.

2. You and your student colleagues can share information and learn from each other if you each present a different type of case and discuss the cases in a sort of case-presentation seminar. Each patient case you present should contain the following information:

   Patient background and demographics

   A general description of your patient, including name, age, race, sex, height, weight, blood pressure, pulse, and respiration

   Other information about your patient that is important for understanding the special condition

   A statement describing the significance of these data for planning and providing dental hygiene care

   Medical history

   A definition of each medical problem with an explanation of its significance to the delivery of dental care

   A description of your patient's ASA level

   A statement of the physical and oral manifestations of your patient's conditions

   A note about the anticipated complications associated with patient management during dental hygiene care

A statement of the anticipated complications or potential emergency situations that are related to your patient's medical history

A description of the actions needed to prevent complications and emergencies during dental hygiene care

Pharmacological and therapeutic considerations (Hint: Refer to a Physician's Desk Reference *or other accepted drug information reference as a guide)*

Identification of specific medications your patient is taking currently and how they relate to the medical history

A list containing the commercial and generic name of each drug, class or mechanism of action, usual dosage, indications for use, and anticipated adverse side effects for dentistry

An evaluation of your patient's local anesthesia considerations

Dental hygiene care delivery considerations

A description of the general physical and oral manifestations of your patient's condition that affect dental hygiene care

A description of your patient's ADL and IADL levels

A description of your patient's OSCAR considerations

Identification of and rationale for modifications to standard dental hygiene treatment procedures needed to meet your patient's special needs during dental hygiene care

Identification of and rationale for modifications in providing oral hygiene instructions

Identification of and rationale for modifications of oral hygiene aids

A description of behavioral and psychosocial considerations for planning and providing care for your patient

Identification of communication issues and needed actions to ensure that your patient is fully informed before he or she consents to the planned dental hygiene treatment.

3. Use information you gathered from a literature and/or developed for your patient case presentation to prepare a table clinic summarizing the dental hygiene care considerations for patients with the condition you have studied. (*Hint:* Check out the American Dental Hygienists' Association website http://www.adha.org for information and guidelines for constructing and presenting a table clinic.)

4. Go to your local pharmacy, grocery store, or department store and find different brands and types of pacifiers available for parents to select for their baby. Use the criteria listed in Chapter 49 of the textbook to determine which brand and type of pacifier you will recommend.

FOR YOUR PORTFOLIO

1. Include your written responses to the Everyday Ethics questions from any of the chapters in this section.

2. It is likely that while you are a student, you will develop many dental hygiene care plans for a variety of patients with a wide range of special needs. Include all of these written care plans in your portfolio. Also include the care plans you developed using the patient-assessment data summaries when completing the competency exercises in this workbook; be sure to indicate which care plans were developed for practice patient cases and which were developed for individuals for whom you provided dental hygiene care in your school clinic.

3. An effective way to document your growing knowledge about planning patient care is to include a written reflection that describes, in detail, how the care plans you developed later in your student career are different from the care plans you developed when you were first providing patient care.

   Cite specific examples from your earlier and later care plans to document your increased competency in planning individualized, patient-specific dental hygiene care. The examples should show how your later plans are more complete, more comprehensive, and more professional than your earlier plans.

4. If you develop and present a table clinic, include your presentation outline, along with any PowerPoint presentation or handouts you created to accompany the table clinic. Or include a photograph that shows you and your coauthor colleagues presenting your table clinic in a professional setting. A brief written reflection of what you learned from the experience of preparing and presenting the table clinic will add depth to your documentation.

Crossword Puzzle

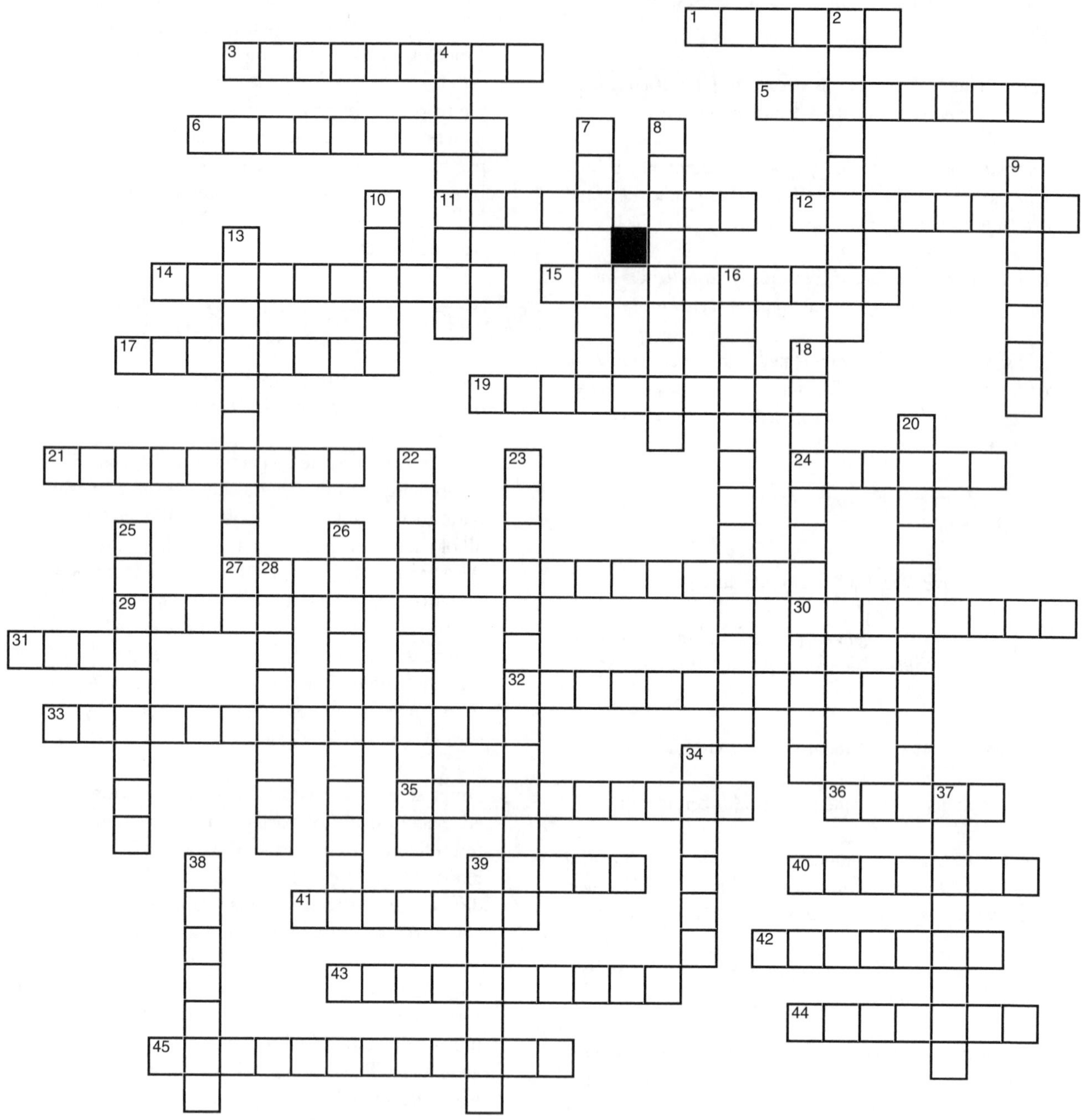

Puzzle Clues

Across

1. Screening and classification; sorting and allocating relative priority for patient treatment.
3. Type of tumor that has the properties of anaplasia, invasiveness, and metastasis.
5. Symptom that indicates the onset of a disease or condition.
6. Habitual psychologic and physiologic dependence on a substance.
11. Bony projection extending beyond the normal contour of a bony surface.
12. Hearing a constant noise such as ringing or buzzing.
14. Artificial replacement of a body part.
15. Another name for a bruise.
17. Loss of cognitive function that is sufficient to interfere with daily functioning.
19. Restriction in performing an activity; the result of an impairment.
21. Affording relief, but not cure.
24. Pertaining to the eye.
27. Healthcare team comprised of specialists from many disciplines.
29. Persistent patterns of heavy intake of substances, causing health consequences.
30. Coexisting or simultaneously existing disease processes.
31. To discontinue bottle or breast feeding.
32. The concurrent use of a large number of medications or drugs.
33. Pertaining to, or arising through the action of, many factors.
35. Loss or abnormality of structure or function.
36. Sudden, involuntary contraction of a muscle or group of muscles.
39. Beginning abruptly with marked intensity.
40. Developing slowly and persisting for a long period of time.
41. Temporary loss of consciousness caused by sudden fall in blood pressure.
42. Within the womb (two words).
43. Fold of skin characteristic near the eye of a person with Down syndrome.
44. Disturbance of trigeminal nerve causing spasms of masticatory muscles and limiting the opening of the mouth.
45. Involuntary muscular contraction; in the heart muscle can be a cause of cardiac arrest.

Down

2. Inflammation of the tongue.
4. Refers to baldness or hair loss.
7. Minute reddish spot on the skin or mucous membrane caused by hemorrhage.
8. Difficulty in swallowing.
9. Hemorrhage into the tissues, produces petechiae and ecchymoses.
10. Abnormal fluid accumulation.
13. Tendency of biologic systems to maintain internal stability while continually adjusting to external changes.
16. Pertaining to the jaws and face.
18. Abnormally low blood glucose.
20. Pain in the tongue.
22. Slow heartbeat.
23. Failure to carry out prescribed healthcare recommendations.
25. Nodular inflammatory lesion containing macrophages and surrounded by lymphocytes.
26. The study of the aging process.
28. The period immediately following birth.
34. Absence of oxygen.
37. A combination of symptoms that are related to a single cause or occur commonly together.
38. Diminished availability of oxygen to body tissues.
39. Loss of ability to communicate.

APPENDIX A

ADEA Competencies for Entry into the Profession of Dental Hygiene

CORE COMPETENCIES (C)

C.1 Apply a professional code of ethics in all endeavors.

C.2 Adhere to state and federal laws, recommendations, and regulations in the provision of dental hygiene care.

C.3 Use critical thinking skills and comprehensive problem solving to identify oral healthcare strategies that promote patient health and wellness.

C.4 Use evidence-based decision making to evaluate emerging technology and treatment modalities to integrate into patient dental hygiene care plans to achieve high-quality, cost-effective care.

C.5 Assume responsibility for professional actions and care based on accepted scientific theories, research, and the accepted standard of care.

C.6 Continuously perform self-assessment for lifelong learning and professional growth.

C.7 Integrate accepted scientific theories and research into educational, preventive, and therapeutic oral health services.

C.8 Promote the values of the dental hygiene profession through service-based activities, positive community affiliations, and active involvement in local organizations.

C.9 Apply quality-assurance mechanisms to insure contiuous commitment to accepted standards of care.

C.10 Communicate effectively with diverse individuals and groups, serving all persons without discrimination by acknowledging and appreciating diversity.

C.11 Record accurate, consistent, and complete documentation of oral health services provided.

C.12 Initiate a collaborative approach with all patients when developing individualized care plans that are specialized, comprehensive, culturally sensitive, and acceptable to all parties involved in care planning.

C.13 Initiate consultations and collaborations with all relevant healthcare providers to facilitate optimal treatments.

C.14 Manage medical emergencies by using professional judgement, providing life support, and utilizing required CPR and any specialized training or knowledge.

HEALTH PROMOTION AND DISEASE PREVENTION (HP)

HP.1 Promote positive values of overall health and wellness to the public and organizations within and outside the profession.

HP.2 Respect the goals, values, beliefs, and preferences of all patients.

Reprinted with permission from American Dental Education Association (ADEA). Competencies for entry into the allied dental professions (As approved by the 2010 House of Delegates). *J Dent Educ*. 2010;74(7):769–775.

HP.3 Refer patients who may have a physiological, psychological, and/or social problem for comprehensive evaluation.

HP.4 Identify individual and population risk factors and develop strategies that promote health-related quality of life.

HP.5 Evaluate factors that can be used to promote patient adherence to disease-prevention or health maintenance strategies.

HP.6 Utilize methods that ensure the health and safety of the patient and the oral health professional in the delivery of care.

COMMUNITY INVOLVEMENT (CM)

CM.1 Assess the oral health needs and services of the community to determine action plans and availability of resources to meet healthcare needs.

CM.2 Provide screening, referral, and educational services that allow patients to access the resources of the healthcare system.

CM.3 Provide community oral health services in a variety of settings.

CM.4 Facilitate patient access to oral health services by influencing individuals or organizations for the provision of oral health care.

CM.5 Evaluate reimbursement mechanisms and their impact on the patient's access to oral health care.

CM.6 Evaluate the outcomes of community-based programs, and plan for future activities.

CM.7 Advocate for effective oral health care for underserved populations.

PATIENT/CLIENT CARE (PC)

Assessment

PC.1 Systematically collect, analyze, and record diagnostic data on the general, oral, and psychosocial health status of a variety of patients using methods consistent with medicolegal principles.

PC.2 Recognize predisposing and etiologic risk factors that require intervention to prevent disease.

PC.3 Recognize the relationshops among systemic disease, medications, and oral health that impact overall patient care and treatment outcomes.

PC.4 Identify patients at risk for a medical emergency, and manage the patient care in a manner that prevents an emergency.

Detnal Hygiene Diagnosis

PC.5 Use patient assessment data, diagnostic technologies, and critical decision making skills to determine a dental hygiene diagnosis, a component of the dental diagnosis, to reach conclusions about the patient's dental hygiene care needs.

Planning

PC.6 Use reflective judgment in developing a comprehensive patient dental hygiene care plan.

PC.7 Collaborate with the patient and other health professionals as indicated to formulate a comprehensive dental hygiene care plan that is patient centered and based on the best scientific evidence and professional judgement.

PC.8 Make referrals to professional colleagues and other healthcare professionals as indicated in the patient care plan.

PC.9 Obtain the patient's informed consent based on a thorough case presentation.

Implementation

PC.10 Provide specialized treatment that includes educational, preventive, and therapeutic services designed to achieve and maintain oral health. Partner with the patient in achieving oral health goals.

Evaluation

PC.11 Evaluate the effectiveness of the provided services and modify care plans as needed.

PC.12 Determine the outcomes of dental hygiene interventions using indices, instruments, examination techniques, and patient self-reports as specified in patient goals.

PC.13 Compare actual outcomes to expected outcomes, reevaluating goals, diagnoses, and services when expected outcomes are not achieved.

PROFESSIONAL GROWTH AND DEVELOPMENT (PGD)

PGD.1 Persue career opportunities within health care, industry, education, research, and other roles as they evolve for the dental hygienist.

PGD.2 Develop practice management and marketing strategies to be used in the delivery of oral health care.

PGD.3 Access professional and social networks to pursue professional goals.

APPENDIX B

Patient-Specific Dental Hygiene Care Plan Template

Patient-Specific Dental Hygiene Care Plan

Patient name____________________ Age ____ Gender: M ☐ F ☐

Provider name ____________________ Date ________

Chief complaint:

Initial therapy ☐
Maintenance ☐
Re-evaluation ☐

Assessment Findings

Medical History	At Risk For
Social and Dental History	
Dental Examination	

Periodontal Diagnosis/Case Type and Status:	Caries Management Risk Assessment (CAMBRA) level: Low ☐ Moderate ☐ High ☐ Extreme ☐

Dental Hygiene Diagnosis

Problem	Related to (Risk Factors and Etiology)

Planned Interventions (to arrest or control disease and regenerate, restore, or maintain health)		
Clinical	Education/Counseling	Oral Hygiene Instruction/Home Care

Expected Outcomes		
Goals	Evaluation Methods	Time Frame
1		
2		
3		
4		

Appointment Plan (sequence of planned interventions)		
Appt #	Plan for Treatment and Services	Plan for Education, Counseling, and Oral Hygiene Instruction
1	Quadrant	
2		
3		
4		

Re-evaluation Findings

Retreat ☐ Refer ☐ Continuing care interval ____________

Description of posttreatment outcomes:

APPENDIX C

Example Dental Hygiene Care Plan

Patient Specific Dental Hygiene Care Plan

Patient name *Mrs. Lorna Patel* Age *49* Gender: M [ ] F [X]

Provider name *D.H. Student* Date *Today*

Initial therapy [X]
Maintenance [ ]
Re-evaluation [ ]

Chief complaint: *Gum tissues bleed when brushing and flossing. Mouth is dry all the time*

Assessment Findings	
Medical History	**At Risk For**
History of high blood pressure managed by medication *Cholesterol managed by medication* *Mitral valve prolapse* *Allergy to penicillin* *Zocor 20 mg 1 per day* *Caltrate 1 per day* *Enapril 10 mg/hydrochlorothiazide 25 mg 1 per day* *Multiple vitamin 1 per day* *Clindamycin 2.0 g taken 1 hour before appointment* *ASA II* *ADL level 0*	*Heart disease and stroke* *Xerostomia* *Postural hypotension* *Inappropriate antibiotic prescription*
Social and Dental History	
1.5 years since last recall *Localized 4-5 mm probing depths* *Flosses daily* *Rinses with Listerine* *Mouth dry all the time* *Uses mints and candy for dry mouth* *Uses bottled water with no fluoride content*	*Increased incidence of dental caries and periodontal conditions*
Dental Examination	
Moderate dental biofilm along cervical margins and proximal surfaces *Generalized supra- and subgingival calculus* *Light yellow stain* *Posterior gingiva red and bleeding on probing* *Generalized moderate attrition (evidence of bruxism)* *Numerous faulty MOD amalgam restorations* *Localized 4-5 mm maxillary and mandibular probing depths*	*Increased incidence of dental caries and periodontal conditions* *Increased risk for TMJ problems*

Periodontal Diagnosis/Case Type and Status:	**Caries Management Risk Assessment (CAMBRA) level:**
Generalized biofilm-induced gingivitis with localized chronic slight periodontitis	Low ☐ Moderate ☐ High ☐ Extreme ☒

Dental Hygiene Diagnosis

Problem	Related to (Risk Factors and Etiology)
Unnecssary pretreatment antibiotic prophylaxis	Lack of knowledge about current prophylactic premedication protocols
Current gingivitis and periodontitis	Inadequate dental biofilm Faulty restorations that provide trap for biofilm
Increased caries risk	Xerostomia and use of mints and candies Inadequate biofilm removal and fluoride intake Faulty restorations
Risk for TMJ problems	Attrition (evidence of bruxism)
Management of positioning during dental hygiene procedures	Medications (potential for postural hypotension)
Increased risk for heart disease and stroke	Periodontal infection History of hypertension and high cholesterol

Planned Interventions
(to arrest or control disease and regenerate, restore or maintain health)

Clinical	Education/Counseling	Oral Hygiene Instruction/Home Care
Scaling and root planing Selective polishing Fluoride application	Importance of current prophylactic premedication protocols Importance of management of xerostomia Increased risk of dental caries because of faulty restorations Increased risk of dental caries because of lack of fluoride and use of sugar-based candies Correlation of risk for heart disease and periodontal disease	Reinforce sulcular brushing technique Review flossing technique Discuss the use of Listerine vs nonalcoholic mouthwash (because of xerostomia) Frequent use of water and/or saliva substitutes Use of Xylitol gum/candies Reinforce the need for further dental intervention to manage faulty restorations and attrition

Expected Outcomes		
Goals	**Evaluation Methods**	**Time Frame**
1 *Eliminate gingivitis/ control periodontitis*	1 *Reduction of dental biofilm, gingival redness, gingival bleeding, and periodontal probing depths*	1 *4 week re-evaluation* 1a *Reassessment at maintenance appointment (3 months)*
2 *Increase use and frequency of sugarless mints and gum*	2 *Patient discussion*	2 *4 week re-evaluation*
3 *Increase fluoride exposure; use of daily fluoride rinse and fluoridated water*	3 *Patient discussion*	3 *4 week re-evaluation*
4 *Reduce attrition*	4 *Refer for night guard fabrication*	4 *4 week re-evaluation* 4a *Reassessment at maintenance appointment (3 months)*
5 *Eliminate faulty restorations*	5 *Refer for restorative dental care*	5 *4 week re-evaluation* 5a *Reassessment at maintenance appointment (3 months)*
6 *Maintain patient comfort and safety during dental treatment throughout treatment*	6 *Patient discussion*	6 *At all appointments*

Appointment Plan
(sequence of planned interventions)

Appt #	Plan for Treatment and Services	Quadrant	Plan for Education, Counseling and Oral Hygiene Instruction
1	*Assessment, scaling/root planing*	X (upper left), X (lower left)	*Importance of managing xerostomia* *Systemic impact of periodontal disease* *Importance of biofilm removal* *Reinforce sulcular brushing technique*
2	*Complete scaling/root planing, selective polishing, fluoride treatment*	X (upper right), X (lower right)	*Importance of fluoride* *Importance of managing xerostomia* *Importance of biofilm removal* *Demonstrate flossing technique* *Importance of follow-up for management of attrition and faulty restorations*
3	*Re-evaluation assessment – in 4 weeks*		

Re-evaluation Findings

Re-treat ☐ Refer ☐ Continuing care interval *3 months*

Description of post-treatment outcomes:

APPENDIX D

Understanding the Motivational Interviewing (MI) Approach to Patient Counseling

The purpose of all patient education and counseling is to help your patient adopt healthy behaviors that ensure positive health outcomes.

Motivational Interviewing is a patient-centered, goal-directed approach to communicating that:

- Engages the patient
- Provides continuous support and feedback
- Encourages an exchange of information
- Stimulates the patient's own motivation for change
- Leads to development of a commitment to healthy behavior change.

Brief motivational interviewing (BMI) uses the MI tools during short conversations (5–10 minutes) during patient care.

The Spirit of MI	Guiding Principles
P Partnership **A** Acceptance **C** Compassion **E** Evocation	**R** Resist righting reflex **U** Understand **L** Listen **E** Empower

Four processes of the MI approach
• **Engaging** the patient's attention and interest • **Focusing** the discussion • **Evoking** the patient's own responses about health goals, reasons for, and ambivalence toward change • **Planning** behavior change for health

To implement the MI approach, use the following MI tools:		The MI approach offers continuous support and feedback to help your patient:		
Core skills that lead to good information exchange: **O** Open-ended questions **A** Affirmations **R** Reflective listening • Simple • Complex **S** Summary	Components that facilitate **information exchange:** • Ask permission • Elicit, provide, elicit • Agenda setting • Use of MI core skills	**Explore ambivalence:** **Sustain talk vs. change talk** (Readiness ruler) **Decisional balance** (pro/con matrix)	**Initiate change talk:** **Preparatory change talk** Patient expresses the *desire, ability, reasons, or need* for change (DARN) **Mobilizing change talk** Patient expresses *commitment, actions, or steps taken* toward change (CAT)	**Express commitment** through development of a plan: • Clear plan • Several clear options • Brainstorming

APPENDIX E

Evaluation Rubric for Competency Exercises

Competence is the ability to apply knowledge and skills in a relevant way to solve problems, answer questions, or make decisions.

Objectively evaluating a learner's ability to recall factual information is relatively easy. Evaluation of student responses to exercises/learning activities that are intended to assess competence is often significantly more difficult. Competence is a complex interaction of skills that begins with an understanding of basic facts (*knowledge*) and incorporates the *analysis* of all relevant factors in a specific situation and *synthesis* of information in order to answer questions or solve problems. Competence also includes being able to *support* or clearly explain the rationale for decisions and as well as effectively *communicate* the plan for action.

An academic grading rubric provides objective criteria useful for evaluating student work that has been submitted to demonstrate competence. The assignment of points for each of the criteria stated in the rubric will aid the faculty member in providing an objective grade or score. When the evaluation rubric is provided along with instructions for the assignment, students receive a guide to faculty expectations. When the finished assignment is graded, focused feedback will help the student understand errors or omissions that result in a lower score or grade for the assignment.

The example evaluation rubric on the next page can be used as a template for evaluating student responses to all of the competency exercises, including those related to Factors to Teach the Patient and Everyday Ethics, in each chapter of the Student Workbook.

EVALUATION RUBRIC FOR COMPETENCY EXERCISES			
CATEGORIES	EXCELLENT 3 points	ACCEPTABLE 2 points	UNSATISFACTORY 0–1 points
Knowledge Familiarity with and understanding of concepts and information. Points ________	Student includes relevant and accurate information from the main chapter. And Student includes relevant information from related chapters in the textbook.	Student includes relevant and accurate information from the main chapter.	Significant relevant information from the main chapter is missing. Or Misunderstanding of one or more basic concepts is evident.
Analysis Breaking down a complex topic into its component parts. Points ________	All components of the question, case scenario, or patient assessment data are considered in the student's answer.	Only minor details or components of the question, case scenario, or patient assessment data have not been addressed in the student's answer.	At least one major component has not been addressed.
Synthesis Combining ideas to form a complex, cohesive whole using logical reasoning and deduction. Points ________	Connections or comparisons made between factors, concepts, and facts/knowledge from the textbook chapter are very clear.	Connections or comparisons between factors, concepts, and facts/knowledge from the chapter textbook are apparent, but not completely explained.	Important or obvious connections are missing from the students answer.
Support Providing rationale for statements. Points ________	Student provides clear explanations that support conclusions, statements, or connections made. Examples: • Linking basic information and intended actions or conclusions drawn • Explaining personal perspective • Defining controversy that requires further investigation.	Explanations are provided that support conclusions, statements, or connections, but could be more completely or clearly explained.	Little evidence is provided to support conclusions, statements, or connections.
Communication Conveying information. Points ________	Meets professional writing standards for: • Grammar • Spelling • Appropriate use of either a formal or "patient-friendly" writing style (based on the focus of the exercise).	Minor errors in professional writing standards for: • Grammar • Spelling • Appropriate use of either a formal or "patient-friendly" writing style (based on the focus of the exercise).	Errors in spelling or grammar. Or Writing style is too casual/conversational for professional writing. Or Inappropriate professional jargon is used for a patient discussion.
Total points ________ / 15 possible points **FACULTY FEEDBACK:**			